# The Women's Health
# BIG BOOK *of*
# PILATES

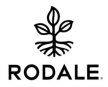

RODALE

D1286759

© 2013 by Rodale Inc.

Rodale books may be purchased for business or promotional use or for special sales.
For information, please write to: Special Markets Department, Rodale Inc., 733 Third Avenue, New York, NY 10017.

Women's Health is a registered trademark of Rodale Inc.

Printed in the United States of America
Rodale Inc. makes every effort to use acid-free ⊗, recycled paper ♻.

Book design by Laura White

All photography by Beth Bischoff, with the exception of photos on pages 6 to 9 that were provided by Gratz Industries, LLC
and the photo of Joe Pilates on page 2 © Getty Images/Susan Schiff Faludi
Stylist: Marysol Ortiz
Hair/Makeup: Anja Grassegger and Misuzu Miyake

Library of Congress Cataloging-in-Publication Data is on file with the publisher.

ISBN-13: 978-1-62336-092-4 trade paperback
ISBN-13: 978-1-62336-100-6 direct hardcover

Distributed to the trade by Macmillan

2 4 6 8 10 9 7 5 3 1 paperback

2 4 6 8 10 9 7 5 3 1 hardcover

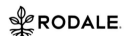

**RODALE.**

We inspire and enable people to improve their lives and the world around them.
rodalebooks.com

To those who value love as an everyday practice:
I dedicate this book to you who uplift others
by living through integrity, truth, and compassion.

To those who recognize laughter and tears as everyday practices:
I dedicate this book to you who value emotional expression
and who listen deeply to yourself
and others with an open, warm, and humorous heart.

To those who appreciate the monumental importance of
accountability as everyday practice:
I dedicate this book to you, who are digging deep and awakening
to the physical, mental, emotional, and spiritual,
allowing you to organically take care of the world around you.

Do your work. Never stop doing your work.

# Contents

# Acknowledgments

To the remarkable natural talents of Michele Promaulayko for her impeccable taste in authors ;) and her Pilates prowess. (Special thanks to Lauren Borden for the faith and introduction.)

To Kathryn Budig for awakening me to the bliss of chia seed pudding.

To Caryn Karmatz Rudy for the hand-holding and cheerleading—the secret ingredients for any great agent.

To Sarah and her team at SHPNY, best PR in the biz!

To my editing powerhouse Ursula Cary and all "sports bar" references.

To Jess Fromm for always greeting me with high-wattage smiles and positivity.

To the sharply tuned creative direction of George Karabotsos and Laura White (and an added nod to the optimistic idea that sticky rice might be a solution to something on a photo shoot.)

To Nancy Bailey, Sara Cox, Chris Krogermeier, Debbie McHugh, Carol Angstadt, Amy King, and the rest of the team at Rodale for their work in making this book possible.

For the fab photo shoot, I thank Ayla Christman, Beth Bischoff, Marysol Ortiz, and Misuzu Miyake.

To my beautiful, talented, hardworking Pilates models Amber Stone, Katie Yip, Belissa Savery, and my adoptive niece Zoe Ross-Nash, all of whom epitomize grace in motion.

Gravity-defying gratitude and love to my soul sister Kathi Ross-Nash, for so many reasons I would need to write another book to cover them all.

To the multitude of heroes of the musculoskeletal and organic health world, Joe Muscolino, Leslie Kaminoff, Lou Granirer, etc., for their information and inspiration as I wrote this book.

Without my network of loving friends, family, and special supporters, there would be no book in which to write acknowledgments. To my incredible and inspirational brothers, Eric, Todd, Paul, and Matt, for cheering me on with never-ending support. Extra-special love to Joan Block, Delia Garica, and Sherma Karim for nurturing and bolstering me along the way. Thanks to Ariana "A-Ray" Rabinowitz for "fit-friend Fridays" and so much more.

To my fellow Authentic Pilates Union board members and the PTA of P.S. 59 for supporting my off-duty efforts this year.

To the patience and understanding of my re:AB Pilates team.

To my tolerant and loving husband, Mevin, with whom I continuously learn and grow. It just keeps getting better.

To my amazing and BEST (!) little teachers, Sebastian and Matteus. Thank you for your understanding when I needed to write and for all the incredible love you've given me along the way—I am the luckiest mamma!

One last thank-you to my brilliant Pilates mentors and colleagues who tirelessly do what they do for the love of the work. We are blessed!

*"I slept and dreamt that life was joy. I awoke and saw that life was service. I acted and behold, service was joy."*
—Rabindranath Tagore

# Introduction

The importance of health and fitness was instilled in me in childhood. I was the youngest of six incredibly sporty siblings, and my father was listed in the US almanac for his track-and-field prowess—physicality was a given in my house. The fact that my dad also worked in the field of medical electronics and talked passionately daily about the body's ability to heal itself made a strong impression on me, too. I learned from a very young age that our bodies are miraculous entities that sometimes need our help and guidance, and, at other times, simply need us to get out of their way and let them do their thing.

When I was 11, my mother was diagnosed with progressive multiple sclerosis. Our next 26 years together allowed me to see the "other" side of health and fitness. We spent years in alternative treatments, countless hours in physical therapy offices, and, in her last years, doing sporadic Pilates sessions together. Even though my mother couldn't move her left leg, had very little control over her left hand, and had such severe scoliosis that her lower right ribs sat on top of her hip bone, we were always able to craft creative Pilates sessions that illuminated her strengths (great abs!) and aided in facilitating her limited circulation. Best of all, they made her feel stronger, both physically and mentally. These sessions were deeply rewarding for us both and gave me confidence in recognizing the power of the human spirit.

As a product of these two incredible humans, my genetics are a mixed bag. On the one hand, I have the athleticism and physique from my father's side of the family, but darn it if I didn't also get asthma, allergies, poor circulation, and a connective tissue disorder from my mom's side. I see each side as bearing its own unique gifts, and my Pilates practice has helped me live with and appreciate both. I'm a big believer that we're given what we need in this lifetime. If you struggle with elements of your own body, health, or life, it is critical to embrace those struggles as what my brilliant spiritual teacher calls "uncomfortable opportunities for growth." This is not to deny any pain involved—but when you look at obstacles as opportunities, their entire paradigm shifts! Pilates can help you do this.

I discovered Pilates in my midtwenties. I was a self-proclaimed "gym rat": Strong and healthy, I loved weights, treadmills, and step classes. But I was humbled by the challenges Pilates offered. Suddenly, I was working from a deep, mysterious place called the "powerhouse," and it proved tricky and entertaining. Since I couldn't afford private Pilates lessons on the exotic and tantalizing equipment,

I relegated myself to taking as many group mat classes as possible.

A few months in, already feeling a giant transformation, I ended up on the doorstep of Drago's Gym in the hands of the grande dame of Pilates herself, Romana Kryzanowska. Already in her seventies, Romana taught faithfully from 7:00 a.m. to 1:00 p.m. daily. Having been Joe Pilates's chosen protégée (he called her "my most conscientious disciple"), Romana was full of knowledge, stories, zest, and zeal. I knew I was exactly where I was supposed to be. Drago's became my home for years, and I shadowed Romana and absorbed as much of her passion and dedication as I possibly could.

What I learned about Pilates from Romana goes well beyond using props like springs and straps. Romana taught me about authenticity, loyalty, playfulness, diligence, taskmastering and nurturing, tapping into intuition and imagination, commanding with kindness, pushing with positivity, and being creatively compassionate. All of these qualities are also how I would describe my personal Pilates practice, and they are what I hope you will find in yours by using this book!

I will let you in on a little secret: We all struggle with our bodies. As a Pilates teacher, I feel extra pressure to look "perfect." In fact, I don't know one model, dancer, or instructor who isn't hard on herself or hasn't had some form of body dysmorphia. Whether we are skinny, ripped, or neither, we all have "stuff" we're working on. We're all works in progress. Where you are now is neither where you were nor where you will be. It is simply now. The more in touch we can become with that idea, the easier it is to let go and have some fun. Whether or not you end up with a "perfect" body doesn't really matter—don't get too attached to the outcome, and you might be surprised at your own transformation!

I have often said, "Pilates is only as good as its teacher," and guess what—that teacher is actually you! My role is your guide, your cheerleader, and, hopefully, your inspiration. Pilates has helped me through asthma, two pregnancies (and births), one heart surgery, and the emotional roller coaster of life. It's the glue that holds me together. I feel as passionate about Pilates as I did in my first mat class—maybe even more so. I am beyond honored to meet you as you begin your own journey. With Pilates, you'll move toward your individual goals with strength, humor, compassion, and a lot of sweat! Your body is an incredible, adaptable canvas: If you empower yourself to take the brushes in your hand, then there is little in the way of creating and discovering the true masterpiece that you are. —*Brooke*

*Be strong then, and enter into your own body; there you have a solid place for your feet.*

*Think about it carefully!*

*Don't go off somewhere else!*

*…just throw away all thoughts of imaginary things, and stand firm in that which you are.*

—Kabir (mystic poet, 1440–1518)

# CHAPTER 1

# What's Pilates?

*"You can say what Pilates
is in these words:
Stretch with strength and control.
And the control part is the most important
because it makes you
use your mind."*
—Romana Kryzanowska,
Pilates elder

# Y

ou've heard great things about Pilates, seen the toned tummies, and read the buzz in magazines. Pilates has become a fitness darling. Every celebrity on the planet has tried it and endorsed it. Every supermodel has used Pilates to get back on the runway practically minutes after giving birth. Every athlete and sports team has incorporated Pilates into their winning training regimen. Bottom line: Pilates is hot! But … what is it?

# *What's Pilates?*

When I was introduced to Pilates in the early 1990s, it had already been around for 70-odd years. Its initial heyday included a studio opening in the famous Henri Bendel department store in New York City in the midsixties. But in 1994, I had never heard of it (neither had 99 percent of the population, except for maybe dancers). I spent my first years as a Pilates instructor mainly teaching people who wanted to do what they called "the Pilates."

"It's a man," I would say. "It's the founder's name: Joseph Pilates." (And just "Joe" or "Uncle Joe" to those in the know.) I have always known it to be pronounced as *Puh-la-teez*. I admit to being amused by the variations I've heard over the years. "Pie-lat-ees?" Um, no. "Puhladies?" Nope. "Pie-lates?" Sorry, no. And now, in an ironic twist, Joe's own niece, Mary Pilates, has come forward to say it is actually pronounced Pi-LOTTS. Don't I feel silly! It just goes to show that the learning process never ends. However, so long as Americans continue to call croissants "cruh-sonts," I may also go right on calling it *Puh-la-teez*. (Apologies to the Pi-LOTTS family!)

Today, the word *Pilates* is generally used to describe movements involving your core. The class you take at your local gym or studio may be some variation of Joe Pilates's original program. When people tell me how much they love Pilates, I smile and nod politely, wondering just what they're actually doing! To be fair, I am happy for them, whether I consider their regimen to be Pilates or not. If it gets you moving intelligently and your body is changing for the better, then by all means, keep doing it! But I can usually spot a true Pilates body at 10 paces. It's not just about tone and proportion: A Pilates body has energy and a particular strength to it. While there are many ways to position the body and call it Pilates, there is only one authentic philosophy.

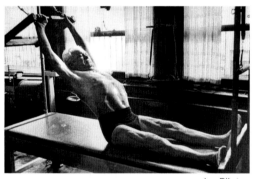

Joe Pilates

## The Man behind the Method

The more I read about Joe's ideology and character, and the more I watch his movements in archived films, the better I am able to embrace the soul of his unique method. There is a special lore that surrounds Joe and his work, and I've compiled a brief history based on years of stories from my teacher, Romana, as well as other Pilates "elders" (for more about these teachers, see the "Pilates Elders" section on page 25 in Chapter 2). Hopefully what follows will shed light into the force behind this multifaceted man and how he came to develop what's known today simply as Pilates.

Joseph Hubertus Pilates was born in Germany in 1883. As a child, he was plagued by ailments such as asthma and rickets (soft bones due to lack of vitamin D) and often teased by other boys due to his lack of physical strength. Like the quintessential "98-pound weakling," Joe was determined to man up and better himself physically—he took to the pursuit of sports, particularly gymnastics, wrestling, boxing, and self-defense. As the story goes, a family physician gave him a discarded anatomy book, and Joseph set about learning the muscles in the human body and studying the movements of animals. It's said that he worked his body to such an ideal extent that he was asked to model for the anatomy charts that hung in his New York City studio many years later. Redemption!

Nearing his 30th birthday, Joe moved to England to continue his boxing pursuits and, according to some, he even worked as a self-defense instructor for detectives in Scotland Yard. By 1914, he was touring England with his brother, Fred, putting his ideal physique to good use by performing a Greek statue act in a German circus troupe. At the outbreak of the First World War, Joe was interned as an "alien enemy" at a German nationals' work camp in England. Never deterred, he continued to teach wrestling and self-defense inside the camp and began developing a sequence of exercises known today as "the Pilates matwork"—which Joe called "Contrology." (He later claimed that his students left the camp stronger than they came in, and that not one of the camp internees who followed his Contrology regimen contracted influenza during the pandemic of 1918 that killed an estimated 50 million people worldwide!)

Joe was transferred to another camp, but he continued to work with fellow internees. He found work in some sort of hospital setting and became something of an exercise therapist to bedridden soldiers. By attaching the bedsprings to the bed frames themselves, Joe devised a way to support the patients' limbs while helping to strengthen and mobilize them, without their ever leaving the bed. This inspired spark of genius was the cornerstone of Joe's intricate Contrology system and the beginning of his use of apparatus.

Joe spent the next 6 years back in Germany, using his Contrology method to train military police as well as boxers, including an up-and-coming superstar named Max Schmeling (who won the world heavyweight championship in 1930! Not too shabby). Joe moved to New York City in 1926, likely on the advice of his powerful boxing friends, who wanted Joe to share his revolutionary method. He settled into a boxers' gym in midtown Manhattan near the original Madison Square Garden and also near the training studios of many athletes and dancers. Famous choreographers and dancers not only studied with Joe but also began to send him their injured dancers for rehabilitation. Romana Kryzanowska, a Balanchine dance standout at the tender age of 17, came to be healed by "Uncle Joe," and not only was she transformed but she also eventually inherited his studio.

# *What's Pilates?*

## A Lasting Legacy

Part of the reason Pilates has endured is that Joe faithfully documented his work with photographs, text, and film footage (he was particularly fond of before-and-after photographs and films of his students showing the improvement of their "deformations"). The other reason is the dedicated work of Joe's students (and lucky teachers like me!), who have proudly carried on his legacy.

From the time Joe arrived in New York until his death in 1967, Joe and his gal Friday, Clara—along with a revolving cast of students-turned-teachers—have trained countless clients, students, and teachers in the remarkable method of mind and body reformation that we now simply call Pilates. Joe always had reason to puff up his chest with pride, but like so many genius artists, he is only being fully recognized postmortem! Except for brief stints of popularity, Joe spent his first 45 years in New York City as an underground mastermind known mainly to broken dancers and performers.

And while Joe died without ever truly seeing the fruits of his labor utilized and appreciated to the degree he wished, he absolutely knew that one day the world would "get it."

So let's not end the history of dear Joe by dwelling on the ignorance of our past; instead, let's carry on by celebrating the exciting progress we've achieved in health and wellness over the last 40 years. I'll raise a glass to Joe—I'm so glad he was right!

## "Contrology"—The Ideology behind the Movement

While Joe developed his method over the course of his lifetime, he referred to it as the art and science of Contrology, a term he coined to describe its mind-control-over-muscle-control decree. Contrology principles govern all exercises in the Pilates system, whether performed on equipment or not. And while this book focuses largely on the non-spring-centric part of Joe's system, the mission of all Contrology exercises remains the same: to develop every muscle in the body "properly and scientifically" in order to improve blood circulation, boost muscle power, and build endurance. He said this could be done by "gaining the mastery of your mind over the complete control of your body"—uh, easier said than done! But it's possible.

Joe published a book in 1945 called *Return to Life through Contrology* that he hoped would serve as an antidote to the "dreadful" conditions of living in the modern age. In the book, he laid out the 34 exercises of his Contrology mat series that could be learned and practiced "right in your own home" (very much like the exercises in this book!). Joe didn't expect people—nor want them—to swallow his beliefs unquestioningly. Instead, he challenged us all to investigate his claims for ourselves ... and for humanity! Yes, he was that impassioned.

Remember that Joe threw down the gauntlet by strengthening his own sick and frail body through self-study and conscious movement. He proved it could be done. Contrology is a method of strength and fortitude and winning over adversity. It was not conceived as a meditative medium, nor as a system of gentle stretches, as many people often incorrectly assume. The thought behind each move absolutely elevates the work of Pilates beyond that of mere repetitive exercise and into its own branch of physical culture.

Contrology was devised as a method of reconditioning both body and mind to work at peak efficiency. Pilates is meant to be the sound physical foundation on which all your other activities are built. Whether you're looking to boost energy throughout the day or up your athletic game, Pilates will take you to the next level. Joe's vision was to empower you to take care of yourself. He favored intelligence over brawn. He wanted the body to move in every direction a body can move, but with control. He wanted us to work from our fingers, toes, and the crowns of our heads, with long, flexible spines and strong, stable centers. He wanted us to increase our circulation to energize and revitalize us and keep us from becoming ill. He wanted us to pay attention to how we breathed and moved and slept and sat. He wanted our commitment to self-study, our insight into our bad habits, and the understanding of our inherent skill to change what isn't working. Nothing was to be left out of Contrology, and, if studied diligently, his promise was that it would create truly efficient minds, bodies, and lives. So get ready for a serious workout!

# Tools of the Trade: Pilates Apparatus

When I first started teaching solo, I had a few of the larger pieces of Pilates equipment in the living room of my tiny apartment. One day, a client remarked, "What do the guys you date think when they come over?" I replied, "They think they've found the right woman!" To this day, there's nothing more entertaining than watching the reaction of a new student entering the studio and seeing Pilates apparatus for the first time. With beds and pulleys and springs and straps and names like the Guillotine and the Electric Chair, they seem more like torture chamber devices or S&M tools! It's a leap of faith, but rest assured the Pilates playground is full of fun and function.

My teacher Romana never referred to the apparatus as machines because, as she was quoted in the *New York Daily News*, "They don't work you. You work them." Joe Pilates was a certificated member of the Chartered Institute of American Inventors, and he would design new pieces to accommodate the needs of his students. All in all, he designed more than 20 different apparatus and furniture pieces, many of which still circulate today. Gratz Pilates continues to be the official Pilates equipment maker for Romana and thousands more. The company's popularity comes from its commitment to maintaining Joe's (and Romana's) standards and stipulations, producing authentic apparatus that truly support, strengthen, and improve the body dramatically.

Many of Joe's apparatus use springs of varying size and tension attached to poles, bars, and hooks at different heights and angles. This gives each apparatus a unique amount of resistance. Some pieces allow for total body movement, while others require the stabilization of one part while coordinating the movement of another. The non-spring pieces are arcs (or "barrels") of varying heights and degrees of curvature that support your body through ranges of spinal flexibility with an emphasis on safe extension (back bending). In a world where we increasingly find ourselves hunched over a computer (I'm guilty!), a little back bending goes a long way.

# *What's Pilates?*

The apparatus were designed to help support and strengthen the body so that the student could perform the matwork exercises as daily maintenance. In this book, I've designed the exercises and sequences so that you can perform all of them at home, but I encourage you to seek out a studio with authentic Pilates apparatus and try them for yourself. It's worth the experience! In the meantime, here's a quick rundown of the apparatus so you can get to know them better. Envision yourself using them as you work through the sequences for even greater control and precision.

## UNIVERSAL REFORMER

Romana calls it "your moving mat." Many of the exercises from the Reformer can be adapted to your matwork routine at home.

- Up to 100 pounds of spring resistance connect you to your muscles.
- The carriage glides on special wheels.
- Exercises can be done lying, sitting, kneeling, standing, and jumping.
- "Less is more": The greatest challenges on the Reformer are often performed with one spring (or even no springs).

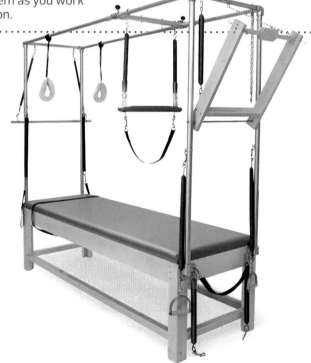

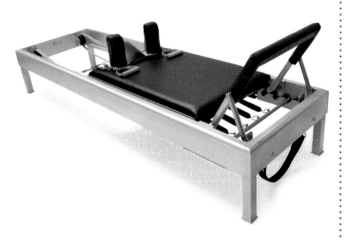

## CADILLAC, AKA TRAPEZE TABLE

The best of its kind in its time, so named by Joe's clients who remarked upon entering the studio, "I see Joe has a new Cadillac!"

- Exercises can be performed in every direction, including upside down.
- Strategically placed hooks and variable-size springs allow you to work at varying levels of tension.
- Push-through bar provides a stable frame to help isolate articulation for the spine.

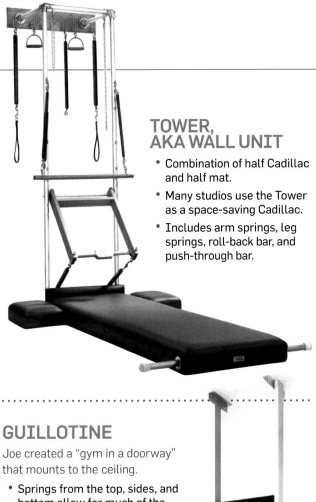

## TOWER, AKA WALL UNIT

- Combination of half Cadillac and half mat.
- Many studios use the Tower as a space-saving Cadillac.
- Includes arm springs, leg springs, roll-back bar, and push-through bar.

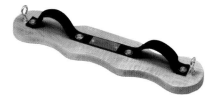

## AIRPLANE BOARD

- Used with the leg springs, this board closes the kinetic chain.
- Illuminates imbalances in muscle strength from side to side of the body.

## GUILLOTINE

Joe created a "gym in a doorway" that mounts to the ceiling.

- Springs from the top, sides, and bottom allow for much of the Cadillac/Tower work to be performed here.
- Vertical spring angle allows for different muscle action than its apparatus counterparts.

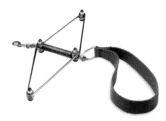

## NECK STRETCHER

Joe worked with boxers (and was one!) and needed to create strong neck muscles that could withstand hits to the head.

- Hook attaches to any of the leg or arm springs from the Cadillac, Tower, or Guillotine.

# *What's Pilates?*

## MAT AND ACCOUTREMENTS

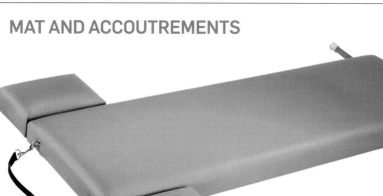

### HIGH MAT WITH HANDLES

- Foot strap helps anchor the lower body.
- Handles help stabilize the upper body.

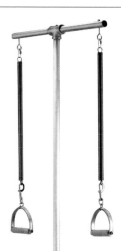

### MAGIC CIRCLE

Lore tells that it was crafted from beer keg hoops!

- Portable tension ring intensifies the Contrology mat exercises through resistance and stabilization.

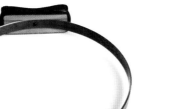

### PEDI-POLE OR PED 'O PULL

- Acts as a wobbly wall with springs to teach balance and upright powerhousing.
- Creates reference points for your spine that a wall can't.

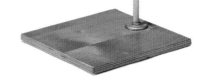

## SANDBAG

* This wrist and forearm strengthener can be made with a pole, a rope, and a bag of sand. Ingenuity made simple!

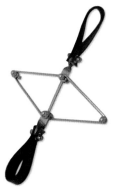

## WEIGHTED POLES

* Used in conjunction with Pilates mat-work to add weighted resistance and to provide a gauge for alignment.

## TOE EXERCISER

No part of the body is left out!

* Strengthens feet and toes, alleviates bunions.
* Connects feet to the powerhouse—especially glutes!

## PUSHUP HANDLES

* Help neutralize wrist pain.
* Allow for larger range of movement and ability to access more musculature.
* Can be used acrobatically for handstands and swing-throughs.

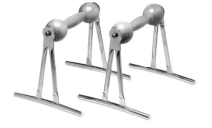

## FOOT CORRECTOR

Genius at work! Pilates works from the ground up!

* Strengthens and mobilizes the muscles of the feet.
* Corrects and connects the feet to legs to knees to hips and on up.

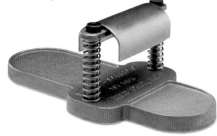

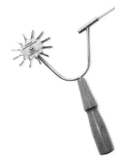

## BREATH-A-CISER

Formerly an asthmatic child, Joe carried the importance of breath into his method of Contrology with breathing devices like this one.

* Try blowing through a straw as you roll forward and you'll have an idea of the power of this pinwheel.

# *What's Pilates?*

## PILATES CHAIRS

Because of the constrained proportions of the chairs, most every exercise is more easily directed into the powerhouse.

### WUNDA CHAIR

* This apparatus can be flipped on its back to become super comfortable (and perfectly aligned) seating!

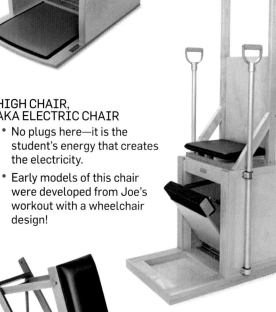

### HIGH CHAIR, AKA ELECTRIC CHAIR

* No plugs here—it is the student's energy that creates the electricity.
* Early models of this chair were developed from Joe's workout with a wheelchair design!

### ARM CHAIR, AKA BABY CHAIR

* The moveable back helps provide a stability challenge.

## PILATES BARRELS

The arcs of the barrels provide support for safe and effective extension.

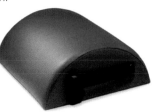

### SMALL BARREL

* Its small size makes it the most portable of the barrels, but it doesn't scrimp on function.

### SPINE CORRECTOR

* The entire matwork sequence can be performed with (and on!) this marvel, designed to support and encourage your curves.

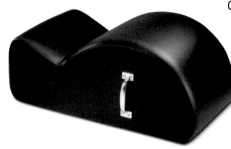

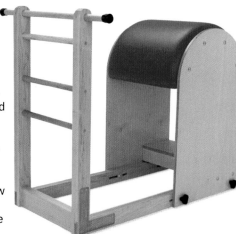

### LADDER BARREL

* Standing, hanging, bending, and climbing are all possibilities on the Ladder Barrel, whose unique height and design allow for incredible, supported range of motion.

# How Pilates Will Change Your Life

Over the years, I have been fortunate enough to teach many, many hundreds of clients. I have been awestruck as I've watched as their commitment to themselves transforms not only their bodies but their entire sense of self. I have seen students develop the courage to make major life decisions that would not have been possible had they not been bolstered by their strong Pilates bodies. It seems strange to say, but I can attest to the life-altering power of a few well-executed flips and twists! Here's what you have to look forward to.

## You'll Transform Your Body

When I began taking Pilates classes, I already felt strong, and I was in tip-top cardiovascular shape to boot. But I was also 6 feet tall, and all those muscles I'd built in the gym only served to make me feel big and clunky, if not a little masculine. The amazing thing was, the more Pilates I did, the stronger I felt, but I added grace, coordination, and responsiveness to my body's résumé. Like a badass Baryshnikov, I felt light on my feet and able to leap tall buildings in a single bound. There was a new quickness to the way I could move my body, and, best of all, I was completely in charge of it.

In a positive and important way, Joe Pilates called us out on our s#*t. He was baffled by our submission to a sedentary "modern" lifestyle and our mental complacency in the responsibility for our self-care. I shudder to think what he would say about the junk food–video game generation! Self-care means exercising control over your body, and to have that, you need awareness—that is, you must listen to your body and understand what it's trying to tell you. The more you practice this art, the better you become at deciphering its messages. I always think of aches and sensations in my body as messengers at the door: First they tap, then they beat, then they knock you off your feet! (Warning: Not listening to your body may be bad for your health.)

By moving in specific ways and paying attention to how your body reacts, you'll gain strength, tone your shape, and be able to notice stress, tension, indigestion, headaches, aches, pains, stiffness, and low energy—all signs that identify possible health issues. The more you practice, the more in "control of" and at ease you will feel in your body. It's not what the scale (or your boss or your partner) says about you—you'll be empowered through your own body awareness.

*"A good session will massage your entire body from the inside out. You should feel refreshed and invigorated at the end. You will feel better, look better, and sleep better. Pilates is more than a method of exercise; it is a way of life."*

*—Jay Grimes, Pilates elder*

# *What's Pilates?*

## You'll Transform Your Mind

Pilates helps you use three Cs to sharpen your mind and take you anywhere you want to go in the fitness world: concentration, control, and commitment.

### CONCENTRATION

The beauty of Pilates is that even though you're using your mind intently, you're also on a little mental vacation from the cares of the world. During your practice, nothing is more important than the task at hand. Pilates becomes its own "moving meditation," and your mind will become calmer when you give it permission to focus on 1 or 2 tasks rather than 20. Make no mistake, it's still a working vacation. The precision of the movements requires full brainpower, but working on the coordination to accomplish the movements is great fodder for your mind. When teaching and practicing Pilates, I find it instrumental to carry the images of Joe's boot camp–style videos (now happily available to all on YouTube) in my mind. It reminds me that this is an athletic pursuit of muscle mastery that requires tough mental focus.

### CONTROL

I've never been big on skiing; I don't like freezing my tail off while trying to brush up on technique. But one time, I agreed to go to Utah on a ski trip with cousins. Day one was, well, bad. It wasn't so much the cold as my absolute awkwardness, with my skis and gloves and poles flailing about. I caught my pole on the ski of my chairlift companion and, on exiting, sent that poor stranger right into the woods. (If you're out there, I'm so sorry!) That night, I went to sleep tired and frustrated and vowing to spend more time at the lodge the next day, but something strange happened. I dreamed that I skied—and liked it. I was comfortable and capable, swishing over the slopes with ease. I woke up excited, and guess what? I could ski! I'm not saying I was Olympic-grade material, but my cousins took me down some black diamond runs and I actually enjoyed myself—because I could!

Pilates changes the way you think about movement. As you progress, you recognize that your mind can make your muscles respond like little soldiers, in the exact manner you wish! That's a whole lot of power. But first you must click your heels together three times and believe that you can. Pilates says: You want that body? You make that body. Yes … you … can!

Are you building some strength in your ocular muscles by rolling your eyes at my optimism? Good, it's working!

### COMMITMENT

To all you commitment-phobes, hello and welcome! I'm in recovery myself and will readily admit that my love affairs with new things, while passionate, have often been short term. However, here I am, nearly 20 years after my first Pilates lesson, and more committed to Pilates today than ever. How did that happen? Well, I'm a very determined person. Once I've set my mind to something, I'm not so easily deterred (just ask my husband!). Commitment starts with the determination to succeed—when positive results follow, you're hooked.

When you decide to go out with someone, you're open and positive and full of the hope for the future. Of course, that all starts with the first date—if it goes well, you commit to another, and another, and your relationship deepens. So now the question is: Will you go out with Pilates? Consider this Joe's unofficial proposal: "Make up your mind immediately that you will perform your Contrology exercises for 10 minutes per session without fail. Amazingly enough, once you travel on this Contrology road to health, you will subconsciously lengthen your trips from 10 to 20 or more minutes before you even realize it."

He asked for your commitment of four times a week for 3 months so that you'd be able to truly experience the benefits of the method. Basically, he'd really like you to get to know Pilates. It's hard to realize just how much better you can feel until you try Pilates. Once it's taken hold of you, it's even harder, if not impossible, to ever let it go completely. And as your commitment grows, your results increase exponentially.

# You'll Transform Your Spirit

You may be surprised to see the word *spirit* in a Pilates book because you thought Pilates was just about your abs and, hey, this isn't yoga, after all. While the spiritual element of Pilates often takes a backseat to the physical, Joe absolutely intended for us to work our inner beings as well as our cores. He believed that the trinity of physical well-being, mental calm, and spiritual peace allowed us to achieve happiness.

## SO HOW DOES PILATES ENLIGHTEN US?
### Connection

While the practice of Pilates is indeed a physical one, it is also a mental, emotional, and deeply intuitive one, if you allow it to be. The time I've spent practicing Pilates on my own mat has become a sacred way of tapping into myself and checking in with my feelings and sensations. Before my heart surgery, I used Pilates as a daily moving meditation to get clear in my head and work through any stray fears lurking in my body. Why do Pilates instead of sitting in meditation? I find the movements of Pilates to be both energizing and comforting. My familiarity with the exercises allows me to turn off my messenger brain and connect to my emotional one. Joe Pilates asked that the movements of the matwork be practiced to the point of mastery on a subconscious level so that our connection to our bodies need not detract from but can make room for our connection to the rest of the world around us. Ultimately, we connect to one another, as well as with ourselves, in many ways, not just physically. The commitment we've made to our health and well-being connects us all in a universal spirit of humanity.

*"In my experience, both in Joe's studio and in my work, the method works for the people who are willing to make a mental commitment. The principle goes back to Joe, to a contrology, which meant the mind controls the body. If a person does not want to involve the mind, they don't get much more out of it than they get out of anything else. The real benefits come to the person who is willing to make a commitment to the work. As the body improves, the whole spirit seems to improve, the whole sense of adjustment to themselves and therefore to the world, gets better."*
—Pilates elder Bruce King, who studied with Joe from 1955 onward

# *What's Pilates?*

## Breath

I love the uncanny relationship of spirit and breath. The Latin word for spirit—*spiritus*—actually means "breath," and I liken inhaling to inspiring yourself with air. If you've never thought about your breath before, you're not alone. I listened to a radio show that discussed "10 tips to feel happier this year." One tip was to concentrate on breathing for 1 minute a day. One of the hosts groaned, "Oohhh, I'll never do that one; I'm just not that Zen." I couldn't help but laugh at the absurdity that breathing—the thing we do somewhere in the region of 20,000 times a day—is too Zen! Guess what, it's not Zen; it's fitness! It's life!

I confess that it was only when I began to study anatomy at an educational nonprofit known as the Breathing Project (yes, a real place!) and learned the true extent to which breath governs movement (terribly ironic for an asthmatic fitness professional) that I gave myself permission to delve into its deeper connections. Breathing is not just about flooding our bodies with oxygen to help us twist and flip into various positions. I believe our reluctance to focus on breathing stems from a sneaking suspicion that it will bring up unresolved emotions like fear, grief, anxiety, or disappointment. Those emotions get trapped in our bodies through muscular patterns of tension, and we may be really good at ignoring their signs.

Focused breath, combined with movement or not, can be like a flashlight illuminating the dark corners of our subconscious patterns, whether they're physical, mental, or emotional. In turn, combining an awareness of our breath with an awareness of our movements and emotions becomes an incredibly powerful vehicle that propels us toward a deeper connection with our spirit.

## Happiness

If mastering our breath can better connect us with ourselves and the outside world, then happiness comes from accepting ourselves—either just as we are or maybe by recognizing that it's time for us to change. When Joe Pilates said, "Physical fitness is the first requisite of happiness," he wasn't talking about fitting into skinny jeans. When you're not feeling well in body, mind, or spirit, how much peace and happiness would you say you feel? Not much. Health and fitness go hand in hand with happiness. Nothing quite lifts your spirits like feeling fit and healthy—inside and out.

# Are You Ready?

One of my all-time favorite quotes of Joe's is this: "Physical fitness can neither be acquired by wishful thinking nor outright purchase." In other words ... you've got to do the work!

Are you ready to get started? Be honest with yourself about what you really want to gain (or lose) from Pilates and/or your fitness plan in general. Going into a program with intention is a huge part of achieving real results.

# Before You Begin

**1** What do I currently like about my body?

**2** What aspect of my body or my current health situation makes me unhappy but could be positively affected by a regular exercise program?

**3** What about my body do I want to change and why?

**4** Am I willing to give up current bad habits or routines to make that change?

**5** Am I motivated to make that change?

**6** In my previous experience with health/fitness/behavior change: What worked? What didn't?

**7** My fitness/health goal (stated positively) is:

**8** This goal is important to me because:

**9** To achieve my goal, I will:

**10** Potential roadblocks to reaching my goal are:

**11** Strategies to overcome these roadblocks are:

**12** Three important action steps to reach my goal include:

**13** My goal is both realistic and challenging because:

**14** Fitness and health-oriented things I am good at include:

**15** Fitness and health-oriented things I need to work on include:

**16** My plan to improve is:

**17** If my plan doesn't work then I will:

**18** I'll know if my plan is working when:

**19** My reasons for wanting to improve are:

**20** People who will help me to improve are:

*"A goal is not always meant to be reached, it often serves simply as something to aim at."* —Bruce Lee

# *All Your Questions Answered*

*"As to methods there are many,
but principles are few.
The man who grasps the principles
can select his own methods."*
—Ralph Waldo Emerson

# *W*hat's my "core"? *When you*

hear the term "core," do you think of the core of an apple? The earth? Any bit in the middle of something else? Well, you're pretty much on target. Most fitness folk use "core" to mean your abdominals. The thing is, there are lots of collaborative muscles down there, so I'll give you the Pilates version of your core—which we call your "powerhouse." Think of the powerhouse like a girdle extending from the base of your sternum (breastbone) down to your pubic bone in the front, and wrapping around your back with parts of your bottom and inner/outer thighs included. The musculature involved inside this "girdle" will be what is used to stabilize (and also to mobilize) your spine and pelvis when needed. Your core is the power center of your body, like its electric company; before you proceed with Pilates, the powerhouse switch must be flipped to its On position! Every move in Pilates includes this core group of muscles. It's not Pilates without them.

# *All Your Questions Answered*

## Am I strong enough to do Pilates? Is Pilates easy or hard?

What's great about Pilates is that it's a progressive technique with many, many movements so there'll always be some things you can do easily, and you work toward the rest. The series runs the gamut from basic to difficult movements in terms of strength, flexibility, and coordination; depending on your unique talents, you may be stronger than you think. Pilates prefers to work in low repetitions (under 10) and focus more on moving your body in a wider range of ways. So instead of three sets of 50 × situps, you will do 3 to 5 each of 10 different situp-type moves. It involves many more muscles and requires coordination, control, and flexibility to work similar muscle groups in a variety of ways.

Is Pilates hard? Depends on what's hard for you. I find mindless repetitions hard. I find running hard. Hard to me is not having concrete, focused goals as I move. Here's what I hear in my head when I'm at the gym: "One, twoo, threee, foour . . ." Here's what I hear when I'm running: "Ow, ow, ow, ow . . ." To me, Pilates is the good kind of hard. It involves creativity and imagination, it's not repetitive, it has levels and goals, it has strategy, it keeps me attentive. The more energy and focus you put into the work, the harder it becomes but also the more satisfying. You choose how much effort you're willing to expend, and that determines the challenge level. I've often heard the statement "Pilates is easy . . . until you learn to do it correctly," and that is all too true. But Pilates is also great fun. It's an art based on practice. The more you do, the better you get.

## Will I lose weight with Pilates? How many calories does it burn?

Ah, the fateful question. The short answer: Yes! If you do Pilates consistently, you will lose weight. Pilates, however, was not designed as a weight-loss plan. That's just a happy by-product of this multifaceted system. Pilates works on the ideal of moving the body in such a way that circulation is optimized. It is impossible to optimize circulation and not reap the benefits of better digestion and a more efficient lymphatic system. These are critical factors in healthy weight loss. That said, I have strapped on a heart monitor a time or two and had at the Pilates system to determine its calorie expenditure. Performing the advanced matwork, without stopping, I was able to burn 300 calories in 30 minutes. That rivals a solid gym workout in terms of calorie expenditure. You will need to learn the exercises, order, and transitions well enough that you can keep your heart pumping in the weight-loss zone (see "Cardio Goals," opposite), but I have had many satisfied clients happily shop for new wardrobes!

# Is Pilates cardio? Will I sweat? Do I need to do a gym workout, too?

I used to be a gym junkie (still love it) before I entered the world of Pilates. In the 1980s, it was all about cardio. Fitness and cardio are synonymous in my mind, and Pilates is both. It may surprise you to know—or find out—just how athletic Pilates really is. It has a funny rap of being either slow, stretchy movements or physical therapy. Well, just look at its founder, Joe Pilates— I don't think you get that ripped without a vigorous workout!

I, for one, love to sweat in my workouts, but how much I choose to drive myself to sweat each time is a different story. There are times when I need to let my inner Thoroughbred loose and foam at the mouth and other times when a gentle trot with a damp sheen will suffice. I've learned to gauge what's right for that moment with what my teacher would call, "an elegant sufficiency." It's really up to you.

Pilates is tailored to varying levels of difficulty so that anyone can find success within its scope. What you need to figure out next is just how much cardio you need (see "Cardio Goals," right). And while I love the gym, with Pilates, you don't need a fancy membership in addition to your practice. That said, if you're already a gym member, then your Pilates training will definitely boost the efficiency of your other workouts.

# Will Pilates make me taller? Will I look like a supermodel?

Well, not exactly. What Pilates does is find all the places in your body where there should be space or length and help you create that space or length. If you are chronically stooped over your computer all day, your spinal musculature has gotten comfortable in this position—but Pilates can reverse this by stretching through the fascial layers that have attached themselves to your bad habit. As you build the musculature (including mental muscles) necessary to keep the pattern from returning, you will indeed stand taller from each and every place in your body. So, yes, you may "grow" an inch or so. Thing is, that inch was there all along; you were just constricting it.

Many celebrities and supermodels practice Pilates for its amazing effects. However, if you're not 6 feet tall or with the money and time to work out constantly, it's not worth comparing yourself to the women you might admire in magazines. Many celebrities base their entire careers and lives around the way they look and have an army of people to help them achieve their goals.

While it's perfectly fine to use Pilates to improve your physique, I'd love to encourage you to practice because it makes you feel fantastic, whether you're on a runway or not. Fitness is about feeling great and boosting the quality of our lives.

## CARDIO GOALS

To roughly calculate your maximum heart rate, subtract your age from 227 (for women) or 220 (for men). Then use the following guidelines to calculate your target heart rates, depending on your goals:

- GENERAL HEALTH: Exercise approximately 30 minutes per day at 50 to 60 percent of your maximum heart rate.
- WEIGHT LOSS: Exercise approximately 60 minutes per day at 60 to 70 percent of your maximum heart rate.
- AEROBIC: Exercise approximately 20 to 40 minutes per day at 70 to 80 percent of your maximum heart rate.

# All Your Questions Answered

## Can I do Pilates if I'm injured?

It depends on the severity of and time since the injury. I have had clients work out with casts on arms and braces on knees because we've been able to adapt exercises to work for their body in the moment. The first thing you'll need is your doctor's clearance. If a doctor or physical therapist has cleared you to move, then a Pilates routine can be adapted to fit you. However, Pilates is definitely not a "no pain, no gain" technique. It should challenge you and make you sweat—but you should definitely not feel pinching, aching, overdoing, or any kind of sharp pain! There is a big difference between effort and pain. When you're out of shape, your body's receptors may send signals to your brain saying, "Holy crap, this is hard!" and "Man, my glutes are burning!" But as you get stronger, your body will acclimate to the work, and soon you may find yourself looking for that sensation again. Happily, Pilates always has ways to accommodate your increasing might.

## Can I do Pilates if I'm not flexible?

You can and you should! Pilates is a wonderful way to balance the body so that what's locked and inflexible can have the opportunity to move. Circulation needs movement, and when areas of your body are "stuck," you not only are at risk for injury but are also negatively affecting the internal workings of your system. You may feel sluggish, tired, stressed, or uptight because of unconscious tension held in your body. Moving is the key, and everything in your body that can move, should! For a little extra mobility mojo, refer to Chapter 7, Pilates Props.

## Can I do Pilates if I'm pregnant and/or nursing?

If you've been practicing Pilates for at least a few months before pregnancy, then yes. If you've never done Pilates before, now is not the time to start. In Pilates, we work from your deepest core muscles, the ones surrounding the very area where you're trying to grow a baby. Pregnancy is generally not the time to start to get in shape, although that is often the answer I get when I ask, "Why now?" I feel that the first trimester, in particular, is just not the period to go abs crazy. It's a matter of "better safe than sorry." That said, I've seen clients continuing their advanced workouts up until their due dates. The beauty of the Pilates system in an authentic studio is that the apparatus is designed to support body weight and help you move in ways that are conducive to your changing body. During pregnancy, we look to maintain your level of fitness, help with any discomfort that may arise, and cheer you along the way and across the "finish" line.

While you're nursing, the relaxin hormone is still in your body and therefore your joints are looser and more susceptible to injury. Work on balance and strength more than flexibility during this time. You may also want to avoid exercises where you are lying prone (facedown) due to breast sensitivity.

## Should I eat before or after my workout?

Since Pilates involves moves that are concentrated around your center and also sends your legs overhead with certain frequency, big meals are not recommended beforehand. But don't come empty either. The amount of food you'll need depends on the intensity of the workout you're planning. When I do my 6:00 a.m. workouts, I rarely feel the need to eat beforehand because I happen to be a late-night snacker, so there's still enough fuel in my system to get me through a 30-minute mat session. If I'm planning a longer or more intense workout, especially on the apparatus or with weights, then I definitely make sure I get fruit and nut butter in me. (My faves: bananas and walnuts or a slice of brown rice bread with almond butter.) You want carbohydrates to provide the majority of the fuel for your workouts, so if you're someone who works out later in the day, just make sure that lunch contained some sort of healthy carbs. And I definitely try to eat as soon after a workout as possible—within 30 minutes. That's when your body is looking to replenish glycogen (a type of carb stored in the muscles) lost during the workout. A combination of carbs and proteins is the best way of replacing glycogen, and many fitness pros turn to shakes (instead of whole foods) to get the nutrients back into the body more quickly.

## When is the best time of day to practice?

This one is totally subjective. You want to find a time of day that works for you so that you create a sustainable habit of doing Pilates. Personally, I'm a morning gal. I like to roll out of bed and onto my mat super-early, before I know what's hit me. It helps me to start the day before anyone else is awake so that I can make the workout "me" time. I'm usually so proud of myself for making time for self-care that I go through my day with more confidence and consciousness.

If you work out in the morning, when your body temperature is lower, allow yourself a little extra warmup time. If you work out late at night, beware: Since exercising raises your heart rate and temperature, you may have trouble getting to sleep. Try to leave enough time between your workout and bedtime to downregulate your system.

## How many days a week should I work out?

Joe Pilates asked that you "faithfully" perform your Contrology exercises four times a week for 3 months to find your body approaching the ideal. I think we may have to give a wide berth to the word "ideal." I like to pose the question this way: If you were setting out to learn a new language (which you are, by the way!) and you were tutored for only 1 hour a week, how long do you think it would be before you were speaking fluently? Now, if you were to go to that tutor four times a week plus practice throughout the day (at work, in the car, on the street, in your head), how much faster do you think you'd see results? The beauty of Pilates is, just like a language, once you've gotten it into your system, you'll never lose it. It may wane with lack of practice, but you and your body will always remember how to speak Pilates!

## What do I wear?

Well, if you were Joe Pilates (and most of his students pictured in his archives), you wore as little as possible. And I mean *little*. Joe is famous for his uniform of tight, white . . . well, were they shorts? A bathing suit? I'm still not sure, but he was very fond of them because they let his pores breathe. In the interest of relative discretion, I advise you to wear comfortable, supportive clothes that are not too restrictive yet are as form fitting as you are willing to go. Avoid clothes with zippers, snaps, and pockets. Bedazzled numbers won't work either. Much of the work is done lying on your back or your stomach, so anything that protrudes from your clothing will eventually embed itself into you! I avoid clothing that is too loose either in the leg (the pants fall when your legs are up in the air, which they are right from the start) or in the body (I've had a shirt slip right over my head when I was upside down). You can always tuck things in, so if bigger is better for you, don't let my advice stop you.

## Do I need a mat?

Not necessarily. In all honesty, I know I won't be getting any sponsors by saying that, but the truth isn't always so marketable. When traveling, I simply lay a towel or two down on a carpeted floor or rug and get going. If you're on hardwood floors and/or are someone with a sensitive or particularly bony body, you might want to invest in a thick (½-inch-plus) mat or stack two yoga mats together. Since we roll on our spines and our hips, it's important that your bones be protected from a hard surface. Joe Pilates liked to work out outside on the ground or in the snow to get the most fresh air—or "nature's tonic"—as possible. I've tried the ground a few times, and all I can say is . . . sticks and stones really do break bones!

## Do I need other props?

Joe Pilates was very creative and created accessories from springs, wood blocks, metal pipes, and even keg supports. In Chapter 7, Pilates Props, we'll work with various items that can intensify your practice. For now, here's a brief list of the props you may want to try. The Resources section at the back of the book lists companies I recommend, but for those on a budget, I try to suggest homemade alternatives to almost all the props so you don't need to spend to gain!

**Magic circle/Tensatoner:** These resistance tools act as a way to maintain inner-thigh engagement for better low-abs connection. If you can't afford these options, try an 8-inch playground ball or maybe even a well-stuffed pillow.

**One- to 3-pound hand weights:** These will feel much heavier during Pilates than you think, so don't be a hero and try to go heavier.

**Ankle/wrist weights:** These are good tools if (a) you cannot hold a weight or (b) you want consistent added resistance throughout your workout. These props are not required by any means.

**Stability balls:** Every size ball has a different function, but for our needs a Swiss ball/stability ball will be best. Here's a general guide:

**Under 5 feet tall:** Try an 18-inch ball

**5 feet 1 inches to 5 feet 7 inches:** Use a 22-inch ball

**5 feet 8 inches to 6 feet 2 inches:** Use a 26-inch ball

**Taller than 6 feet 2 inches:** Use a 30-inch ball

Considering only your overall height doesn't take into account your leg-to-torso ratio—if you have particularly long or short legs, you might need to go up or down a size.

**Stretchy bands:** Resistance bands come in many different tensions (usually distinguished by color, depending on the brand). Find one that isn't so loose that you can't rely on it for support nor so tight that you have to strain to pull it apart. To properly set up for the "bands as springs" section in Chapter 7, you'll want to invest $6 in a door anchor.

**Pads/pillows:** When lying on your back, pillow placement should work to align you so you're pain free during exercise. For pain from a flat neck (loss of cervical curve), placing a small pillow (or rolled-up hand towel) under your *neck* might alleviate discomfort and keep you in proper alignment. If you tend to feel pain when you move your head back (extension of the neck), placing a small pillow (or folded hand towel) under the very back of your *head* might be the answer.

**Three-foot pole:** Holding a weighted pole—a broom handle may do—can provide good visual feedback for alignment and tactile feedback for finding weakness on one side. Plumbing pipe works nicely, too, and comes in all different weights and circumferences for your grip.

# Will I be sore? Do I need to rest my muscles between workouts? And if so, how often?

If you're not used to moving in a Pilates workout, then yes, you'll probably be sore in the beginning. And anytime along the way that you kick it up a notch, or work something in a new way, you may be sore again. This is due to "delayed onset muscle soreness" from the microtears in the cells of the muscle fibers that help build stronger muscles, so that every time you perform that exercise it gets easier on your body. Clever body, no? "Resting" your muscles is about allowing the cells that tear to repair themselves. Bodybuilders try to build as much muscle as possible and therefore continually increase the intensity and weight of their workouts, tearing many muscle fibers in the process. "Healing" time is necessary for the muscle tissues to repair. During that process, the muscles are weaker, so it can take days until the muscle is capable of exerting similar force again.

# *All Your Questions Answered*

Since Pilates is interested not in building as much muscle as possible but as much muscle as is *needed* to live easily, there is less tearing and repairing necessary. Therefore, depending on the intensity of your workouts, you could do Pilates daily. If you find you're *very* sore after a session, you can give your muscles 2 or 3 days of recovery. In the meantime, change your definition of "rest" to include a nice walk in the fresh air.

## What's the difference between Pilates and yoga?

Pilates and yoga are like third cousins once removed. They share a few traces of family traits, but they are different tribes. First, Pilates is named after one specific man, its founder, Joseph H. Pilates (1883–1967). Originally called Contrology, Pilates was developed as a way to attain mastery and control of the body rather than prepare it for long seated meditations. The full Pilates system is performed on apparatus, most of which are spring based in their resistance and offer up to approximately 100 pounds of weight. In Pilates, no moves are held for longer than a count of about three, and so if you were to compare the Pilates matwork to yoga, it would be most akin to Vinyasa flow. Much of Pilates is performed on the back so as not to put undue stress on the organs, and there is a strong focus on the core muscles of the body. Pilates teaches from the ground up—lying, sitting, kneeling—and there are fewer standing exercises in the system than you would find in a yoga class. Pilates asks for

dynamic movement, often against resistance, and thus it requires the abdominals to remain pulled "in and up" throughout its execution to support and stabilize the spine. Since the abdominals are to remain taut throughout, the breathing in Pilates is spherically isolated to the movement of the ribcage so the chest, side, and back body expand on an inhalation but the waist does not. In contrast, certain yoga styles strongly emphasize complete relaxation of the body, and the yoga breathing allows for the expansion and relaxation of the abdominal cavity and is often called "belly breathing." Both Pilates and yoga are wonderful at accomplishing their goals.

Pilates has its roots in the physical. Although Joe's beliefs and aims of Contrology were curative in nature, his desire and ability to emulate the Greek vision of "ideal" physical specimens are what has brought the most attention to this method: in particular, world-class abs and functional strength designed to facilitate daily living in this modern age. However, if you continue to scratch the surface of this method, there are riches to be found, such as yogalike intentions of mental calmness and spiritual peace.

## Like yoga, there seem to be so many "types" of Pilates. Which one is right for me?

Yoga has many branches of teachings and movement styles based upon who learned from whom and when. Pilates has followed a similar path into the modern day—different styles of Pilates represent different interpretations of Joe Pilates's work, based on the "elder" who learned it. We call them elders because they're usually first-generation Pilates teachers who studied with Joe himself and then took on the work of teaching Contrology. Because many of the elders were given lessons for their own bodies—not necessarily taught one consistent method—much of the work became dominated by the modifications and variants they made for themselves. Only a few were with Joe long enough, or thoroughly enough, to be deemed true teachers of his work.

Many people "study" Pilates not knowing they're getting a much different version than the one Joe intended. My opinion is that the "right" kind of Pilates is the one that is right for you; the one that brings out the best in you and your body while remaining as true to Joe's philosophy of Contrology as possible. However, these core principles should not be sacrificed: controlled movement, opposition, athleticism, spinal flexibility, focus, breath, resistance, hard work, and taking personal responsibility for one's health. Now, whether you choose to work out in a tiny white bathing suit like Joe is really up to you!

# Pilates Elders

Who are these "elders" I keep talking about, anyway? Well, in Pilates, they're the first-generation teachers who studied directly with Joe and Clara Pilates. In other words, they learned firsthand the techniques and principles of the method. You may see quotes or references to them throughout this book—they're highly respected by those in the field. Many people helped bring Pilates to life, but here's a little more about some of the key figures:

## ROMANA KRYZANOWSKA

Joe Pilates called Romana his most conscientious student. Romana began studying with Joe and Clara in 1941, at the age of 17, when George Ballanchine brought his young dancer to "Uncle Joe" to work around an injured ankle. After leaving for Peru in 1944 to raise her children, Romana taught Pilates from her home and corresponded with Joe and Clara by mail. In 1959, Romana returned to the United States and taught Contrology (and ballet) until, in 1970, she became the director of the Pilates Studio. She worked alongside Clara until Clara's passing in 1976 and has continued to keep the work alive ever since. Her loyalty to Joe's vision has made her the grande dame of the Pilates method and the most respected Pilates teacher in the world. (My teacher!)

## CAROLA TRIER (1913–2000)

A dancer, acrobat, and most notably a roller-skating contortion-ist, Carola experienced a devastating back injury that brought her to Joseph and Clara Pilates. Her injury was so severe, she thought she'd be using an orthopedic support for the rest of her life. After she began working with Pilates, she regained her strength and stability. In the late 1950s, with Joe and Clara's help, she opened her own Contrology studio. Carola stressed Joe's philosophy that uniform development was a key to fitness and later furthered her anatomical knowledge at New York City's Lenox Hill Hospital, where she aided Dr. Henry Jordan with patient rehabilitation and research.

# *All Your Questions Answered*

## EVE GENTRY (1909–1994)

Eve was a master of modern dance and movement who worked with Joe Pilates for more than 20 years after developing knee and back pain from extensive dancing. Eve was quoted as saying, "I'll never forget this sensation—after Joe had worked with me, all of my pains were gone, back pains and knees—everything. It was the first time in 3 years that I had not had pain, and I felt wonderful." Based on her work with Joe, Hanya Holm, and Rudolph von Laban, Eve developed her own body-conditioning technique. In 1968, Eve opened the Pilates Method Studio in Santa Fe, New Mexico, where she developed a strong rehabilitation practice.

## KATHY GRANT (1921–2010)

Kathy was a Broadway and television dancer, chorus girl, and choreographer before she suffered a knee injury. She became a longtime student of Joe Pilates, and she was one of only two people to receive official Pilates certification through a federally subsidized program of instruction approved of and supervised by Joe himself at the New York State Division of Vocational Rehabilitation. Kathy taught at Carola Trier's studio and later managed the Pilates studio in the famous Henri Bendel department store from 1972 to 1988. From then until her passing, Kathy taught Pilates at New York University's Tisch School of the Arts.

## RON FLETCHER (1921–2011)

Ron began working with Joe and Clara on and off from 1948 after a knee injury sidelined him early in his dance career. Joe put him to work on the Reformer, allowing him to avoid undue pressure on his knee while focusing therapeutic strengthening and lengthening exercises on the surrounding muscles. After a personal hiatus, Ron returned to work with Joe and Clara Pilates in 1967; though Joe died later that year, Ron continued to work with Clara. In 1971, with Clara's blessing, he opened the Ron Fletcher Studio for Body Contrology in Beverly Hills. By the early 1980s, Ron was training instructors in Ron Fletcher Work, which he called "a marvelous organic recipe"—flavored with the teachings of dance masters Martha Graham, Gertrude Shurr, and Yeichi Nimura as well as Contrology. Ron developed a number of new floor-based adaptations of Joe's equipment exercises and other techniques he called "towel work" and "percussive breathing."

## JAY GRIMES

Jay began studying with Joseph and Clara Pilates in 1964 while he was a professional dancer working with ballet companies and on Broadway. He danced professionally for 18 years and was injury free during that time, which he attributes to his Pilates conditioning. Jay was "sent" out to Los Angeles in 1974 by Clara to help bring Pilates to the West Coast. Jay continues teaching the traditional methods and techniques he learned directly from Joe and Clara in workshops and seminars for teachers and their students, conducting master classes around the world.

## LOLITA SAN MIGUEL

During her distinguished career in dance, Lolita suffered a debilitating injury and was sent to Carola Trier's studio in the late 1950s. According to Lolita, she trained as Trier's client "on and off" for 7 years. Eventually, Carola asked whether she would consider teaching Pilates. She became the only person Carola ever certified. One of Trier's assistants was Kathy Grant, who took Lolita to meet Joe and Clara. After diligent study with Joe, Clara, and their assistants, Lolita San Miguel and Kathy Grant became the only two Pilates practitioners who were officially certified by Joseph Pilates. They received their certificates from a state university in New York on February 2, 1967.

## JONATHAN WINTERS

A theater pipe organist, John served in the army during World War II. He was referred to Joe after gaining 30 pounds, despite going to a gym. He became a regular at Joe and Clara's studio and eventually became second in command under Romana after Joe passed away.

## MARY BOWEN

Mary began her studies with Joseph Pilates in 1959 and studied with Joe and Clara for 6 years. She has been a Jungian psychoanalyst since 1970 and has taught Pilates since 1975. Bowen recalls that around the age of 65, her two professions—Pilates instructor and Jungian psychoanalyst—began to merge. She called the approach that emerged Pilates Plus Psyche and refers to it as "her special contribution to the Pilates community."

## BRUCE KING (1926–1993)

Modern dancer Bruce King had his first lesson with Joe Pilates in 1955. To maintain his dance career, he took one or two lessons weekly. After a few years of study, Bruce was offered the opportunity to learn to teach Pilates. Clara became his main teacher and inspiration. By 1966, Bruce was living in the Pilates's building, where he had a small studio. A fire in the building left Joe and Clara's studio damaged and Bruce's destroyed. He taught at the Pilates Studio and, after Joe's death in 1967, he assisted Clara.

He received accolades as a dancer, choreographer (he established the Bruce King Dance Company in the 1970s), and respected author. In 1972, Bruce bought a Reformer from Joe and Clara's studio and taught Pilates out of his apartment, as well as traveled to teach workshops, until his passing.

## BOB SEED (1921–1987)

A Marine lieutenant colonel in the Korean war, Bob's war wounds were extensive—they included a steel plate in his skull and shrapnel in his intestines. He had been paralyzed and had to learn to walk again, exploring the Eastern philosophies of yoga, meditation, kung fu, karate, and sumo wrestling to do so. His own infirmaries led him to the attitude of exercise, and he became a registered nurse and self-practiced acupuncturist, a skill he had learned well in Korea. Bob met Joe a few years after the war. Not much is known about their time together other than a falling out that sent them their separate ways. Practically across the street from one another for years, Bob developed a following that likely aggravated Joe's famous ego. When people left the Seed studio, Bob would say, "Carry on."

## MARY PILATES

In the 1940s, when she was just 18, Mary's parents put her on a bus for New York. She said, "My dad had the [Pilates] studio in St. Louis, but I never paid that much attention to it until I got sent to New York [to live] with Uncle Joe." For most of the following 3 years, she learned the Pilates way and led clients through their workouts at her uncle's studio. Mary relocated to South Florida in the 1960s and still likes to show people the "right way" to do the Hundred. See page 64 to try it yourself!

CHAPTER 3

# *How Pilates Gets You Fit*

*"We delight in the beauty
of the butterfly,
but rarely admit the changes
it has gone through
to achieve that beauty."*
—**Maya Angelou**

# Pilates is a unique methodology

that improves both your mind and body—here's how!

Pilates is usually perceived as being just like yoga or a mat-only technique. It's not! It's a unique methodology that offers a host of benefits that improve both your body and mind, including: a rock-solid core, improved posture and flexibility, and toned muscles. Not only that, it reduces stress and toxins and teaches you overall body awareness and control. Here's how it works …

# *How Pilates Gets You Fit*

## You'll Boost Your Brainpower

The latest research in the world of neuroscience now says that exercise does more for thinking than thinking does for itself! Did you get that? Joe sure did. Back in 1934, he put forth the idea that the longer we go without learning proper control of the body, the more our vitality diminishes and our mental capacity wanes and the closer we are to becoming "animated clothes racks." Great image! (Admit it; you've met some!) Pilates's effect on brain building, Joe explained, happens by reawakening thousands of dormant muscle cells, which then activate thousands of dormant brain cells—stimulating increased mind power and function. Sounds good to me!

Joe was way ahead of his time. In 2011, a team of researchers at the University of Illinois put four groups of mice in various living arrangements—one group had delicious food and lavish cages, one had standard kibble and no embellishments, and two other groups had the same setups with the addition of a running wheel. The scientists tested the mice and discovered that the only thing that made a difference in their cognitive improvement was the wheel. The mice that exercised had healthier brains and performed significantly better on cognitive tests than the other mice.

## You'll Become Stress Savvy

It's hard to pick up a health magazine these days without reading that exercise is good for stress reduction. Did you know, though, that exercise not only reduces your stress but it actually prepares you to better cope with *more* stress? Researchers at the Society of Neuroscience found that when rats were subjected to stress, the ones that had been allowed to run beforehand reacted better than the rats that didn't run. Exercise appeared to effectively rewire their brains to better cope with negative stress. All the conscious breathing, the releasing of muscle tension, as well as the releasing of "happy hormones" (endorphins, serotonin, dopamine) during your workouts make Pilates the perfect stress-busting workout!

## You'll Get a Rock-Steady Body

The archetype of strength has always been the meaty muscle-bound bodybuilder with the bulging muscles, but really, what good is all that strength if you can't move and groove with it? The more mass you have, the harder it is to get going and the harder it is to slow down, stop, or change tack. If you wanted to tango, would you choose the Hulk or Spiderman as your dancing partner? Which one of them could get in a car faster? Sprint up a flight of stairs to catch a train or more easily scratch their own back? These are the qualities of movement that are of actual value in our daily lives.

Pilates creates this balance of muscle and movement by treating the center of the body—the powerhouse—as the meeting point of all your extremities. A body with a stable center is much more adept at withstanding the sudden shifts and twists that come from exercise, sports, and life. Pilates partners a strong center with a broader base by helping to create more effectual feet (imagine being bumped while wearing 6-inch stilettos versus standing on your bare feet) and a balanced spine created by perfecting your posture. Who's the superhero now?

## You'll Feel Bulletproof

Bad habits trap us in repeated patterns of movement (sitting with your right leg crossed over your left, carrying your bag on the same shoulder every day, sitting stooped over a keyboard for hours on end), overdeveloping some muscles and locking down others without any counter-movements to offset their eventual, unfortunate effects. When the body becomes overly imbalanced, some of your muscles bear the brunt of the work while others wither away. This is when injury happens. You've heard "If you don't use it, you lose it," but injury from imbalance is more like "What your muscles don't share, you'll have to repair."

Pilates builds the strength and length of your large and small muscles uniformly, and balanced muscles create bodies that are agile, coordinated, flexible, and less prone to injury.

## You'll Defy Gravity

If we have Father Time and Mother Nature, then perhaps gravity is our grand-parent, slowly sinking us deeper toward the ground. We can't avoid gravity. It acts on us every moment of every day, and if we're not working against it, we're unwittingly working for it.

As gravity presses down, our spinal disks—which we need for shock absorption—are the first in the line of fire. Compression causes our intervertebral disks to lose moisture each day, which, although replenished at night, is never restored 100 percent. Over the course of a lifetime, you can lose a few inches of precious height.

Romana loved to say that Pilates defied gravity. Nothing ever goes down in Pilates! Even as we lower ourselves to the floor, we are always lengthening UP at the same time. By doing this, we call on the musculature of the body—in particular, the powerhouse muscles—to help take some of the compressive pressure off our disks and organs. Pilates shakes things up by working the body in all positions to allow blood to travel in new directions, especially when our legs are overhead. And many of the "reclining" exercises were designed to maintain proper organ placement and take undue pressure off the heart.

## You'll Stay Slick

You may have seen or heard of the term ROM—which stands for range of motion and is most often used in the context of your body's joints. The more limited a joint's ROM, the stiffer and more limited your movements. Conversely, the more free a joint's range, the more mobility at that junction (sometimes too much, called hypermobility). There are "normal" degrees by which doctors and specialists

*"Extend from your center, return to your center."* —Buddha

# *How Pilates Gets You Fit*

may measure your joint ranges to determine their functionality. Happily, Pilates movements work your joints through their full, "normal," and comfortable range of motion for where you are, increasing range where need be and limiting it when need be.

Here's how: Wrists, shoulders, hips, knees, elbows, ankles, etc., all have joints where articular cartilage (the white bits at the ends of the bones that allow them to glide on one another) is covered with a liquid called synovial (Latin for "egglike") fluid that both nourishes the bones and greases the joint. These joints rely on synovial fluid to stay healthy. The less active you are, the thicker and less mobile the fluid in your joints becomes. Medical researcher, biochemist, and chiropractor Dr. David Williams says: "Joint motion increases the production of lubricin [a protein in joint fluid]. That's why activity—specifically, exercises for joint mobility—is so crucial to maintaining joint health."

## You'll Beef Up Your Bones

While density is not a quality we want in most areas of our body, when it comes to bones, density is aces! Bones are actually porous, but there's a limit to how porous we want them to be. If they become too porous (think osteo-*por*-osis), the bones weaken and break, so maintaining "full" bones is critical to their health—especially as we age. Bones are always changing, breaking down and building back up. Activity, particularly resistance exercises like those in Pilates,

increase the physical stress on bones, which is a good thing. The forces the muscles elicit when pulling on the bone creates the necessary stress to stimulate the bone rebuilding process. Isn't it great to know, then, that one of the best ways of maintaining bone density, especially when weight bearing, is through Pilates!

## You'll Breathe Easy

When you picture your lungs, do you picture balloonlike objects full of air, expanding and contracting with each breath? Well, that's partially correct. The truth is, the lungs themselves don't do the expanding alone, they are "breathed" by external forces acting upon them. Lungs are actually dense tissue through which oxygen and gases are exchanged and air is literally sucked into, and pushed out of, by the change in volume within the chest and abdominal cavities. The more expansive you can make the area around the lungs, the greater the volume and force of air you can affect within them.

Pilates exercises do this by stretching and strengthening the respiratory musculature of the ribs and abdominals through articulated movements and full inhalations and exhalations, freeing up space and allowing the bloodstream to function at its peak. Joe said that the benefits of breathing properly and filling your entire body with fresh oxygen was like the heat generated in your boiler and distributed by radiators throughout your house.

# You'll Keep Your Best Interest at Heart

Your heart is the great and mighty Oz behind the curtain of your cardiovascular system. Its steady pumping supplies every part of your body with the oxygen and nutrients necessary for things to run properly. Healthy circulation is paramount for your body to operate at its full potential; it's how you combat weakness and fatigue as well as stave off disease. According to Dr. David Katz, associate professor in public health at the Yale University School of Medicine, poor circulation plays a role in almost every disease, from dementia to diabetes, influenza to cirrhosis. Joe wrote that Pilates was conceived with the very idea of "exercising every muscle in your body in order to improve blood circulation." And how grateful we are that he was so thorough in his approach!

Good circulation also helps boost energy, and Pilates makes this happen tenfold! I can't think of a single time a client hasn't remarked on just how much more energy he or she feels after taking a session with me. Pilates stirs the system up and makes you feel energized and alive. The title of Joe's book, *Return to Life through Contrology,* is no exaggeration—it's a clever nod to the full benefits of the method.

# You'll Be Nontoxic

The lymph system is like an eco-cleaning service for our bodies—it eliminates bacteria, toxins, and cellular waste through your lymph nodes and then deposits fresh, clean immune cells where they're needed to protect you from disease. Joe referred to this *circulation effect* as "bodily house-cleaning" and likened it to an "internal shower." The lymph system works in tandem with your cardio system to balance blood and bolster immunity in the body, but it needs some prodding to stay motivated.

One of the main organs of the lymph system is the thoracic duct, which lives right behind the breastbone and in between the lungs. Inhaling and exhaling cause the lungs to act by compressing and releasing it like the bulb of a turkey baster, pulling more lymph fluid from its vessels and stimulating its movement through the body. I'm not surprised that Joe insisted that to breathe correctly, we must "completely exhale and inhale always trying very hard to 'squeeze' every atom of impure air from [our] lungs."

Since the lymph fluid is actually squeezed from the blood through smaller and smaller conduits, called capillaries, it can be influenced by stimuli like exercise, gravity, breath, and pressure. Romana used to tell us, "Pilates is an internal massage for your body." Indeed, the dynamics of rolling on the front, sides, and back of our bodies; the undulating and articulating movements; and the complete breathing we employ in Pilates are all perfect modes of stimulation for the lymphatic system.

CHAPTER 4

# Pilates for Your Plate

*"What we think is
electrochemically transduced
into physiological responses.
Thinking, therefore,
is a nutritional choice.
Author your relationship
to food and hence author the
chemistry of the body."*
**—Marc David,
author of *The Slow-Down Diet***

**P**eople love to peg fitness folk as naturals in the food department. We think our trainers can't understand food struggles because their bodies appear fitter than ours or they appear more disciplined than we are. And maybe they are. But keep digging, because there's almost always more to the story. The fitness world is chock-full of pros who have struggled, or are still struggling, to figure "it all" out for themselves. How many great trainers' stories begin with "I was overweight as a kid" or "I found fitness after stress left me sick and unhealthy"?

# *Pilates for Your Plate*

If healthy habits haven't been trained into us at an early age, most all Americans—fitness pros included—have suffered the same Doritos and Ding Dongs temptations. No one is safe from the onslaught of marketing jargon and food styling that bombards our senses daily. I find myself regularly schooling my children on the truth behind that "blue raspberry" candy or that talking cereal creature beckoning my innocent child to a land of Fruity Pebbles. Even my husband is taken by images of "butter" being sumptuously poured over "fresh" lobster tails on TV. I have to remind him of my friend who styled food for these ads and what he needed to do to that "food" to make it tempt our taste buds. It's gag-worthy.

No real foods sparkle, and few come in rainbow colors ('Rainbow' chard being a notable exception!). The bottom line is that most of us are simply trying to make better choices for ourselves and to move toward one healthier meal, movement, and lifestyle at a time.

## My First Taste of Nutrition

At the age of 19, I was referred to a nutritionist to help determine the cause of skin flare-ups that had plagued me throughout high school. At the time, I had absolutely no idea what a nutritionist was! I simply trusted my friend's recommendation and made my appointment. I was given an extensive food and health questionnaire to fill out, and the doctor ran a blood test. Results in hand, the doctor showed me my substantial food intolerance list—the culprits behind my skin problems. I was shocked. Oysters? But I'd never even eaten an oyster!

Right then and there, I was put on my first elimination diet, where I had to cut yeast, cow's milk, egg yolk, and 20 other of my favorite, yet inflammatory, foods from my diet. I cried at every meal. I felt deprived and hungry and sad to be me. But then something happened. I began to feel better. Not only did my skin clear up, but I felt a direct connection to the food I put in my mouth. I also began to recognize how each of my taboo foods affected me if I cheated. Some symptoms were stronger than others. Some came or went away faster. I began to recognize the power I could exert over how I felt by manipulating what foods I chose to put in my mouth. So despite the initial sting of restriction, the return on my nutrition investment has left me wiser and better equipped to practice self-care.

## The Way We Do Food Is the Way We Do Life

In the years since, I've taken a number of courses in sports and women's nutrition and been on fitness retreats where lessons in eating healthy were a main feature. From all that I have learned, I believe that you can absolutely, 100 percent heal, energize, and bulletproof your body with the right balance of foods.

My ideal world plan for eating would be all-organic, fresh, chemical-free, cruelty-free, whole foods all day every day. While I don't always manage that,

I never give up! Like any normal person, I struggle to balance healthy eating with my schedule. Gone all day without eating only to binge ravenously at night? Been there. Eaten all day flat in bed for days on end? Check. Went running for a taxi with a "protein bar" hanging from my mouth? Yep, that was me. Stuck diligently to a clean and healthy eating pattern for months on end? Yes! That too!

I like to change things up often, and part of my life's work is striving to balance these extremes. I know when I've gone too far. I hear my gut even if I don't always listen to it. I push the edge of the envelope but not without awareness that these are my choices. I accept the inconsistencies in myself because in the end it's about progress, not perfection. One of my favorite quotes—and my mantra most days—is this one from John Lennon: "Everything will be okay in the end. And if it's not okay, it's not the end."

# A Pilates Body Needs Nutrition

When we exercise, we're looking to move our bodies in healthy ways that promote energy and well-being. We want to feel great and enjoy living well in our bodies. Wouldn't it make sense, then, to eat for the same purpose? Eating to feel good means understanding what it is about our food (other than the psychology of it) that keeps our bodies functioning and feeling in top form.

In the same way that we want to work all of our muscles in a balanced way through Pilates (the large ones, the small ones, and the mental ones), we also want to create balance in the properties of our foods so that we're able to flex any and all of our nutrient muscles when needed. Let's look at the assets in our foods that help make our bodies happy and healthy.

## MACRONUTRIENTS

- **Proteins** are necessary for building the tissues in the body, including all the muscles, organs, skin, and parts of the immune system. The body also uses protein for energy or converts it to fat.

- **Fats** are needed to support the membranes that surround all the cells in the body, for normal brain and nerve function, and for signaling hormones. Extra fat can be used as fuel for the body or can be stored as fat.

- **Carbohydrates** like sugars and starches are needed to provide the energy that the body must have to function every day. Extra carbohydrates are converted to fat.

## MICRONUTRIENTS

- **Vitamin A** supports healthy eyes, keeps the immune system healthy, regulates the expression of genes, and creates healthy red blood cells.

- **B vitamins** help the body break down foods and use the energy more efficiently, and some help in formation of red blood cells. (There are eight in the B complex: $B_1$/thiamin, $B_2$/riboflavin, $B_3$/niacin, $B_5$/pantothenic acid, $B_6$, $B_7$/biotin, $B_9$/folic acid, and $B_{12}$.)

# *Pilates for Your Plate*

- If you usually eat in 5 minutes, stretch that to 10. Time yourself. Remember how long it feels to sit and enjoy your food.

- Eat sitting down, preferably at a nice spot where you feel comfortable and relaxed.

- Commit to no distractions—especially to not tapping away on your laptop!

- Concentrate on your food as you eat it. Think about the taste and texture.

- **Vitamin C** helps produce collagen for connective tissues and bones, repair tissues, and heal wounds and protects the cells from damage caused by negatively charged particles in the body.

- **Vitamin D** promotes calcium absorption (vital for bone density), regulates cell growth, supports the immune system, and reduces inflammation.

- **Vitamin E** is important for immune function.

- **Vitamin K** plays a crucial role in blood clotting and also helps the bones effectively use calcium (essential for bone density).

- **Macro minerals** build strong bones, help to transmit electrical impulses between nerves, help produce digestive juices, and clean waste products from the blood. They include calcium, chlorine, sodium, potassium, phosphorus, magnesium, and sulfur.

- **Trace minerals** perform a variety of functions like producing proteins, transporting oxygen, stimulating the growth of cells, or helping to repair damaged cells. The body needs only small amounts, less than 100 milligrams, of things like chromium, zinc, manganese, copper, iron, fluorine, cobalt, tin, iodine, selenium, vanadium, nickel, molybdenum, and boron.

## PHYTONUTRIENTS

"Phyto" refers to plants, and many of these chemical nutrients are found only in the colorful skins and flesh of fruits and vegetables. Some of them may function as antioxidants that protect the cells in our bodies from free radical damage and boost immunity.

Overall, phytonutrients are said to help slow down the aging process and may protect against a host of illnesses and diseases like some cancers, heart disease, high blood pressure, and other chronic health conditions.

A couple of phytonutrients that may be more familiar than others are carotenoids and flavonoids.

- **Carotenoids** (e.g., beta-carotene) basically give fruit and vegetables their red, orange, and yellow coloring. These compounds are believed to protect against certain cancers, heart disease, and even vision loss. See if you can eat at least five different-colored foods every day. The brighter the color, the better. This will help fuel your body with the essential nutrients it needs.

- **Flavonoids** have anti-allergenic, anti-inflammatory, and anticancer properties, and some (found in red wine or dark chocolate) may improve bloodflow and heart health. Other flavones are naturally found in parsley, celery, and citrus peels.

## Creating a Plan for Positive Change

Many people come to my Pilates studio wanting to "lose weight" when, in fact, what we discover along the way is that they really want to feel *good* in their bodies. The number on the scale is not the problem so much as what is going into their body, why it's going into their body, and how it's being used by their body. Ultimately, it's a question of how to love ourselves and get healthy with practical self-care. We've already discussed the ways that Pilates moves us to feel great and own our bodies, and it's those same values and principles that we can look to for help in the food department. If you are eating well and working out consistently, you'll find that looking good and weight loss are happy accidents.

Let's see how we can apply the Pilates principles of concentration, control, breath, fluidity, and commitment to our plate.

## CONCENTRATE ON YOUR PLATE!

Let's face it, most of us are so busy working down our to-do lists that eating becomes just another tick on a list. We eat without thinking about what we're eating while we're eating it. We don't look at it, smell it, taste it, or even remember it! I admit sometimes I've forgotten whether I've eaten lunch or not. Now that's scary.

So many Americans eat while driving or watching television or staring at their computers. Researchers at the University of Massachusetts found that people who watched TV during a meal consumed 288 more calories on average than those who didn't. But here's the real kicker: Thirty to 40 percent of how our bodies respond digestively to food is directly affected by our full attention to our meal.

This means that not only are we consuming more calories, we're also inefficiently digesting the food we ate because our body is not 100 percent sure that we even ate it!

The brain must fully cycle through the sensations of eating (like taste, smell, enjoyment, and satisfaction) before it can fully commit to breaking down our foods properly. It needs the assessment period of eating with attention to determine the best course of action for what will go where and then to tell us we're full. If it doesn't have your full attention, it will not register the food—and you will remain consistently hungry.

As with the practice of Pilates, the more awareness you bring to the table, the better your weight-loss results will be.

Rule number one is to start paying attention to what's going into your mouth from this moment forward. Be curious about your meal. Ask yourself questions like: Can I distinguish each of the ingredients in my meal? What are the textures of the food in my mouth? How many bites does it take before I swallow? Can I feel the food go down my throat and into my stomach? How much of this plate do I need to eat before I feel full? These questions are not only helpful in slowing us down so we can savor our food, but when we focus on almost any area of the body, we can increase bloodflow to that area—and better bloodflow means more oxygen, which means better digestion!

## CONTROL: THINK AHEAD, PLAN AHEAD

So many of my bad food habits rise up like a rash when I am short for time and caught unprepared (for example, convincing myself that an energy bar is an okay choice, when I would much prefer a fresh, wholesome meal). It's so tempting

*"If we're operating on automatic pilot . . . we are not sensitive to how we're being influenced by what we eat, where we live, the way we work, and our actions, thoughts, and emotions. When we're not aware of these connections, we also remain baffled why we're sick, tense, in chronic pain, or depressed."*
—Mirka Knaster, author of *Discovering the Body's Wisdom*

# *Pilates for Your Plate*

**STRESS-REDUCING FOODS:**

- Almonds
- Avocados
- Berries
- Lemons
- Swiss chard
- Walnuts
- Yams

to tell ourselves, "This time it's going to be different," only to end up disappointed when we enter the danger zone. We need to be prepared.

First things first. I found a deal on a professional organizer who came to my apartment and helped me organize my desk and my kitchen (it cost about $75 for 3 hours—a worthwhile investment). You could ask a friend to help you. I started by getting rid of all boxed or canned food with more than five ingredients, any food items I purchased with great intentions that never came to fruition, and anything with high-fructose corn syrup or chemicals. I then arranged my cabinets and fridge by food groups (sauces, gluten-free pastas, snacks, etc.) and then *labeled* them. (Labeling has made all the difference in keeping a sane

kitchen—we can see exactly what we have and what we need.)

Once I had an idea of our staples, I simply switched them all out for their healthier counterparts. Pasta became organic and gluten free, wheat flour became almond and brown rice flours, and everything in the cupboard that could be organic became organic—most of it gluten free to boot.

Here's my new routine: Every Monday after I drop my kids off at school, I go to the grocery store. I pick up fresh, organic produce and staples that need replenishing. I then come home and do any food prep: washing fruits and veggies, slicing or shredding cheese, dicing protein, separating egg whites. I place water bottles strategically around my house. On any given week, I make pesto, almond

---

## BREATHE MORE TO EAT LESS

Did you know that oxygen is the key nutrient to maximizing your metabolism? Well, it is! The efficiency with which your body metabolizes food is dependent upon having enough oxygen to burn calories. The greater your capacity to take in oxygen, the better calorie-burning you'll achieve.

But you must actually be breathing to make it work. Unfortunately, we're all so stressed that our bodies tend to go into fight-or-flight mode too often. When that happens, our digestive system switches off. The solution is to begin breathing with consciousness and changing the stress pattern of shallow and arrhythmic breath into the Pilates breath pattern of slow and complete breaths. Quite simply, breathe between forkfuls! Researchers at the University of Rhode Island found that consciously slowing down between bites decreased a person's calorie intake by 10 percent—and that's not counting the

added burn from a boosted metabolism.

Breathing doesn't just help you eat less, it's literally a fat-burning exercise! The body uses oxygen more efficiently when paired up with body fat as fuel. So open a window or get outside and start breathing, because the percentage of oxygen in outdoor air is

actually greater than that of indoor air. Joe Pilates said, "Fresh air is nature's tonic!" How right he was.

Most of us know that exercise boosts our oxygen quotient, but did you know that eating does, too? Chlorophyll is a biomolecule in the green pigment of vegetables (like spinach, broccoli, and kale) that allows blood to

transport more oxygen to our cells. Complex carbohydrates like fruits, vegetables, whole grains, and legumes can also significantly improve the blood's ability to transport oxygen to cells. Juices extracted from vegetables and fruit offer another way to put antioxidants into the bloodstream to enhance oxygen

*"You can survive for 4 weeks without food, 4 days without water, but you can last only 4 minutes without oxygen."*
—Marc David, author of *The Slow-Down Diet*

uptake into our cells, because antioxidants help the body use oxygen more efficiently. Foods rich in nutrients such as iron (beans, artichokes), $B_{12}$ (fish, cheese, eggs), and copper (chocolate, nuts, sunflower seeds) can boost oxygen levels and help maintain good blood status for delivering oxygen to working muscles.

butter, or hummus. None of these things take more than 10 minutes to prepare in a food processor! I've gotten my prep time down to a minimum, and it helps me stay focused and healthy throughout the week.

## FLUIDITY

Your body's need for water is second only to that of oxygen. It lubricates your joints and serves as a building material for every cell in your body (your muscle cells are 70 to 80 percent water). So why is it such a challenge to stay properly hydrated? Many people don't recognize the signs of dehydration because hunger can mask thirst. We reach for food when we really need fluid. Then, too, drinks like cappuccinos and cocktails can act as diuretics, and slugging them dehydrates us further.

Because water plays a vital role in the removal of waste and the transportation of nutrients, your body perceives any lack of water as a major stress—and one of the body's defence mechanisms is to preserve fat and water. Once you've reached the point of thirst, you're already on your way to dehydration. Headaches and dizziness, dry mouth, or muscle twitching can all be signs that you're dehydrated. Not sure how dry you are? A good self-monitoring method of your state of hydration is to look at your urine (I know, gross). The darker your urine, the more dehydrated you are (and vice versa).

If you don't love drinking water, don't worry. The solution to dehydration is to

consume electrolytes—which can be found in enhanced water but also in fruit, veggies, soup, and smoothies.

I like to add lemon, fresh mint, or naturally flavored electrolyte tablets to my water. Lots of fitness folk love to pack their fluids with as many vitamins and minerals as possible. People often ignore the amount of water that occurs naturally in food—take a look at the lists of fruits and veggies on page 43 that are packed with vitamins and nutrients to boot.

## MAKING THE (GULP) COMMITMENT

If you could have all of your meals and snacks made for you on the spot from fresh, organic, chemical-free, nutrient-dense ingredients, would you still choose the drive-thru window? If you knew that the "food" in fast food was not nearly as sabotaging as the "fast," would you slow down and pay attention to your food as it goes into your mouth? Self-care is about making the best choices for you—even if, at first, it seems like a sacrifice.

Here are five ways to commit to healthier eating habits:

1. Clean out your kitchen, pantry, or wherever else you stash low-quality food. Chemical additives are antinutrients. That means they're not only putting bad stuff into you but also taking good stuff out!

2. Make a list of high-quality foods you love (or like well enough to eat regularly) and find creative ways to work with them daily.

## A LITTLE "CONTROLOGY" IN YOUR KITCHEN

When you are so focused on a task, other things can fall by the wayside. Preparing for that eventuality is your smartest bet. This is what preparedness might look like in your kitchen:

- Clearing and organizing your fridge and kitchen cabinets

- Shopping and prepping before the week starts so you can make sure you have everything you need

- Taking a minute each morning to plan out your lunch and snacks for the day

- Keeping fast, healthy breakfasts on hand that you can take out the door with you

# Pilates for Your Plate

Eating quality foods is important. But the precise timing of when you consume those good foods plays a major role in your digestive health, too.

When you wake up each morning, your body temperature begins to rise, indicating that your metabolic fire is ready for stoking. Try adding food fuel to the fire between 6:30 and 9:30 a.m. to get energized.

Since our metabolic peak is between 12:00 and 1:30 in the afternoon, this is the best time to consume the largest meal of the day.

Between 2:00 and 5:00 p.m., our fire starts to dwindle, and we usually feel a touch of laze take over. (If only we could take siestas each day!)

Somewhere around 4:00 to 6:00 p.m., the fire begins to rise again, so this is a great time to enjoy a nice dinner. By 9:00 p.m., the metabolism slows in preparation for sleep. Although millions of us find ourselves ravenous around this hour, if you eat now you'll interfere with sleep and weight loss because your body will be busy digesting when it should be resting, rebuilding, and repairing.

3. Keep a food journal and acknowledge what you're putting in your mouth. Pilates teaches us accountability and how to connect to our bodies so we can better care for ourselves and, therefore, others. It teaches us awareness so that we can notice our bad habits and change them to good ones. By doing these things, we empower ourselves. It's not about getting it "right" all the time but working on making better choices a little at a time.

4. Embark on a safe elimination diet (usually about 28 days without the usual suspects—dairy, gluten, yeast, soy, corn, etc.) with the assistance of a nutrition professional to help clean out, wipe the slate clean, and start over to see what ails you.

5. Slow down and smell the coffee. Commit more time to sitting and eating with awareness and pleasure. Try to find a rhythm to your eating that works within the stoking framework of your metabolic fire.

## Eating for Your Mind: Alertness, Mental Energy, Vitality

When you eat until you're stuffed, your body needs to boost its metabolism to digest all that food. To do so, it pulls bloodflow from the head and extremities. This makes us feel tired and sluggish. To prevent these doldrums, choose foods that release energy more slowly and give you a gradual boost of long-lasting energy. Avoid foods mainly made with white flour, sugar, or other simple carbohydrates (high-glycemic foods) that deliver an immediate, short-lived boost but ultimately leave you feeling sluggish and tired. Some great slow-release foods to try are:

- Nonstarchy vegetables including asparagus, broccoli, cauliflower, cucumber, kale, onions, spinach, and tomatoes.

- Apples, berries, cherries, melons, pears, and plums. (Avoid quick-release carbs like fruit juices, dried fruits, and canned fruits.)

- Sweet potatoes are a super-energy trade-up for white potatoes!

- Nuts and nut butter contain very few carbohydrates, and because of their high fiber, protein, and healthy fat content, these carbohydrates are digested at a very slow pace.

- To replace your daily bowl of breakfast cereal with slow-release carbohydrates, choose steel-cut oats or quinoa instead.

Sugary foods deplete the body of the B vitamins it needs for energy. Sugar exhausts the thyroid, pancreas, and adrenals (the glands that produce true energy). When sugar is eaten, the pancreas is forced to produce excess insulin, which lowers blood sugar below healthy levels. This puts a stress on the adrenals, which must produce a hormone called cortisol to bring blood sugar back to normal. Years of eating sweets and refined white flour products weaken both the pancreas and the adrenals, leading to hypoglycemia (low blood sugar) and fatigue. The moral? Eat foods high in B-complex vitamins (all B vitamins help the body turn carbohydrates into glucose, a sugar the body requires for energy) as well as vitamin E and iron.

**IRON-RICH FOODS**
- **Animal protein**
- **Artichokes**
- **Chickpeas**
- **Dark, leafy greens (collards, spinach)**
- **Egg yolks**

**Tip:** If you eat foods that provide plenty of vitamin C at the same time you eat iron-rich foods, your body can better absorb the iron.

**B-COMPLEX-RICH FOODS**
- **Almonds**
- **Beans**
- **Beets**
- **Brown rice**
- **Carrots**
- **Citrus fruits**
- **Eggs and meat**
- **Green leafy veggies (broccoli, Brussels sprouts, spinach)**
- **Lentils**
- **Wild rice**

**VITAMIN E–RICH FOODS**
- **Almonds**
- **Cooked spinach**
- **Dried apricots**
- **Dried herbs (basil, oregano)**
- **Paprika**
- **Peanuts**
- **Pickled green olives**
- **Pine nuts**
- **Sunflower seeds**

Healthy fats also play a huge role in helping you manage your moods, stay on top of your mental game, fight fatigue, and even control your weight. Our bodies use fat to make tissue and manufacture hormones. Fat is also one of the fuels used by the body to make energy. Good fats include:

- Avocados
- Fatty fish (salmon, tuna, mackerel, herring, trout, sardines)
- Flaxseed
- Nuts and nut butters (almonds, walnuts, macadamia nuts, hazelnuts, pecans, cashews)
- Oils (olive, canola, sesame)
- Olives
- Organic dairy products from grass-fed animals
- Organic free-range eggs
- Sunflower, sesame, and pumpkin seeds

Here's something to keep in mind: Omega-3 fatty acids (found in oils, fish, and flaxseed) are highly concentrated in the brain. Research indicates that they play a vital role in cognitive function (memory, problem-solving abilities, etc.) as well as emotional health. Getting

## HYDRATING FRUITS AND VEGGIES

**VEGGIES MORE THAN 85 PERCENT WATER:**

Bell peppers
Broccoli (raw)
Carrots
Celery (more efficient than water itself at hydrating you!)
Cucumber
Romaine lettuce (has less water than iceberg but three times more folate, six times more vitamin C, and eight times more beta-carotene, making it a great choice)
Spinach (raw)
Tomato
Zucchini

**FRUITS MORE THAN 80 PERCENT WATER:**

Apples
Blueberries
Cantaloupe
Grapefruit
Mango
Oranges
Pears
Raspberries
Red seedless grapes (great to freeze and pop as snacks in summer—plus their skin contains the powerful antioxidant resveratrol)
Strawberries (organic)

# Pilates for Your Plate

more omega-3 fatty acids in your diet can help you battle fatigue, sharpen your memory, and balance your mood. Studies have shown that omega-3s can be helpful in the treatment of depression, attention deficit/hyperactivity disorder (ADHD), and bipolar disorder.

## Eating for Your Body: Weight Loss, Fuel, Lean Muscle, Joint Health

Digestion actually begins in the mind, right when you see or think about food. The same way that you can visualize getting better at a sport and then actually improve at it, thinking about food can add weight without even eating it! How cruel is that!

Like a billion other souls on the planet (but mostly in the United States), I, too, am fairly addicted to sugar and have a persistent Ping-Pong match in my head about whether to eat, or not to eat, "that cookie." But dreaming about food and not allowing yourself to have any, either because of negative self-talk or time restricting, triggers a response in which the body creates insulin in preparation for that food to come. When insulin is created with no food to act upon, it will begin to store fat and inhibit muscle growth.

Weight-loss strategies driven by restriction, fear, and shame can only fail, so the good news is that you'll have to be nutritionally nicer to yourself if you want to succeed at managing your weight! Here are some ways to start the process:

- Eat! Eating too few calories (less than 1,400 per day) is counterproductive to weight loss because the act of eating raises your metabolism, and this is what's needed to burn fat.

- You've heard it before but I'm saying it again—eat breakfast! Reset the rhythm of your day by getting this energizing meal into you before 9:30 a.m. You get one new shot at it every day when you wake up, so keep trying.

- Don't survive on a cup of java. Coffee is not a meal, it's a restrictor! Unless you are looking to put on pounds, especially around your middle, lack of food plus anxiety plus caffeine all create a hormonal stress response in your body that suppresses digestive metabolism and promotes the deposit of weight.

- Energy begets energy. To aid weight loss and build lean muscle, we need fuel, and the B-complex vitamins are very important to help the body convert food into fuel (see page 43 for a list of B-rich foods).

## Eating for Your Spirit: Soothing, Pacification, Cravings, Stress, Pleasure

Stress doesn't just kill your day, it can negatively affect your waistline, too. The brain doesn't distinguish between a real stressor and an imagined one. In the same way that pretending to lift a heavy weight sends signals to your body to build muscle accordingly, any perceived guilt about food, shame about your body, or judgment about your health is immediately translated into the electro-chemical equivalent of stress in the body. If you're frazzled and fried, take a deep breath, put down that doughnut, and start feeding yourself delicious, healthy meals—with a dollop of self-love on the side.

- Enjoy your food! When we shove quick-fix starchy carbs into our bodies, we rationalize that we're eating for pleasure, but in fact we are triggering a stress response that detracts from our actual enjoyment of our food. Taking pleasure in slowly and conscientiously eating food we enjoy raises endorphins (our pleasure hormones), which bring more blood and oxygen to the digestive tract and help to stimulate the burning of fat.

- Slow down! The more slowly you eat, the faster you metabolize. When stressed, the body goes into fight-or-flight mode, and the digestive system shuts down. Unfortunately, our fight-or-flight response is triggered all too often by deadlines, conference calls, bills, breakups, etc. If we can tell ourselves it's important to have a leisurely meal in the middle of the chaos, we might just find we increase our ability to deal with it all.

- Oxygen is the key to lifting depression. Vigorous exercise and oxygen-rich foods will up your maximum $VO_2$.

- Eat potassium-rich foods. By keeping your sodium and potassium levels balanced, you bolster the adrenal functioning in your body. The adrenals send hormonal responses throughout your body that, when overstressed, can lead to feeling fatigued, depressed, anxious, and unable to concentrate. (Calcium, magnesium, and vitamins A, C, and the Bs are also important in stress regulation and adrenal function.)

- Maintain strong bones! Bone loss can compound or cause depression. Women especially are at risk, and studies show that depressed females have bones that are 13 percent less dense than their nondepressed peers. Calcium is an ultra-important mineral. Beware of calcium depleters: caffeine, alcohol, air pollution, cigarette smoke, excess sugar, excess animal protein, and phosphoric acid (found in many colas).

# PERFECT PROTEINS

Protein is the muscle builder of the body—it forms the building blocks for your muscles, blood, immune system, and more. Too little protein in your diet can result in atrophied muscles. But how much is **enough**?

HERE'S A GENERAL GUIDE:
- If you weigh 120 pounds, you need approximately 42 grams of protein a day.

- If you weigh 160 pounds, you need approximately 56 grams of protein a day.

- If you weigh 200 pounds, you need approximately 70 grams of protein a day.

Here's what those grams of protein would look like on your plate:

BEEF
6 ounces >>>>>>> 54 grams
TURKEY, BREAST
6 ounces >>>>>>> 51.4 grams
VEGGIE BURGER
6 ounces >>>>>>> 51.4 grams
TUNA
6 ounces >>>>>>> 40.1 grams
CHICKEN, BREAST
6 ounces >>>>>>> 37.8 grams
SALMON
6 ounces >>>>>>> 33.6 grams
ALMOND BUTTER
2 tablespoons >>>>> 7 grams
EGG
1 large >>>>>>>> 6.3 grams
ORANGE
1 large >>>>>>>> 1.7 grams
BANANA
1 medium >>>>>>> 1.2 grams
CARROTS
1/2 cup >>>>>>>>>>>>0.8 gram

# Pilates Primer: The Technique

*"The first thing I tell
my new students is to forget everything
they've ever learned about exercise.
I tell them they are about
to enter a whole different world
with its own language and
its own way of approaching exercise.
—Jay Grimes, Pilates elder*

# You've learned that Pilates

involves a profound mind-body partnership; now it's time to meet the movements. Unlike weight lifting, where moves are limited to individual muscle groups, or an aerobics class, where the moves are the means to the end, each distinct movement in a Pilates mat series is designed to benefit you in a multitude of ways. As each exercise is learned, the movements are then sewn together in a particular order to keep your body changing direction and level (i.e., lying, sitting, kneeling, standing). Even the transitions between the exercises become part of the process and help maximize the benefits for whatever time you have dedicated to your workout. It may sound complicated, but really, there are only so many ways your body can move.

# *Pilates Primer: The Technique*

Many people have heard of the Pilates principles of concentration, control, center, commitment, breath, fluidity, and precision. But that wording didn't come from Joe. He described the principles of his method as also including leverage, range and limitation of muscle tension and relaxation, equilibrium, gravity, and breath. (Notice breathing is mentioned in both lists. . . . It's important!) *All* these principles, however, are worthy ideals to uphold. The more you think about and apply them, the better equipped you'll be to master the exceptional nuances of this method.

In the beginning, though, simply do your best and remember that the more you put into each exercise, the more you will get out of it!

Why do some people seem to get more from fitness than others? Well, I can tell you with some assuredness that it's not based on their genetics as much as it is their attention to detail. Pilates is a method of precision. In my 20-plus years as a trainer, I consistently see that those who have the mind for the work reap the most benefits. Sometimes, it's the details that escape you, and you may find it hard to believe that little adjustments could make a big difference. The truth is that the devil's in the details! But don't take my word for it, prove it to yourself.

## Pilates Parlance

Joe's thickly accented English was fairly limited and, according to all accounts, his instructional cues were made up mostly of prodding in conjunction with short, sharp commands like: "Pull in zee gut!" and "Long the spine!" In years since, through the creative articulation of its diverse teachers, Pilates has collected quite a lexicon of unique terms and phrases to spur you to action. See page 52 for a chart of the Pilates catchwords and expressions you'll see throughout this book and also hear in studios.

These are more than cute and catchy sayings. They are intended to teach proper muscle engagement, sound form, and use of Pilates movement principles so that you can get the very most out of your workouts. Some phrases may not click right away, but try to translate what you're reading to the actual positioning of your body. If it helps, you can even make up terms of your own! In the end, it's about what works to get your best results and keep you safe in the process.

## Creating a Flow: Transitions, Order, Repetitions, Tempo

In a Pilates workout, you're looking to create flow—or a steady continuation of movement—for a number of reasons. First is that this fluidity keeps your heart pumping at a steady rate, and second, fluidly moving from exercise to exercise challenges your powers of concentration and coordination. "Minimum of motion" is the catchphrase for performing these smooth transitional moves. When implemented properly, the **transitions** themselves become exercises. Watch out for unconscious habits.

For example, if you always flip from front to back by turning on your right side, then turn instead on your left; if you always stand up by pushing off your left foot, then push off with your right. You want to catch these habits as they happen so they don't develop into imbalances in the body.

Transitions become easier and easier as you learn the **order** of the exercises and the reasoning behind them. A bend forward is naturally followed by a bend backward; if you've moved your upper body in one exercise, you'll more than likely move your lower body in the next; if you're on your back for one or two moves, you'll be off it for one or two. The role of this choreography is to move your body in different patterns and planes of movement to practice for real life—well, that was before people decided that "real life" meant sitting in one spot for hours on end, staring into a computer screen. Let's change that, starting now!

People often wonder how performing such a low number of **repetitions** per exercise can have such a great impact. The reason is that you're often cycling through more than 50 separate exercises in a set period of time, so instead of working the same muscle groups over and over in the same way, you are getting at them in different manners from all different directions. Muscles typically get less efficient with each subsequent repetition, which is why doing too many of one move doesn't make sense. Joe knew that too much repetition caused muscular fatigue. In fact, he eventually wanted students to be in such command of their faculties that they could perform the perfect move, in form and function, in just 1 rep!

The **tempo** of a Pilates workout is really up to you, so long as you keep moving with rhythm. (Use the "Cardio Goals" guidelines on page 19 to determine what heart rate you want to target.) Set and follow the rhythm of your own body, breath, and heartbeat when you work out. Anything that might distract you from the goal of mastering the movements, like listening to your favorite tunes, would be unwise, especially when you're just starting out. Plus, there's a lot of Pilates-related stuff to remember and occupy your mind already. Down the road, when the movements have become ingrained in your subconscious, then we can talk playlists!

In the interest of authenticity, I want to mention that when you get to the mat exercises in Chapter 6, you'll see an Abs Series where you're on your back for five consecutive exercises and a Side Kicks Series where you're on your side for at least three or more consecutive exercises. It's important to note that only the first two of the Abs Series and only the first version of the Side Kicks were ever part of Joe's original matwork; the rest came later. Some were added as variations by Joe, postpublishing his original 34 moves in 1945, and some were created by his teachers to add specific movements to the mat.

Use your common sense when practicing and don't linger too long in any one

# *Pilates Primer: The Technique*

## REPS OR CHANCES?

The name of the game here is "Contrology"—knowledge of control—so it would stand to reason that with each repetition, we should be more in control of our bodies. I like to think in terms of opportunities and chances rather than reps. The following game works for my self-competitive spirit. Maybe it will work for yours! Instead of counting the number of times you perform an exercise, give yourself only three to five "chances" to get it right. Each time you perform it is another opportunity to get closer to perfect. Like trying to beat your own best score, try to make each move a little more excellent than the last.

position. If you want to do more of the variations, then make 'em snappy by doing just a few reps and then move on.

## Safety and Modifications

The best way to remain safe and pain free in a Pilates session is to stay focused! Study the "Pilates by Phrase" section (page 52) so that you recognize the cues and their intentions when you see them throughout the workouts. Perform the movements as directed and listen for signals from your body. See also Chapter 12, Pilates Rx, for more information on staying safe while you practice.

Also: A healthy dose of common sense goes a long way in staying pain free! First, make sure you've been cleared for exercise by your doctor or movement therapist. Then, if you come to an exercise where you're not sure if it's right for your body, I offer you this wonderful piece of advice from my very wise teacher Romana: "When in doubt . . . *leave it out!*"

The following are general safety rules to remember as you practice:

* Control is the name of the game! No sloppy movements. Move with care and intention. This doesn't mean you have to go slow; smooth and steady wins the race and is your safest bet.

* Powerhouse! Powerhouse! Powerhouse! Keep your tush, tummy, and inner thigh muscles engaged. When the movements are controlled from a strong center, it is much more difficult to hurt yourself.

* No ballistic or jarring movements. Save the wild stuff for the clubs.

* Stay within the "frame" of your body by limiting your range of motion (ROM). When building strength, you want to keep your joint range under your control and not allow your legs and arms to run away with you.

* Keep your abs firmly lifted to your spine when supporting your back in moves requiring lower-back extension.

* Don't roll onto your neck! There are lots of fun rolling movements and ways to send your legs overhead in Pilates, but make sure that you don't allow your body weight to land or sit on the delicate vertebrae of your cervical spine (neck). Where appropriate, keep your weight distributed on your upper back, shoulders, and triceps instead.

* Know your limits! This is a progressive exercise system, so save the more complicated levels of exercises for a time when you've mastered the foundational ones. It's much more satisfying to progress with safety than to regress from injury.

And here are more specific modifications you can use as you begin your practice, depending on your needs:

### FOR LOWER-BACK SAFETY, MODIFY BY:

* Limiting range of motion. Your lower back should not lift off the mat.

* Folding your knees into your chest instead of holding them up in the air.

* Placing your hands, palms down, under the base of your tail to stabilize your pelvis.

## FOR NECK SAFETY, MODIFY BY:

- Placing your head down on the mat instead of keeping it lifted. Keep the back of your neck long.

- Placing a pillow behind your head or neck to keep it in line with the spine.

- Rolling back instead of up. If lifting your head in order to roll up from the floor hurts, then start lifted and roll back to where you can maintain control from your powerhouse.

## FOR KNEE SAFETY, MODIFY BY:

- Limiting range of motion in flexion (bending). Place a ball or rolled bath towel behind your knees to limit ROM.

- Holding under your knee instead of over your knee (such as during the Single-Leg Stretch).

- Stopping to check alignment. When standing, check that you're not locking in your knees, and check that your kneecaps are facing forward and aligned under your hip bones and over your ankles. When bending, check that you're not letting your knees roll in or out (keep your knee aiming for your second or third toe).

## FOR SHOULDER SAFETY, MODIFY BY:

- Limiting range of motion within the joint. Keep your circles small, and don't lift above shoulder height.

- Stopping to check alignment. When prone, check that your shoulders directly align over your elbows and/or wrists. Check that you're not locking in your elbows on pushups or planks.
  *Tip:* The *insides* of your elbows should turn to face one another.

## FOR WRIST SAFETY, MODIFY BY:

- Getting off them. In almost any exercise that calls for weight on your wrists, you can default to your elbows instead (side bends can be side planks, pushups can be planks on elbows, etc.)

- Make fists. Create straight lines of energy by using fists to inhibit bending at the wrists. When weight is on your fists, make sure to push into the first knuckle to create balance, as the tendency is to sink into the pinky side of the fist, and this is a major no-no! (See "Proper Position" on page 165 in Chapter 6.)

# Pilates by Phrase

| PHRASE | WHAT IT MEANS | WHY IT'S SAID |
|---|---|---|
| "Work from your powerhouse" | Your "core" or power center. Composed of the abs (front to back), glutes, and inner thighs. | The word "powerhouse" is shorthand to trigger all muscles involved. |
| "Stand in Pilates stance"; "Pilates V" | Heels together, toes slightly apart. The natural positioning of the feet as determined by the thigh in the hip joint. | Squeezing the heels together gets you to find your "midline" and engage your inner thighs. |
| "Work in opposition"; "Two-way stretch" | Pull one thing away from another. To move the body in two directions at the same time. | To create dynamic stretch in the body; to utilize all muscles to create a "pulling apart" sensation. |
| "Work with resistance" | Do not move passively: Create an active resistive force with your mind that your body can react to. | To create healthy tension to strengthen your muscles. |
| "Abs in and up"; "Scoop"; "Hollow" | Draw your abs back toward your spine and simultaneously lift them. | To create length in the waist and space for visceral organs and to stabilize the spine. |
| "Articulate your spine"; "One vertebra at a time" | Rolling or unrolling your spine like a wheel, one bit of curvature at a time. | To help gradually restore the spine and increase flexibility. |
| "Work your C curve" | Making the shape of a capital letter C with your spine. | To serve as a visual reference to activate the powerhouse muscles while in flexion. |
| "Lengthen your waist"; "Lengthen your spine"; "Lengthen up through the crown of your head" | Sit up as tall as you possibly can to create vertical/axial extension. | To create space for the organs; to resist gravity. |
| "Soften your elbows" | Do not lock or compress the joints of the elbows. | To keep the work in the muscle; to strengthen around the joint. |
| "Pinch and lift your bottom" | Engage your glutes in such a way as to lift you off your seat (as if stuck by a pin). | To engage the glutes and the pelvic floor as a base of support to the powerhouse. |
| "Squeeze your glutes"; "Engage"; "Fire"; "Turn on" | Muscle activation. | To initiate a sequence of movements with intention. You create the action. |
| "Wrap your thighs" | Slight external rotation of the thigh bones in the hip sockets with simultaneous squeezing together of the backs of the upper inner thighs. | To engage the glutes and adductors more than the quads and flexors. (Don't overwrap!) |
| "Bring your wings down" | Draw your shoulder blades down away from your ears. | To counter the shortening of the upper trapezius. Lengthens and frees the neck. |
| "Pull your navel to your spine" | Draw your belly button up into your back in plank or other prone positions. | To engage the abdominal wall and protect the spine from overextending. |

| PHRASE | WHAT IT MEANS | WHY IT'S SAID |
|---|---|---|
| "Open your chest"; "Chest wide" | Draw your collarbones apart. Deepen your inhalation to expand the chest. | To stop the shoulders from rolling forward and inward. Maintains scapular stability. |
| "Knit your ribs"; "Close your ribs"; "Draw the ribs in" | The act of "pulling" the front ribs, just below the sternum, closer together. | To engage the upper abs and stabilize the spine. |
| "Tail down" | When a greater anterior (forward) tip of the pelvis is needed. | To create additional length between the ribs and hips in the front of the body on specific movements. |
| "Crack a walnut" | Retraction of your scapula (bringing the shoulder blades closer to each other). | To enagage the midback (traps, rhomboids) and open the chest. |
| "Wring out the air" | Continue to forcefully exhale until there is nothing left. | To create muscle action around the lowest portion of the thoracic cavity. Allows for a fuller reflex inspiratory response. |
| "Box square"; "Square your box" | You are aligned and level shoulder to shoulder, hip to hip, and shoulders through hips. | To make sure you are not compensating with one side of the body or another. |
| "Counterstretch" | Take the body in the opposite direction. | To keep muscles balanced. |
| "Work within your frame"; "Within your joint" | Limit your range of motion to equal or less than that of the joint you are working. | To ensure that you have the muscular strength and control to move within a safe range before venturing out. |
| "Pull toward your midline" | The invisible line that cuts vertically down the middle of the body. | To engage the adductors. |
| "Work with a minimum of motion" | Smoothly transition from exercise to exercise. | To keep your heart rate steady and to challenge coordination. |
| "Soften your knees" | Do not lock or compress the joints of the knees. | To keep the work in the muscle; to strengthen around the joint. |
| "Anchor your hips"; "Pin"; "Ground your feet" | Stabilize the body part being described. | By actively stabilizing one point, mobility can be more specifically directed to an adjoining area. |
| "Hinge from your hip"; "Break in the hip" | Fold from the crease of the hip joint. | To maintain a straight spine and instead create flexion at the hip joint. |
| "Keep your eyes on the prize" (a Brooke–ism) | Keep your gaze, attention, and command on the area you are working, usually your center. | To keep your head in correct alignment. |

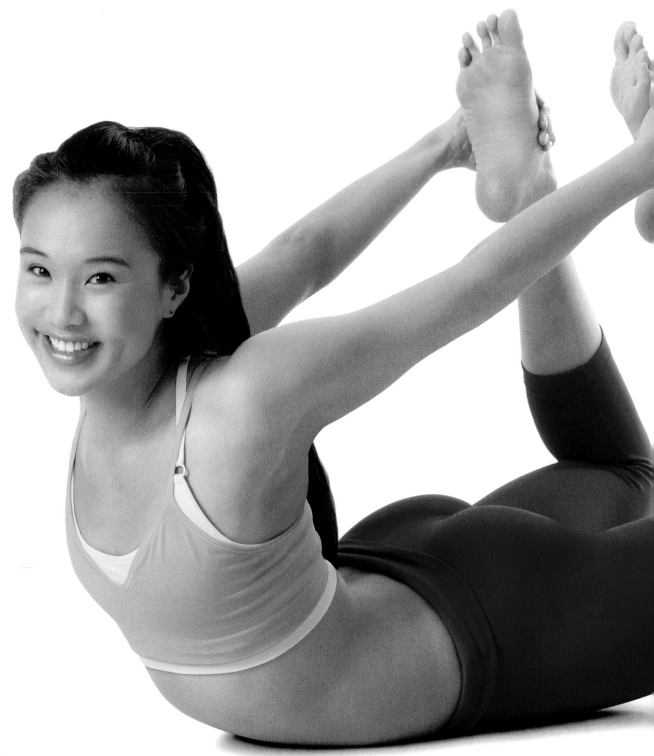

# Pilates on the Mat: The Series

# Find Your Level

Joe Pilates didn't distinguish between beginner, intermediate, or advanced work. He gave you what you needed based on his expert eye, knowledge, and intuition. You did what you could do and worked toward the rest. Today, we still try to teach this way in the studio. When a student comes in for a first visit, we'll chat a little about his or her goals, strengths, challenges, history, and needs—and then we get moving. As a teacher, I don't think of levels, I think of ability. If a student seems coordinated, a good listener, and eager, I may give her "advanced" work right off the bat. With a book, I can't meet you in person, but I can give you basic guidelines—and if you're honest with yourself, you'll get what you need with minimum risk and maximum reward.

Since Pilates is about developing keen self-awareness, it only makes sense that we begin right now with a little awareness test. I've come up with a few questions that I would ask you in our session and that I would use to direct my own exercise choices. Remember that this is designed to help you determine at which level to begin—it's not a judgment nor a prison sentence! As you develop your practice, you can move around the levels depending on how aware, committed, and connected you're feeling.

## Awareness Test

- I'm not so great at concentrating for sustained periods of time.
- I can't usually tell where I'm feeling things in my body.
- When something is physically bothering me, I'm not sure what to do about it.

**Does this sound like you? If so, start with Mat Series Level I.**

- I like to see and feel how my body moves.
- I am aware of how I sit, stand, and walk at points throughout the day.
- I am aware of my breathing during the day and can regulate it at will.

**If this is more your speed, see how Mat Series Level II feels for you.**

- I am a very coordinated person who does not often get hurt (physically).
- I like to challenge my mind with new strategies, and I learn quickly and easily.
- I feel a healthy balance between my strength and my flexibility.

**If this fits you, then try Mat Series Level III. (If it's your first time, go slow and steady through the movements.)**

- Physical challenges that require intense concentration and imagination excite me.
- I am the master of my domain.
- I can hop on one foot while rubbing my head, patting my tummy, and whistling "Dixie."

**Are you this kind of kinesthetic dynamo? Go ahead and try Mat Series Level IV on for size!**

# How to Build Your Workout

In the few instances where no breathing cues accompany the directions, it does not mean hold your breath or stop breathing! Simply breathe naturally through those movements. If there is a direction to inhale where your instinct is to exhale, use the best breathing pattern for you to accomplish your goal at that moment and then come back around to trying that direction another time. If you find that you are mainly mouth breathing (that is, no nose inhalations at all), slow down and work on breaking this breathing habit. Ultimately, if you can breathe through your nose alone, that would be great, but in through the nose and out through the mouth is good, too!

Pilates is a progressive technique. Each move has its own levels from moderate to difficult based on coordination, strength, flexibility, and risk. I have made the movement options progressive, too, so instead of leaving an exercise out completely because it may be too risky, I've subbed in its gentler cousin (labeled as a "I" or a "Prep") to familiarize you with the coming action and to maintain transitions that are as close to the full series as possible.

For all standing exercises, I recommend reading the section "Meet Your Feet" on page 253 before beginning. You can challenge yourself further without needing to change levels in these ways:

- Focus on fluidity by making transitions exercises, too.

- Raise or lower reps.

- Raise or lower tempo.

- Try a variation of an exercise you're already doing from a level up.

The more we understand how we move, what motivates us to move, and why, the richer, more efficient, and ultimately beneficial our workouts become. Joe Pilates spent a lifetime honing these moves, and each time I read his work (easily multiple dozens, at this stage), something else stands out to me. Usually it reflects wherever I am in that moment. Each time you open this book to work out, pick one element of your practice that interests you, and use it in the execution of your workout that day.

*Remember:* Without mental participation, you lose the keys to the kingdom. Turn your attention to the work at hand and don't sacrifice the experience in favor of rushing through. If you're panicking right now because you're the "zone out" type, don't worry too much, because resistance is futile! To climb Mount Pilates, you need a little brainpower—not just to reach the summit but to keep you safe in the process.

I have full confidence in you! I will guide you every step of the way, but ultimately you are your own teacher. Listen to your body when it tells you to back off or push further, pay attention to alignment and form, find the motivation to carry on, and use your imagination and creativity to make the system work for you. If you find a move that looks delicious but you're just not ready for it, look for a way to reap some of the same benefits by altering the move to meet your body where it is right now. Or perhaps it's wiser to omit that move for the time being and come back to it sometime in the future. These choices are yours to make, and they will help you to both master and honor your body.

# Mat Series

## LEVEL I
## > STARTERS

# ROLL-BACK

This is a perfect prep for deep abs, flexion, and articulation exercises—such as Rolling Like a Ball, Roll-Up, Double-Leg Stretch, etc. Whenever you come to an exercise like these and need to modify, Roll-Back will be your go-to move.

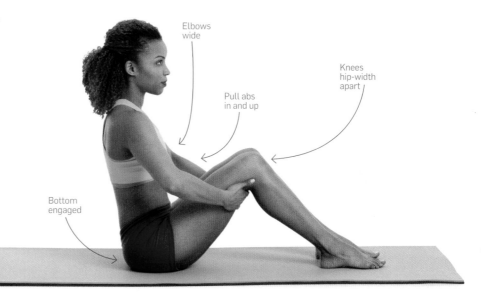

Elbows wide

Knees hip-width apart

Pull abs in and up

Bottom engaged

**A**

• Sit with your knees bent and your feet flat on the floor approximately 2 feet from your bottom. Place your hands behind your thighs with elbows wide.

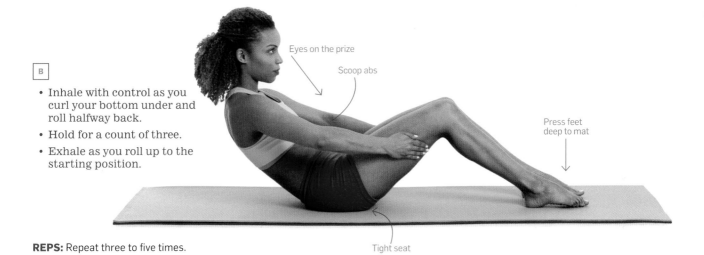

Eyes on the prize

Scoop abs

Press feet deep to mat

**B**

• Inhale with control as you curl your bottom under and roll halfway back.

• Hold for a count of three.

• Exhale as you roll up to the starting position.

Tight seat

**REPS:** Repeat three to five times.

## PELVIC LIFT

This is a great prep for standing since it targets your base support muscles of the lower body (feet, thighs, hips, glutes).

**A**

• Lie back with your knees bent and your feet flat on the floor, with your heels close to your bottom.

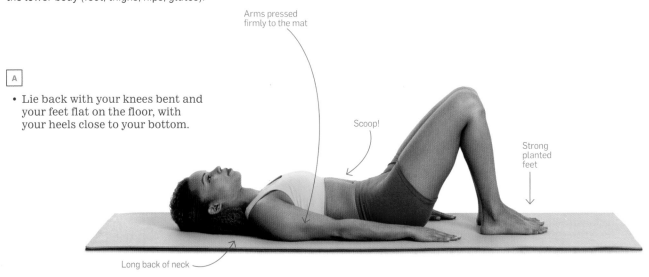

Arms pressed firmly to the mat

Scoop!

Strong planted feet

Long back of neck

**B**

• Inhale with control as you curl your bottom under and roll your pelvis up to a high diagonal.
• Hold for a count of three.
• Exhale as you roll back down to the starting position.

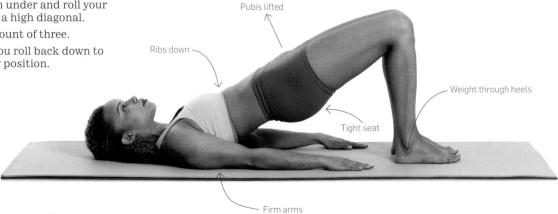

Pubis lifted

Ribs down

Weight through heels

Tight seat

Firm arms

**REPS:** Repeat three to five times.

# MODIFIED HUNDRED X 50

You are warming up your muscles by pumping your heart.

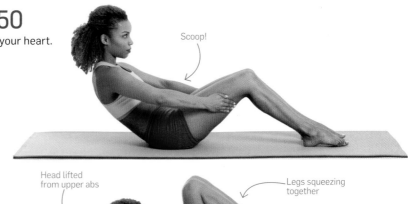

Scoop!

**A**

- Start in the Roll-Back position.

**B**

- Hold there, draw your knees into your chest (head lifted), and straighten your arms.

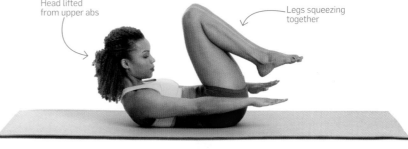

Head lifted
from upper abs

Legs squeezing
together

**C**

- Reach long, strong arms by your sides and begin pumping your arms up and down with energy (reaching past your bottom).
- Your knees remain bent into your chest and squeezed together as one.
- Take a long, steady inhale for five pumps and a long, steady exhale for five pumps.

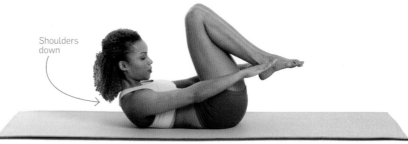

Shoulders
down

**REPS:** Complete five times (50 pumps total).

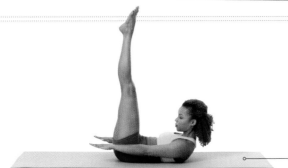

VARIATIONS ON THE THEME

Put your legs straight up at a 90-degree angle to the body and complete the arm pumps.

# Mat Series

## LEVEL I
## > MAINS

# THE HUNDRED

**A**
- Lie flat with your legs squeezed together and long, strong arms by your sides.

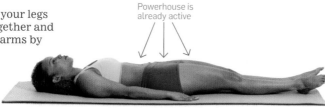

Powerhouse is already active

**B**
- Lift both legs a few inches off the mat, squeeze your buttocks, and scoop your abs.
- Lift your head and look to your toes.

**ASSESS:** WHEN YOU LIFT YOUR LEGS OFF THE MAT, CAN YOU FEEL THE LIFT COMING FROM YOUR POWERHOUSE MUSCLES, OR IS IT DEFAULTING INTO THE HIP JOINTS? SEE IF YOU CAN CHANGE THE WAY YOU LIFT YOUR LEGS TO ORIGINATE FROM YOUR ABS AND THE SQUEEZE OF YOUR GLUTES.

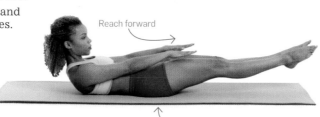

Reach forward

Tight seat

**C**
- Raise your arms over your thighs and pump your arms up and down with energy.
- Take a long, steady inhale for five pumps and a long, steady exhale for five pumps.

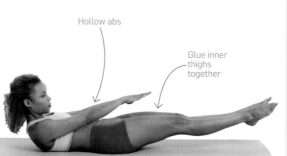

Hollow abs

Glue inner thighs together

**REPS:** Complete two to five sets (one set is 10 pumps) and work up to 100 pumps.

### VARIATIONS ON THE THEME
## Arms by Sides

Instead of pumping your arms over the tops of your thighs, keep your arms as close to the sides of your body as possible and pump the arms up and down with energy, reaching farther and farther past your bottom.

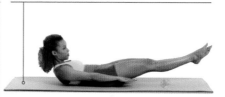

### VARIATIONS ON THE THEME
## With Weighted Pole

**A**

Hold the width of a weighted pole under the backs of your thighs as you pump.

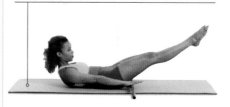

**B**

To challenge the move further, hold the pole over the tops of your thighs as you pump.

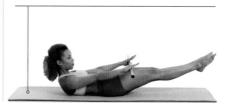

# *Pilates on the Mat: Level I Mains*

## ROLL-UP

**A**

- Lie flat with your legs squeezed together, your feet flexed at the ankles, and your arms reaching back close to your ears.

**B**

- Inhale with control as you bring your arms forward, shoulder-width apart, and plant the backs of your shoulders on the mat. The back is flat.
- Continue inhaling as you lift your head through your arms and begin rolling up and forward, one vertebra at a time.

**ASSESS:** REACH FORWARD TO TRY TO TOUCH YOUR TOES. NOW REACH FORWARD TO TOUCH YOUR TOES WHILE PULLING BACK IN YOUR ABS. CAN YOU FEEL THE DIFFERENCE THAT OPPOSITION MAKES IN THE MUSCULAR RESPONSE OF YOUR BODY? DO BOTH FEEL LIKE STRETCHES? WHICH ONE FEELS MORE "ACTIVE"? OPPOSITION ALLOWS FOR FLEXIBILITY WHILE PROMOTING MUSCULAR CONTROL AND STRENGTH.

**C**

- Exhale with control as you continue forward, reaching your arms across the room and trying to touch your forehead to your knees.
- Reverse the movements as you inhale with control back to position A.

**REPS:** Complete three to five roll-ups.

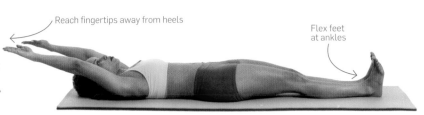
Reach fingertips away from heels
Flex feet at ankles

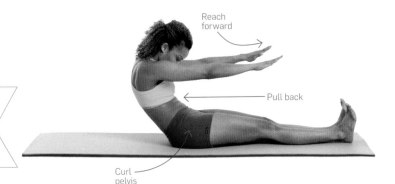
Reach forward
Pull back
Curl pelvis

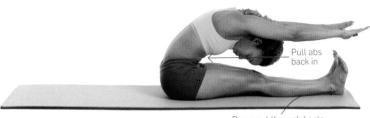
Pull abs back in
Press out through heels

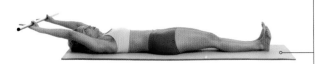

## VARIATIONS ON THE THEME
**With Weighted Pole:** Hold the width of a weighted pole throughout all the movements of the exercise, keeping the bar level. Use the pole as a frame of reference for how you move your body in space, and keep your abdominals scooped away from the bar in opposition at every stage.

# SINGLE-LEG CIRCLES I

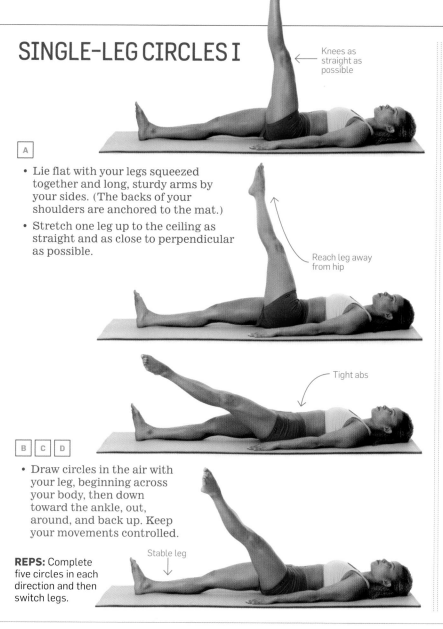

Knees as straight as possible ←

Reach leg away from hip

Tight abs

Stable leg ↓

**A**

- Lie flat with your legs squeezed together and long, sturdy arms by your sides. (The backs of your shoulders are anchored to the mat.)
- Stretch one leg up to the ceiling as straight and as close to perpendicular as possible.

**B** **C** **D**

- Draw circles in the air with your leg, beginning across your body, then down toward the ankle, out, around, and back up. Keep your movements controlled.

**REPS:** Complete five circles in each direction and then switch legs.

## VARIATIONS ON THE THEME
### Prep Stretch

Place a towel, band, or magic circle around the ball of the foot of your lifted leg and deepen the press of your tail into the mat. Now draw the leg gently across your midline and turn the thigh out in the hip. The tail remains grounded.

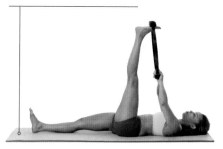

## VARIATIONS ON THE THEME
### Hip Off

Gradually increase the circumference of the circles to the degree that allows your hip to lift off of the mat with control from your powerhouse muscles.

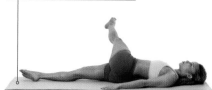

**BREATHING:** TRY INHALING WITH CONTROL TO BEGIN THE CIRCLE AND EXHALING WITH CONTROL TO FINISH IT IN ONE DIRECTION, AND THEN EXHALING TO BEGIN AND INHALING TO FINISH IN THE OTHER. SEE WHICH PATTERN MAKES YOU FEEL MORE STABLE AND PROFICIENT AND STICK WITH THAT PATTERN FOR A BIT.

# Pilates on the Mat: Level I Mains

## ROLLING LIKE A BALL PREP I

The rolling exercises in Pilates are meant as massages. Your back and organs are kneaded by the movements of the abdominal muscles pressing deeply toward the mat as you roll.

**A**

- Sit on the mat with your knees bent, feet together, and your palms under the backs of your thighs.

- Levitate your feet a few inches off the mat and create a high C curve with your spine. Lengthen the waist.

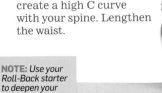

Legs together

**NOTE:** *Use your Roll-Back starter to deepen your understanding of the muscles needed for this exercise. The more connections like this you can find, the easier the coordination of movements becomes.*

**B**

Lift your bottom up

- Look to your abs and begin rolling back and forth from tail to shoulder blades, massaging the back.

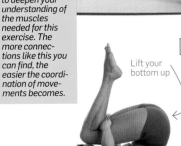

**C**

Eyes on the prize

- Inhale with control to roll back and exhale with control to rock back up to balance.

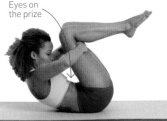

**REPS:** Repeat six times, staying centered on your mat and deepening your abs with each roll. Can you feel each vertebra on the way down and up?

## SINGLE-LEG STRETCH

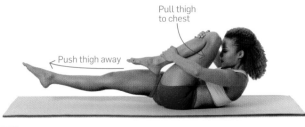

Pull thigh to chest

Push thigh away

**A**

- Roll back from a seated position, clasping one knee to your chest and the other leg extending forward and hovering 2 inches above the mat. Keep your head lifted forward, with your eyes on your abs, and your tailbone down.

- Your abs are scooped, your powerhouse muscles are firing.

- Inhale with control as you pull the bent knee as deeply as possible to your chest.

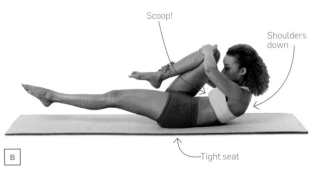

Scoop!

Shoulders down

Tight seat

**B**

- Exhale slowly as you switch legs, pressing your chest to your knee as firmly as possible.

- Maintain alignment of your box by pulling the bent knee directly toward your shoulder and reaching the extended leg directly in line with your hip.

**REPS:** Pull each leg into your chest five times, increasing oppositional tension between the pull of the bent knee and the reach of the straight knee.

# DOUBLE-LEG STRETCH

Pilates elder Jay Grimes likes to say that every Pilates exercise is essentially asking for "two-way stretch with a strong center." Use this exercise to epitomize that theory and remind yourself to maintain a strong core.

**A**

- Hug both knees into your chest with your head lifted forward and your elbows wide.

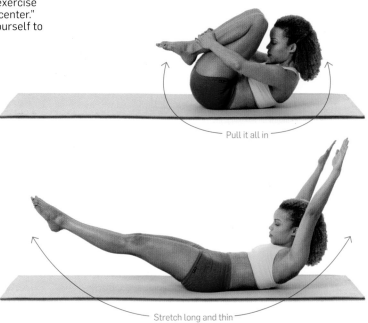

Pull it all in

**B**

- Inhale with control as you reach your legs forward and arms backward—stretching in opposition—and drawing your abdominals in deeply to support your spine.

Stretch long and thin

**C**

- Exhale slowly as you deepen back into your hug position, using the pull of your knees into your belly and chest to expel more and more air from your lungs.

**REPS:** Repeat six times, deepening your breath with each opportunity.

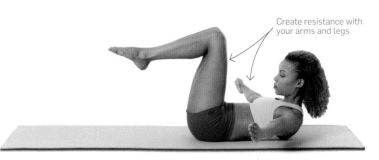

Create resistance with your arms and legs

**NOTE:** *Joe taught this move without the arms extending backward. Instead, the arms stretch straight forward and the palms are pressed firmly against the thighs as the legs extend. The hug position is the same.*

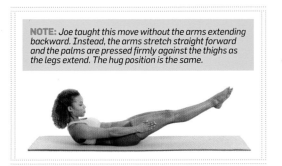

**ASSESS:** PAY ATTENTION TO THAT PELVIS! CAN YOU FEEL WHEN IT'S TIPPING FORWARD OR BACKWARD? AS YOU REACH YOUR LEGS FORWARD, DO NOT ALLOW YOUR PELVIS TO TIP FORWARD AS WELL. CAN YOU SENSE WHICH MUSCLES TURN ON OR OFF TO CREATE THAT STABILITY? IF YES, THEN NOW YOU ARE IN THE CONTROL SEAT OF YOUR POWERHOUSE.

## SPINE STRETCH

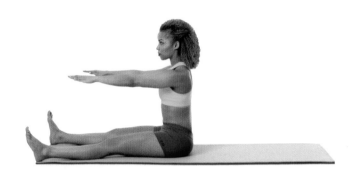

A

- Sit tall with your legs open to the width of the mat and lengthen your spine up through the crown of your head.
- Your arms are extended forward at chest height, your shoulders are nestled back in their sockets, and your feet are flexed.
- Inhale with control, expanding your chest, back, and sides like a balloon.

**ASSESS:** WHEN SITTING UP TALL, ARE YOU ON THE FRONT EDGE OF YOUR BONES OR ON THE BACK EDGE? CAN YOU FEEL THE DIFFERENCE BETWEEN THE TWO? WHICH POSITION CREATES MORE FREEDOM IN YOUR SPINE? WHICH MAKES YOU WORK HARDER WITH YOUR ABS?

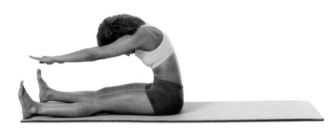

B C

- Slowly exhale as you curl in on yourself, articulating one vertebra at a time and creating a high C curve.
- Resist the temptation to simply lean forward from your hip sockets; instead, pull your abs back in opposition to your arms and keep your pelvis upright.
- When all your air has been expelled, inhale slowly as you begin restacking the vertebrae of your spine and returning to the starting position.

**NOTE:** *Joe taught this exercise with the palms sliding forward on the floor between the legs. This is a great variation for those with shoulder issues.*

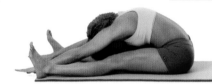

**REPS:** Repeat three to five times, deepening your exhalation with each opportunity.

VARIATIONS ON THE THEME:
## With Arm Circles

Each time you roll up to a tall seated spine, add a lift of the arms to increase the length in your waist and then circle the arms back to the starting position.

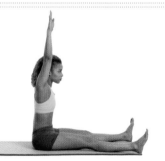

**ASSESS:** WHEN YOU FLEX YOUR FEET, ARE YOU FLEXING FROM YOUR ANKLE JOINTS OR YOUR TOES? WHEN YOU FLEX FROM YOUR ANKLES, YOU CAN BETTER CONNECT TO THE BACK LINE OF YOUR LEG AND UP THROUGH YOUR BODY.

# OPEN-LEG ROCKER PREP I

**NOTE:** *The "pro's" way into this exercise is to round backward from the Spine Stretch position and simply pop both legs up off the mat simultaneously, using your abs to lift your limbs; then grab your ankles and go.*

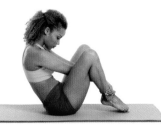

**A**

- Sit on the mat with your knees bent and your feet together, and take hold of your ankles, one in each hand.

- Lift your heels and balance on your tail while hollowing out your belly and lengthening your waist.

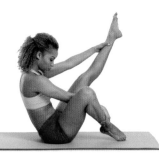

**B**

- Look to your abs and stretch one, or both, legs up in line with your shoulders and with as little movement backward as possible.

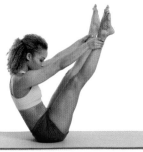

**C**

- Hold this balance as you bend your legs, touching tiptoes to the mat, and then straighten the legs again. Alternately, you can simply hold the balance for a count of three slow, deep breaths.

**REPS:** Repeat three times, getting steadier with each round.

**FUN FACT:** *It is said that Joe would remain perched in this balanced position on the edge of his desk while giving interviews. Talk about making a statement.*

# CORKSCREW PREP I

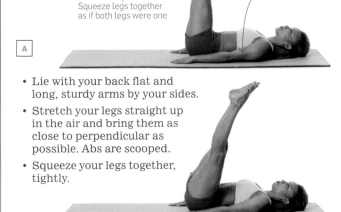

Squeeze legs together as if both legs were one

Arms anchored to mat

**A**

- Lie with your back flat and long, sturdy arms by your sides.

- Stretch your legs straight up in the air and bring them as close to perpendicular as possible. Abs are scooped.

- Squeeze your legs together, tightly.

**B** **C** **D**

No movement in upper body

- Point your toes and begin drawing circles in the air with your legs.

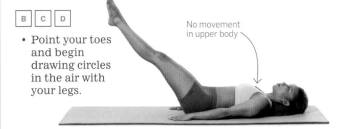

- Inhale with control as you reach your legs to the right, then down away from you, and exhale slowly as you reach your legs to the left and back to center. (This breathing pattern can be reversed.)

**REPS:** Reverse the circle direction each time and complete three sets of circles, deepening the scoop of your abs and stabilizing your spine further with each revolution.

69

# *Pilates on the Mat: Level I Mains*

## SWAN DIVE PREP I

**A**

- Lie on your stomach with your forehead down, the pubis anchored to the mat, and the inner thighs pressed tightly together as if they were one.
- Place your palms down on the mat under your shoulders, finding the connection to a lift in your abs, and press your elbows into your sides.

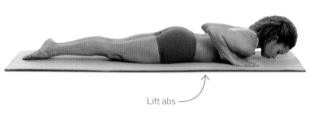

Lift abs

**B**

- Inhale with control as you lift your head and chest forward and up from the mat, searching for a stretch from the pubic bone up through your chest and out from your chin.
- Exhale slowly as you lengthen back down to the mat.

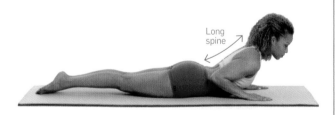

Long spine

**ASSESS:** WHEN YOU ARE IN EXTENSION POSITION (BACK BENDING), ARE YOU OVERARCHING IN YOUR LOWER BACK? YOU'LL KNOW IF YOU FEEL PAIN THERE. SEE IF YOU CAN CORRECT YOUR PELVIC POSITION WHILE IN EXTENSION AND TAKE NOTE OF WHICH MUSCLES YOU USED TO MAKE THAT HAPPEN. (HINT: YOUR POWERHOUSE MUSCLES!)

**REPS:** Repeat three to five times, looking for the chance to create more and more space between your vertebrae with each repetition.

## SINGLE-LEG KICKS

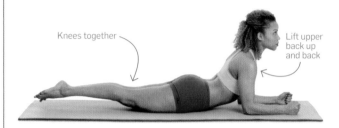

Knees together

Lift upper back up and back

**A**

- Lie facedown with your upper body propped up on your elbows and with tight fists.
- Your arms are shoulder-width apart and your elbows are aligned directly under, or slightly forward of, the shoulders.
- Your chest is lifted high, the pubic bone is anchored to the mat, and the inner thighs are pressed tightly together as if they were one.

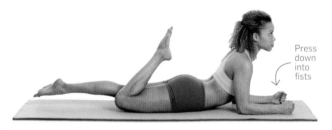

Press down into fists

**B**

- Maintaining this position, lift both knees 2 inches up off the mat and alternately kick your bottom with your heels.
- Switch legs, repeatedly sustaining the stretch of abs up through the chest and out the chin.

**REPS:** Complete six sets of kicks with the goal of incrementally increasing the front-of-body stretch from the tops of the toes to the hips and from the front of the pelvis through the crown of the head.

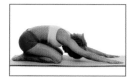

## SIT TO HEELS

This is a counterstretch for your lower back and not a rest position unless you need it to be. Use it whenever you feel you need to counter an extension with a forward flex.

From any exercise on your belly, scoop your abs and press your palms evenly into the mat, lifting your body up backward and bending your knees until you are sitting your bottom on your heels. You can place your forehead on the mat and your arms can stay forward or be brought back to rest alongside your body. When rolling up out of this position, shift your weight back to your heels by pulling back in your abs and rolling up your spine, stacking each vertebra one on top of the next from bottom to top.

# SIDE KICKS SERIES

Body position—maintaining balance on the side edge of the body.

A

- Lie on one side with your body in a straight line from the crown of the head through the spine, hips, and heels.

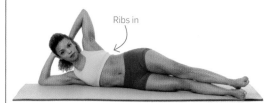

Ribs in

- Bring your legs forward until you have found an angle of stability (depending on your proportions, placing your feet on the front edge of the mat will usually do the trick). The more you wish to challenge your stability, the lesser the angle.
- Lift your head and layer your hands behind the base of your head, elbows wide, head in line with your spine.
- "Crack a walnut" between your shoulder blades and keep the elbows wide.

VARIATIONS ON THE THEME

Your bottom hand is behind the base of your head and your top hand is on the mat in front of the belly.

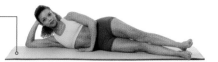

# SIDE KICKS: FRONT/BACK

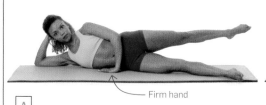

Firm hand

Stable shoulder

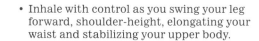

A

- Lift your top leg to the height of your hip, keeping it straight and connected to your abdominals.
- Exhale with control as you swing your leg backward, reaching your toes away from the crown of your head and keeping your knee hip-height. Allow for a shallow extension of the spine in order to open the front of your body.

B

- Inhale with control as you swing your leg forward, shoulder-height, elongating your waist and stabilizing your upper body.

**REPS:** Repeat three to five times, trying to "better your first trial," as Joe wrote, with each swing.

71

# *Pilates on the Mat: Level I Mains*

## SIDE KICKS: UP/DOWN

**A**

- Inhale with control as you kick your top leg straight up to the ceiling.

**B**

- Exhale slowly as you lower it, elongating your waist and stabilizing your upper body. The thigh can be turned out in the hip socket for more attention to the hamstring and inner thigh or it can face forward for more side-hip work.

**REPS:** Repeat three to five times, trying to "better your first trial," as Joe wrote, with each kick.

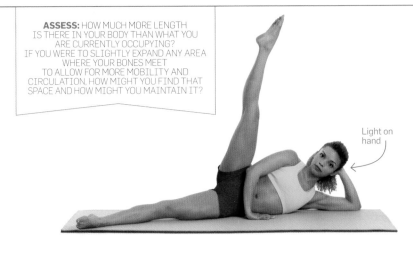

**ASSESS:** HOW MUCH MORE LENGTH IS THERE IN YOUR BODY THAN WHAT YOU ARE CURRENTLY OCCUPYING? IF YOU WERE TO SLIGHTLY EXPAND ANY AREA WHERE YOUR BONES MEET TO ALLOW FOR MORE MOBILITY AND CIRCULATION, HOW MIGHT YOU FIND THAT SPACE AND HOW MIGHT YOU MAINTAIN IT?

Light on hand

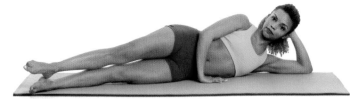

## SIDE KICKS: CIRCLES

**NOTE:** *The thigh can be turned out in the hip socket for more attention to the hamstring and inner thigh or it can face forward for more side-hip work.*

Lengthen neck

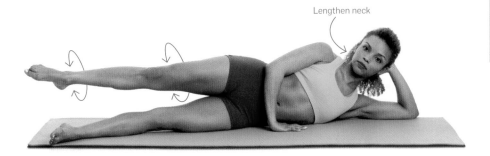

**A**

- Lift your top leg to the height of your hip, keeping it straight and connected to your abdominals.
- Imagine your leg is inside of a long cylinder, about the width of a basketball.

**REPS:** Circle your leg six times forward and six times back, trying to scrape the entire length and width of the cylinder.

# TEASER PREP I

**A**

- Lie back with your knees bent, your feet flat, and your legs squeezing together tightly.
- Reach your arms back overhead with your biceps by your ears and extend one leg in opposition to the fingertips, gluing the knees together.

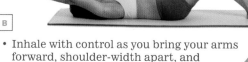

**B**

- Inhale with control as you bring your arms forward, shoulder-width apart, and continue to squeeze the thighs together tightly.

**C** **D**

- When your arms are parallel to your thighs, begin rolling up to a lifted foot, articulating one vertebra at a time.

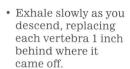

- Exhale slowly as you descend, replacing each vertebra 1 inch behind where it came off.

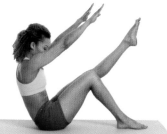

**REPS:** After two chances to deepen through your abs while stabilizing your lower body, switch legs and give yourself two more chances.

# TEASER PREP II

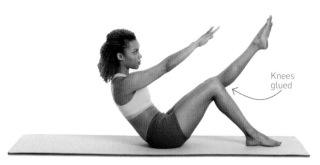

Knees glued

**A**

- Begin in the lifted position of Teaser Prep I.

Twist from the waist

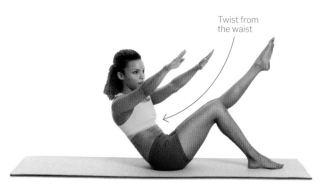

**B**

- Twist your torso (your arms will follow) over the extended leg and then square your box again and roll down to the starting position. Switch legs and repeat the sequence.

**REPS:** You have four chances (two on each side) to find lengthened rotation in the waistline while stabilizing your lower body.

# *Pilates on the Mat: Level I Mains*

## SIDE BEND PREP I

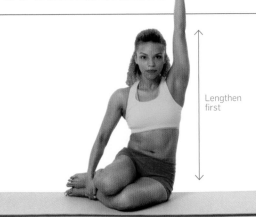

Lengthen first

**A**

- Sit on one buttock with your knees bent to your side and legs stacked knee over knee and ankle over ankle as best as you can.
- Using your leg-side hand, pull your heels close to your bottom and slowly inhale as you raise your opposite arm until your biceps touch your ear.

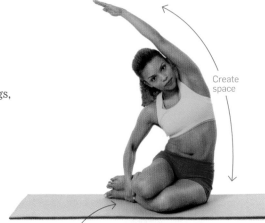

Create space

Pull on ankles

**NOTE:** *This exercise is often called "the Mermaid" and is a modern interpretation of the more rigorous Side Bend. To keep Joe's reputation intact, it might best be labeled "the Poseidon Bend" (Po-Side-on Bend)!*

**B**

- Exhale slowly as you side bend over your legs, stretching up the outside of your body.

**C**

- Return to center on an inhalation and then exhale slowly as you side bend to the other side by placing your hand on the mat in line with your shoulder and bending the elbow toward your waist. One arm is always overhead and connected to your waistline.

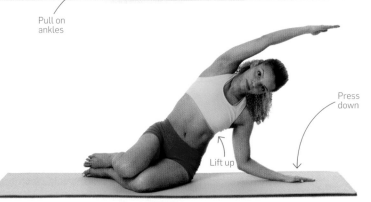

Press down

Lift up

**REPS:** Repeat three breath cycles, with the intention of creating more and more room in and around your ribcage for breathing to take place.

# SWIMMING PREP I

For the shoulder and hip joints

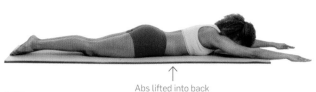

Abs lifted into back

A

- Lie on your stomach with your forehead down, the pubis anchored to the mat, and the inner thighs pressed directly together (i.e., no wrapping). Your navel is pulled to your spine.
- Your arms are stretched forward with the palms down, and your feet are pointed.

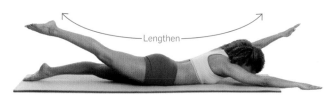

Lengthen

B

- Inhale with control as you lift your left arm and right leg equally off the mat (match the range in your shoulder joint to the range in your hip joint). Exhale slowly as you replace them to the mat.
- Inhale slowly as you lift your right arm and left leg equally off the mat. Exhale slowly as you replace them to the mat.

**NOTE:** *You can choose whether to lift and lower your head with each splash (lifting the head involves the spine). If lifting your head, keep it in line with your spine, and don't lift it if the chest won't lift, too.*

**REPS:** Complete two or three sets (left, right) of these "slow-motion splashing" movements.

# SWIMMING PREP II

For the spinal joints

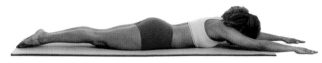

A

- Lie on your stomach with your forehead down, the pubis anchored to the mat, and the inner thighs pressed tightly together.
- Your arms are stretched forward with the palms down, and your feet are pointed. The navel is pulled to your spine.

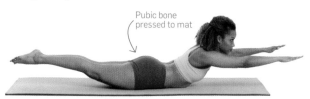

Pubic bone pressed to mat

B

- Inhale with control as you lift your chest, arms, and thighs off the mat, opening up the underside of your body, and hold your breath and position for a count of one. Exhale slowly as you lengthen everything back to the mat.

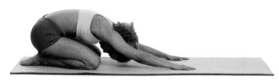

C

- Sit to heels (see page 71).

**REPS:** Repeat three times with the goal of lengthening so much that you might reach your feet past the back edge of your mat while simultaneously reaching your hands past the front edge of the mat. (If you were longer than your mat to begin with, use the perimeter of the room as your gauge instead.)

## SEAL

- Sit on the mat with your knees bent, toes together, and knees apart so you can see your ankles.
- "Dive" your hands between your legs and wind them around to the outsides of your ankles, one palm on the outside of each ankle.

**B**

- Lift your feet off the mat and balance on your tail with your abdominals scooped, inner thighs engaged, and biceps firing. Inhale with control and deepen your abs to initiate rolling back onto your upper back.
- Exhale to roll back up to balance on your tail.
- Try three simple Seals, staying centered on your mat and deepening your abs with each roll. Can you feel each vertebra contacting the mat on the way back and on the way up?

**C**  **D**

- Next add two or three claps of your "flippers" (that is, opening and closing your legs from your deep powerhouse muscles) as you balance on your tail, and add two or three flipper claps as you balance on the backs of your shoulders—never allowing the weight of your body to rest on your neck.

**REPS:** Roll like a Seal six times.

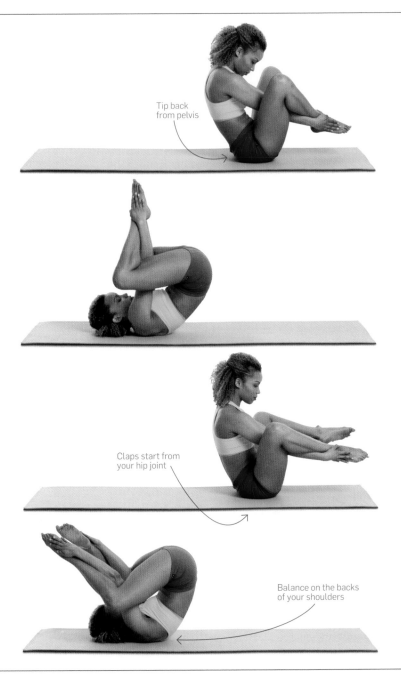

Tip back from pelvis

Claps start from your hip joint

Balance on the backs of your shoulders

# PUSHUP PREP

Rolling down into any Pilates-style pushup from above is akin to the Roll-Up, only vertical!

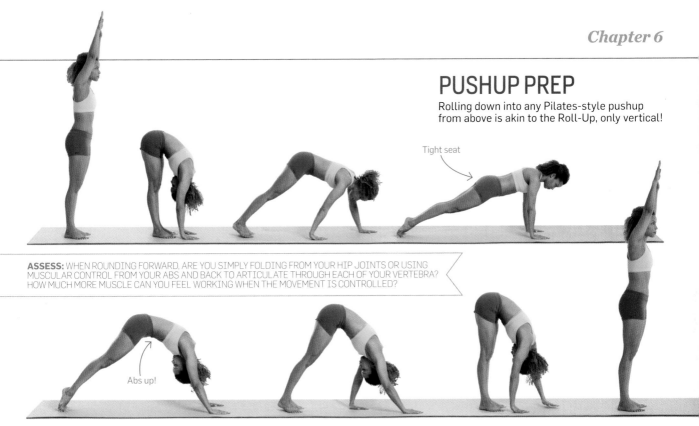

Tight seat

Abs up!

**ASSESS:** WHEN ROUNDING FORWARD, ARE YOU SIMPLY FOLDING FROM YOUR HIP JOINTS OR USING MUSCULAR CONTROL FROM YOUR ABS AND BACK TO ARTICULATE THROUGH EACH OF YOUR VERTEBRA? HOW MUCH MORE MUSCLE CAN YOU FEEL WORKING WHEN THE MOVEMENT IS CONTROLLED?

**A**

- Stand tall, facing the mat at one end.
- Inhale with control as you bring your arms up, lengthening your waist and squeezing the backs of the upper inner thighs together tightly.

**B**

- Exhale slowly as you bring your head and arms forward, shoulder-width apart, and lower your hands to the mat by rolling through your spine (*not* folding at your hips); the abs remain scooped.
- Place your palms on the mat with your head on your knees (bending your knees as needed).

**C** **D**

- Walk your hands forward in 3½ giant steps until you are in a rigid plank position from head to heels with the upper-body weight just past your hands and you are balanced on the tips of your toes.

**E**

- Lift from your powerhouse muscles and fold your chest toward your thighs, like an upside-down Teaser.

**F** **G**

- Lower your heels to the mat and push off your palms, walking your hands (with straight arms) back to your feet in 3½ giant steps. The legs remain as straight as possible until your forehead touches the knees.

**H**

- Reverse the movements and roll your spine back up to standing with your arms and waist lifted.

**ASSESS:** PAY ATTENTION TO WHAT MUSCULAR DIFFERENCES YOU FEEL WHEN YOUR KNEES ARE LOCKED VERSUS UNLOCKED. WHICH POSITION ALLOWS YOU MORE ACCESS TO YOUR POWERHOUSE MUSCLES?

**REPS:** Complete three Pushup Preps, using each as a chance to improve a different step, or two, of the sequence.

# Mat Series

## LEVEL I
## > ENDERS

# WALL: ARM CIRCLES

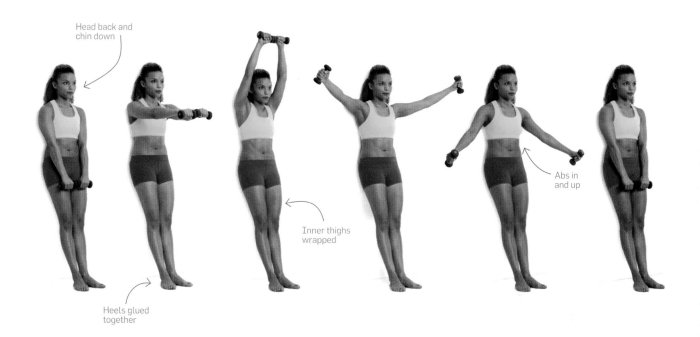

Head back and chin down

Inner thighs wrapped

Abs in and up

Heels glued together

**A**

- Stand with your back flat up against the wall and walk your feet away, as far as needed, to connect the back of your pelvis, your shoulder blades, and the backs of your shoulders to the wall.

- Squeeze your heels together and separate the toes fist-width apart; the thighs are wrapped.

**B** **C**

- Inhale slowly as you lift your arms straight ahead, the heads of the weights touching, as high as possible without losing the connection to your back.

**D** **E**

- Exhale with control as you open your arms as wide to the sides as possible without losing the full connection between your back and the wall.

**F**

- Then bring your arms back down and together.

**REPS:** Repeat the sequence, circling your arms five times forward and then reversing five circles. Use these ten chances to feel how deeply your arms connect to your back and waistline. With each lift and press of the arms, the waistline elongates.

# *Pilates on the Mat: Level I Enders*

## WALLS

I'd like you to officially change your perception about walls and begin seeing them as **vertical mats**! Use similar feedback reference points (the back connected to the mat, the shoulders anchored to the mat, etc.) and the wall becomes a tactile tool for perfecting your upright posture. Your goal is to get as much of your back as close to the wall as possible.

For those with bountiful bottoms, it can be difficult to make contact between the wall and the back of your pelvis (hence Joe's Pedi-Pole apparatus; see page 8), but just do your best to keep your abdominals pulling in and up and your tailbone reaching down toward the floor in opposition.

You may choose to use weights or put them to the side; either way, remain conscious of your wrist alignment and the connection of your arms to your powerhouse.

## WALL: SQUATS

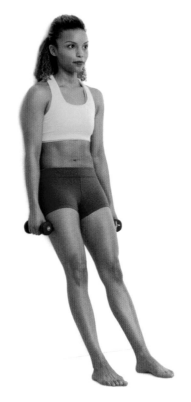

**A**

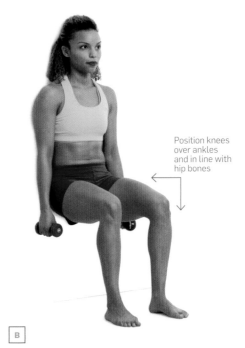

Position knees over ankles and in line with hip bones

**B**

- Open your feet hip-width apart and walk them forward to where, when your hips and thighs are at right angles, your knees will be over your ankles (shins perpendicular to the floor).

- Inhale with control as you slide down the wall until your thighs are parallel to the floor. (If this is too great a strain in your knees, simply slide only halfway down to start and graduate each time you practice.)

- Hold this position and hold your breath for a slow count of three.

- Exhale steadily as you slide back up to the starting position.

- Press your ribs deeply toward the wall and exhale completely, emptying all the air from your lungs.

**REPS:** Try five more squats, increasing the length of time you hold your breath by one count each time.

# THE WALL: ROLL-DOWN

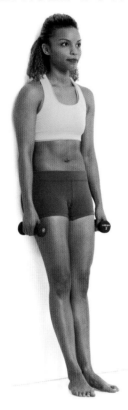

Keep arms heavy, neck relaxed

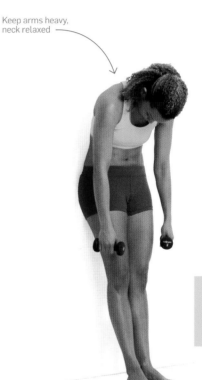

**NOTE:** *You can roll farther down the wall if that's comfortable for your back, so long as you remain scooped in the front and anchored in the back.*

 **A**

- Stand with your back flat up against the wall and walk your feet away, as far as needed, to connect the back of your pelvis, your shoulder blades, and the backs of your shoulders to the wall.

- Squeeze your heels together and separate the toes fist-width apart; the thighs are wrapped.

- Inhale completely and bow your head forward off the wall, looking over your chest and down to your feet.

- Exhale slowly as you begin rolling one vertebra at a time off the wall; use your abs to control the movement.

 **B**

- Stop when the base of your blades are firmly anchored to the wall (like a vertical Hundred position).

- Let your arms hang heavy from your shoulders and allow them to circle, like pendulums, in the sockets. Breathe naturally as you circle them five times in one direction and five times in the other.

- Inhale slowly as you roll back up to the starting position.

**REPS:** You only need to do this once, so enjoy every moment of it. (If you have the time you can always do it again.)

# *Pilates on the Mat: Level I Enders*

## USING WEIGHTS

Arm weights are a way to connect to your power-house in an upright posture. It's all in the posture and attitude. Since we work with light weights in Pilates, maintaining proper form and firing up the imagination are critical factors to achieving the results you want. The movements themselves are simple, but making them work for you can be the challenge. Try these two tips for getting more from your core: Reach your arms out straight in front of you and let your wrists hang limp. Without changing your position, straighten your wrists and reach your fingers long and firm. Can you feel the muscles of your forearms and arms turn on? Can you imagine that the energy coming from deep in your abdominals is traveling all the way out through your fingertips? Applying proper form to your joints will unkink the power lines in your body and stop energy "leaks" from robbing your workout. Now try to imagine that, instead of weights, you are holding handles attached to springs. Depending on the angle of pull, you can imagine the springs are attached to the wall or the floor. Remember, I have awards waiting for the best impersonation of you working with 50 pounds even though you may be holding only 3!

## BICEPS CURLS I

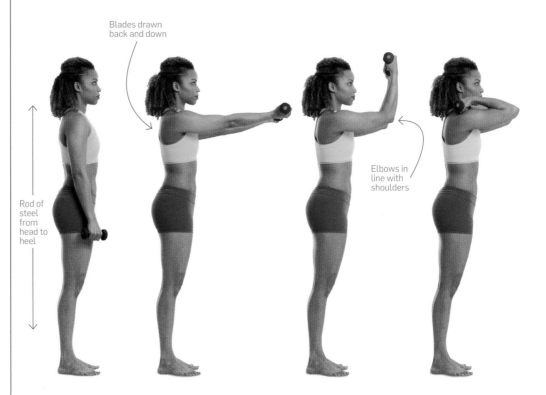

Blades drawn back and down

Rod of steel from head to heel

Elbows in line with shoulders

**A**

- Stand with your heels together and your toes fist-width apart, the thighs wrapped.
- Shift your entire body weight forward from the ankle so that it sits slightly over the balls of your feet and draw the abs in and up.

**B**

- Lift straight arms forward, with the weights faceup, to shoulder-height.

**C**

- Inhale with control as you bend your elbows, bringing the weights toward your shoulders.

**D**

- Hold for a moment, then exhale with control as you reach the weights away.

**REPS:** You have six chances to connect your arms to your back and the curling movement to your powerhouse muscles.

# BICEPS CURLS II

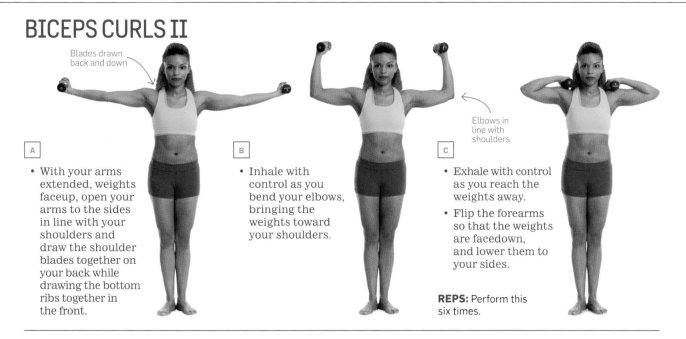

Blades drawn back and down

Elbows in line with shoulders

**A**
- With your arms extended, weights faceup, open your arms to the sides in line with your shoulders and draw the shoulder blades together on your back while drawing the bottom ribs together in the front.

**B**
- Inhale with control as you bend your elbows, bringing the weights toward your shoulders.

**C**
- Exhale with control as you reach the weights away.
- Flip the forearms so that the weights are facedown, and lower them to your sides.

**REPS:** Perform this six times.

# BICEPS CURLS III

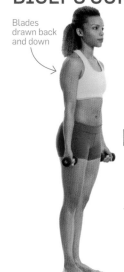
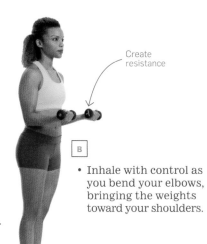
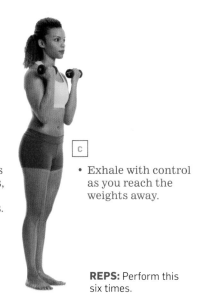

Blades drawn back and down

Create resistance

**A**
- With your arms long and strong by your sides, turn your forearms forward so the weights face front.
- Draw your shoulder blades together on your back while drawing the bottom ribs together in the front.

**B**
- Inhale with control as you bend your elbows, bringing the weights toward your shoulders.

**C**
- Exhale with control as you reach the weights away.

**REPS:** Perform this six times.

# Mat Sequence >LEVEL I

**Start »**
The Hundred
(page 63)

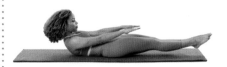

**5** Single-Leg Stretch
(page 66)

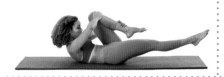

**6** Double-Leg Stretch
(page 67)

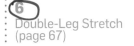

**7** Spine Stretch
(page 68)

**11** Single-Leg Kick
(page 70)

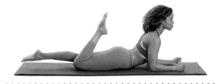

**12** Sit to Heels
(page 71)

**13** Side Kicks: Front/Back
(page 71)

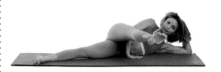

**17** Teaser Prep II
(page 73)

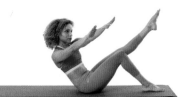

**18** Swimming Prep I
(page 75)

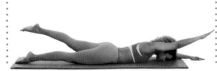

**19** Swimming Prep II
(page 75)

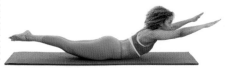

**2**
Roll-Up
(page 64)

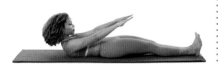

**3**
Single-Leg
Circles
(page 65)

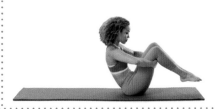

**4**
Rolling like a Ball Prep
(page 66)

**8**
Open-Leg Rocker Prep I
(page 69)

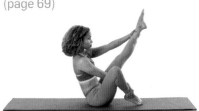

**9**
Corkscrew Prep I
(page 69)

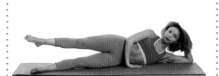

**10**
Swan Dive Prep I
(page 70)

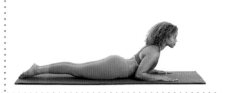

**14**
Side Kicks:
Up/Down
(page 72)

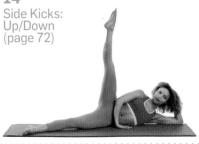

**15**
Side Kicks: Circles
(page 72)

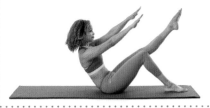

**16**
Teaser Prep I
(page 73)

**20**
Side Bend
Prep I
(page 74)

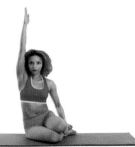

**21**
Seal
(page 76)

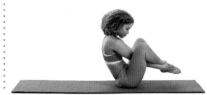

**End**
Pushup Prep
(page 77)

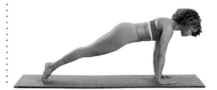

# Mat Series

## LEVEL II
> **STARTERS**

# ELEPHANT PLANKS

Rolling down into any Pilates-style pushup from above is akin to the Roll-Up, only vertical!

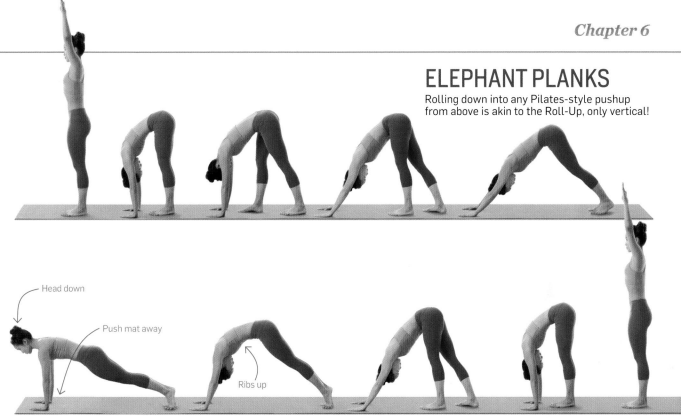

Head down

Push mat away

Ribs up

---

**A**

- Stand tall at the front edge of the mat (facing away) and inhale with control as you bring your arms up, wrapping the thighs together tightly and drawing the abs in and up.

**B**

- Exhale slowly and round forward with control, bringing your palms to the mat. Reach your forehead to your knees.

**C** **D**

- With stiff legs and feet, march your heels backward using just 3½ strides to get you down to a rigid plank position ("steel from head to heels").

**E**

- Hold your plank for a count of three, using the time to broaden the chest and press the mat away.

**F** **G**

- Lift from your powerhouse muscles, draw the ribs in, and fold your chest toward your thighs, like an upside-down Teaser.

**H** **I**

- Lower your heels to the mat and, keeping the knees dead-straight and the feet flexed, walk your feet as far between your hands as possible, scooping your abs to make room for the length of your legs.

**J**

- Roll up to the starting position.

**REPS:** You get five repetitions to appreciate how hard an elephant works in its abs to manage those stiff legs.

# Pilates on the Mat: Level II Starters

## STANDING SAW

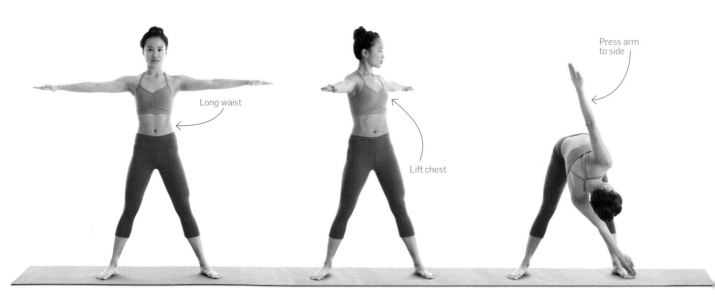

Long waist

Lift chest

Press arm to side

**A**

- Stand sideways on your mat with your arms straight out to your sides at shoulder-height and your legs wider than your shoulders and turned out slightly in the hips, knees, and feet.

**B**

- Inhale with control as you lift your chest and crack a walnut between your blades while rotating your trunk to the left—your hips remain facing front.

**C** **D**

- Exhale with control as you draw the ribs in and round down to your left knee, sending your right hand past your left ankle and drawing your forehead toward your knee. The back arm is lifted in opposition to the crown of your head.

- With the abs scooped, touch your forehead to your knee.

**E**

- Inhale slowly as you roll back up, articulating your spine, to the starting position.

- Repeat the sequence, twisting to the right.

**REPS:** Perform three sets, using every twisting and rounding opportunity to articulate the joints of your spine in preparation for your matwork.

# JOGGING KNEES UP/HEELS UP

The key to anything even remotely impactful on your joints is a strong set of feet and powerful powerhouse muscles to help with pushoff and lift as well as to control your landing.

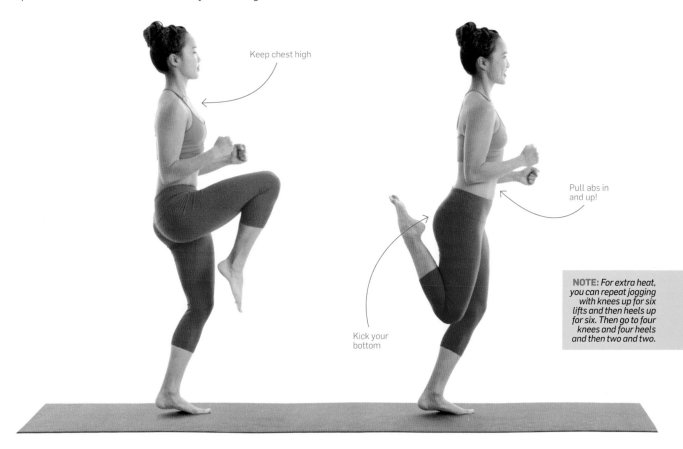

Keep chest high

Pull abs in and up!

Kick your bottom

**NOTE:** *For extra heat, you can repeat jogging with knees up for six lifts and then heels up for six. Then go to four knees and four heels and then two and two.*

**A**

- Stand tall with your chest lifted and your elbows bent to your sides, fists clenched.
- Begin jogging and lifting your knees up as high as possible into your belly (like an upright Single-Leg Stretch).

**B**

- After 10 knee lifts, keep jogging but this time kick each heel up to your bottom for a total of 10 kicks (like an upright Single-Leg Kick).
- The chest must stay lifted as high as possible throughout the entire jogging sequence, and the abs are pulled in and up.

# Mat Series

## LEVEL II
## >MAINS

# TRANSITION: LOWERING DOWN TO THE MAT

If you are suffering from a knee injury, this move is not for you.

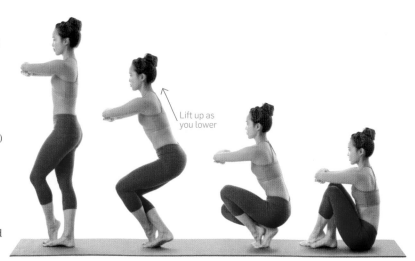

Lift up as you lower

 **A**

- Stand toward one end of the mat, facing away from the center.
- Cross one ankle over the other and fold your arms, like a genie, in front of your shoulders.
- Now switch ankles and switch your arm fold so you use your less comfortable pairing. (Hey, we're here to break habits!)

 **B** **C** **D**

- Exhale completely, emptying your lungs by drawing your ribs together, and then inhale slowly as you lower your bottom to the mat with control. As you lower down, your abs are pulling farther in and up in opposition to the mat.

# ROLLING LIKE A BALL

The rolling exercises in Pilates are meant as massages. Your back and organs are kneaded by the movements of the abdominal muscles pressing deeply toward the mat as you roll.

Keep heels close to bottom

Stay round

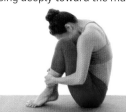 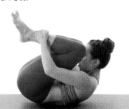 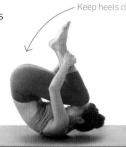 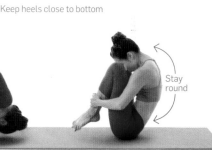

**A**

- Sit on the mat with your knees bent to your chest and your hands wrapped tightly around the fronts of your ankles.
- Tuck your head down between your knees and pull your abs in and up away from the thighs.

**B** **C**

- Roll onto your upper back—never allowing the weight of your body to rest on your cervical vertebrae.

**D**

- Roll back up to balance on your tail. Draw the ribs in.

**REPS:** Try to roll like a ball six to ten times, working on deepening your scoop and bringing your heels to your bottom more and more with each opportunity.

# *Pilates on the Mat: Level II Mains*

## SINGLE STRAIGHT-LEG STRETCH

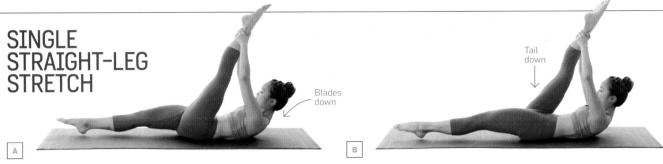

Blades down

Tail down

**A**

- Lie on your back with your head lifted forward, the ribs drawn in, your knees into your chest and your eyes on your scooped abs.
- Straighten one leg to the ceiling and take hold of the ankle or calf with both hands while straightening your other leg forward a few inches above the mat.

**B**

- Inhale slowly as you switch legs twice, focusing on keeping your shoulder blades and tailbone grounded to the mat.
- Exhale slowly as you switch legs twice, maintaining alignment of your box by keeping the lifted leg directly in line with its corresponding shoulder and the extended leg directly in line with its corresponding hip.

**REPS:** Complete three full breath cycles (inhalation and exhalation) or 12 switches total.

## DOUBLE STRAIGHT-LEG STRETCH PREP

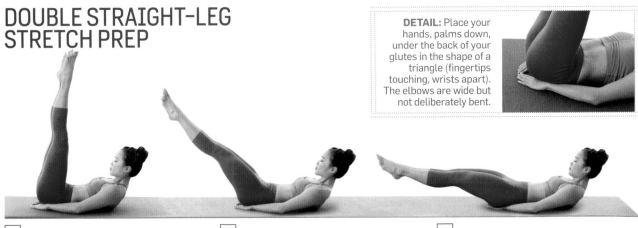

**DETAIL:** Place your hands, palms down, under the back of your glutes in the shape of a triangle (fingertips touching, wrists apart). The elbows are wide but not deliberately bent.

**A**

- Lie on your back with your head lifted and the ribs drawn in.
- Create a "wedge" under your pelvis for stability (see detail).

**B**

- Exhale slowly as you simultaneously stretch your legs away and pull the abs in and up to create oppositional pull.

**C**

- Lower your legs as far as possible while keeping the lower back firmly connected to the mat.
- Inhale with control as you bring your legs back to a 90-degree angle, making sure they remain resolutely straight.

**REPS:** Repeat six times, deepening your bottom ribs and using each stretch as an opportunity to further lengthen your waist. See how much of your upper body you can keep pinned to the mat as you go.

92

# CORKSCREW PREP II

- Lie flat on your back with long, sturdy arms by your sides. (The backs of your arms and shoulders are anchored to the mat.) The abs are scooped.

- Squeeze your legs together, tightly wrapping from the backs of your upper inner thighs, as if both legs were now one, and raise them straight up in the air as close to perpendicular as possible.

- Point your toes and feet and inhale with control as you circle to the right and exhale with control as you come around to the left and back to center. (This breathing pattern can be reversed.)

- As you circle your legs toward center, press the backs of your arms and shoulders firmly into the mat and lift your bottom up until you are balanced in the middle of your shoulder blades and on the backs of your arms (the wrists are flat, the triceps are firing).

- Inhale slowly as you roll back down your spine with articulation, and when your bottom touches the mat, reverse the circle.

**REPS:** Continue reversing the circle direction each time and complete three sets, deepening the scoop of your abs and stabilizing your spine further with each revolution.

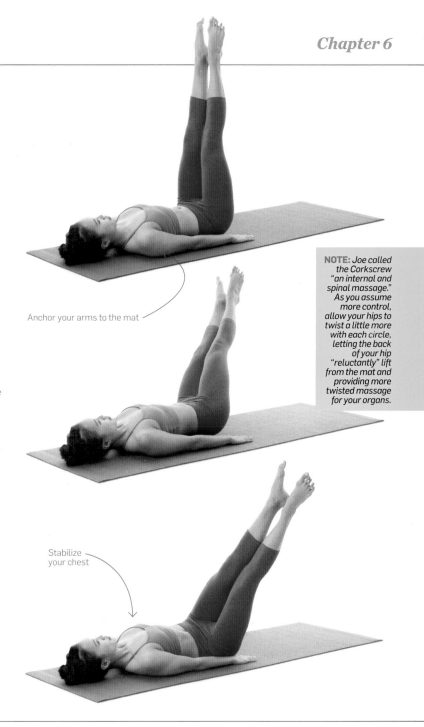

Anchor your arms to the mat

**NOTE:** *Joe called the Corkscrew "an internal and spinal massage." As you assume more control, allow your hips to twist a little more with each circle, letting the back of your hip "reluctantly" lift from the mat and providing more twisted massage for your organs.*

Stabilize your chest

## OPEN-LEG ROCKER PREP II

The rolling exercises in Pilates are meant as massages. Your back and organs are kneaded by the movements of the abdominal muscles pressing deeply toward the mat as you roll.

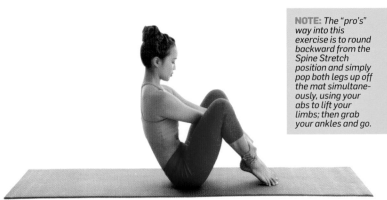

**NOTE:** *The "pro's" way into this exercise is to round backward from the Spine Stretch position and simply pop both legs up off the mat simultaneously, using your abs to lift your limbs; then grab your ankles and go.*

**A**

- Sit on the mat with your knees bent and your feet together.
- Reach between your legs and take hold of your ankles, one in each hand.
- Lift your heels and balance on your tail while hollowing out your belly and lengthening your waist.

**BREATH FOR ROCKING AND ROLLING:** JOE RECOMMENDED INHALING IN THE STABLE POSITIONS AND EXHALING ON THE ROLLING PORTIONS IN ORDER TO "PRESS" THE AIR OUT. FIND THE PATTERN OF BREATH THAT BEST HELPS YOU STABILIZE AND MOBILIZE WHERE NEEDED.

**B**

- Look to your abs ("eyes on the prize") and stretch both legs up in line with your shoulders and with as little movement backward as possible.

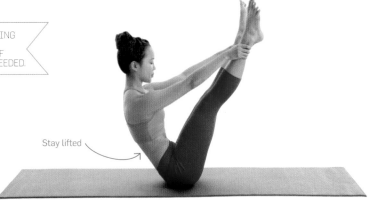

Stay lifted

**C**

- From this lifted, balanced position, deepen the abs in and up along the spine and rock back to the base of the shoulder blades—pressing your palms into the shins and your shins into the palms—and then rock back up to your tail. Your arms and legs remain firmly extended.

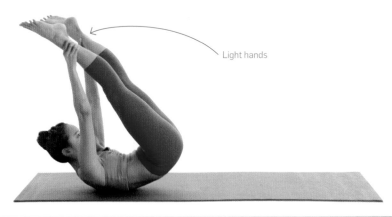

Light hands

**REPS:** Perform four to six sets, getting higher and lighter in your hands to turn on more powerhouse muscles.

# SAW

- Sit tall with a straight back and long waist.
- Open your arms straight out to your sides at shoulder-height and "crack a walnut" between your blades.
- Open your legs wider than your shoulders, flex your feet from the ankles, and anchor your bottom to the mat.

**B**

- Inhale with control as you rotate your trunk to the left and round over your left knee; pressing your right hand against the outer edge of your left foot and lifting your back arm as high as possible, palm down.

**ASSESS:** WHEN PULLING YOUR ABS "IN AND UP," ARE YOU REALLY GETTING THE "UP"? THE WAY TO KNOW IS IF YOU CAN FEEL YOUR BACK FLATTEN AND YOUR RIBS LIFT UP AND AWAY FROM YOUR HIPS, CREATING SPACE IN YOUR WAIST-LINE. TRY TO FEEL THE DIFFERENCE BETWEEN SIMPLY PULLING YOUR BELLY BACKWARD TO YOUR SPINE OR PULLING BACK AND THEN UP YOUR SPINE. WHICH FEELS LIKE IT CREATES MORE SPACE? WHICH FEELS MORE STABLE?

**C**

- Exhale slowly as you slide your right hand along your outer foot in three progressive forward "sawing" motions while drawing back in your right hip to create diagonal opposition for your oblique abs (keep the weight of your lower body even on the mat no matter what the upper body is doing).
- Inhale slowly and return to the starting position.
- Repeat the sequence, twisting right.

**REPS:** Perform three sets using every twisting and rounding opportunity to "wring" more and more air out of your lungs and using the inverse to fill the lungs with new air.

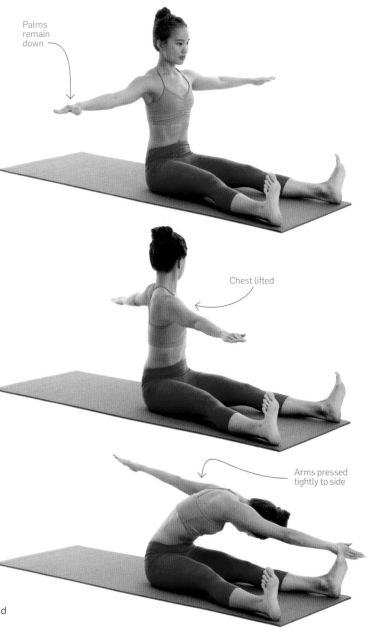

Palms remain down

Chest lifted

Arms pressed tightly to side

# *Pilates on the Mat: Level II Mains*

## SWAN DIVE PREP II

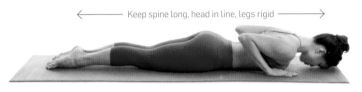

← ——— Keep spine long, head in line, legs rigid ——— →

**A**

- Lie on your stomach with your forehead down, the pubis anchored to the mat, and the inner thighs pressed tightly together as if they were one.

- Place your palms down on the mat under your shoulders, draw your navel to your spine, and press your elbows into your sides.

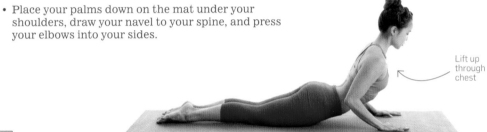

Lift up through chest

**B**

- Inhale with control as you lift your head and chest forward and up from the mat, searching for a stretch from the pubic bone up through your chest and out from your chin.

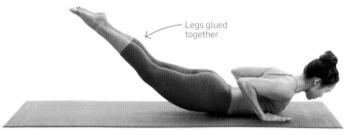

Legs glued together

**C**

- Hold your breath for one count and then rock forward onto your chest, lifting the thighs (as one unit) off the mat behind you and using the movement to "press" the air from your lungs in a deep exhalation.

- End on a lifted inhalation and then exhale with control as you lengthen back down to the mat.

**REPS:** Continue rocking three to six times, looking for the chance to create more space between your vertebrae with each repetition.

## SIT TO HEELS

This is a counterstretch for your lower back and not a rest position unless you need it to be. Use it whenever you feel you need to counter an extension with a forward flex.

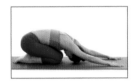

- From any exercise on your belly, scoop your abs and press your palms evenly into the mat, lifting your body up backward and bending your knees until you are sitting your bottom on your heels. Simply rounding your lower back for a moment after being in extension is fine, too.

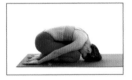

- Should you choose to stay back on your heels, you can place your fore-head on the mat and your arms can stay forward or be brought back to rest alongside your body. When rolling up out of this position, shift your weight back to your heels by pulling back in your abs and rolling up your spine, stacking each vertebra one on top of the next from bottom to top.

# DOUBLE-LEG KICKS

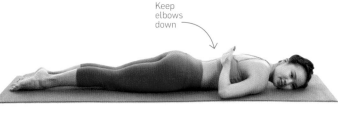

Keep elbows down

**A**

- Lie facedown with one cheek on the mat and your hands behind your back, grasping the fingers of one hand with the other.

- Your hands can be as high up on the back as the elbows can comfortably remain on the mat.

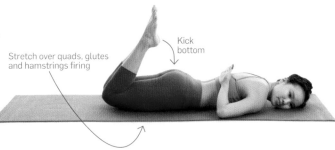

Kick bottom

Stretch over quads, glutes and hamstrings firing

**B**

- Inhale slowly as you lift both legs 2 inches off the mat and, with inner thighs glued together, "kick" your bottom three times with your heels as you exhale.

**C**

- Inhale with control as you stretch your legs back and lift your chest high, reaching your hands (still grasping one another) back toward the heels and hovering a few inches from your bottom.

**ASSESS:** WHEN IN EXTENSION, ARE YOU ARCHING FROM JUST UNDER YOUR SHOULDER BLADES? DON'T! IF YOUR RIBS ARE HANGING OUT IN FRONT, MANAGE THE LINE OF YOUR SPINE BY CREATING EVEN SPACE BETWEEN EACH VERTEBRA IN EVERY POSITION.

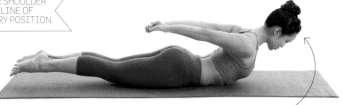

Lengthen through crown

- Exhale with control as you turn your face and place the opposite cheek on the mat. The elbows bend, the hands return to your back, and your knees are still lifted.

**REPS:** Repeat two sets (that is, four times total) with the goal of incrementally increasing the openness of your chest and shoulders in opposition to your feet and hands.

# TRANSITION: JUMP THROUGH TO SEATED

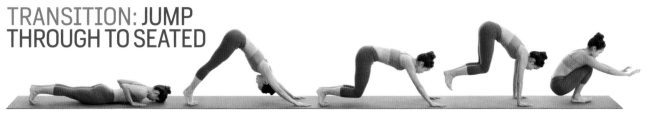

**A**  **B**  **C**  **D**  **E**

- Use the spring of your legs paired with the stability of your arms to smoothly jump your feet to the mat between your hands with bent knees, then have a seat.

# *Pilates on the Mat: Level II Mains*

## SHOULDER BRIDGE

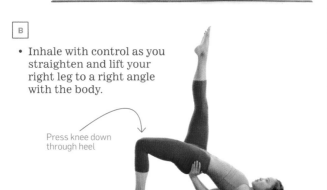

**A**

- Lie back with your knees bent and your feet flat on the floor and long, strong arms by your sides.
- Roll your pelvis up off the mat and position your hands under your pelvis with the fingers facing away from one another.

**B**

- Inhale with control as you straighten and lift your right leg to a right angle with the body.

Press knee down through heel

**C**

- Exhale with control as you reach your right leg away from you, lifting your chest back in opposition and levering the weight of your hips up off of your hands.

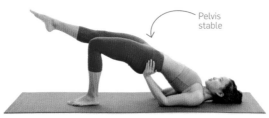

Pelvis stable

**REPS:** Repeat three times with each leg, increasing the lift of the hips with each levered movement of the thigh.

## SPINE TWIST

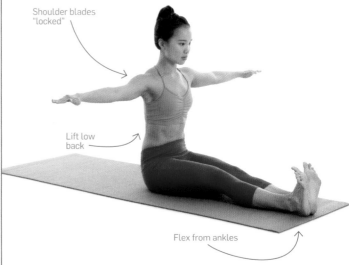

Shoulder blades "locked"

Lift low back

Flex from ankles

**A**

- Sit tall with your legs straight out on the mat at a 90-degree angle to your body and squeezing together tightly.
- Lift in your waist and open your arms straight out to your sides at shoulder-height; "crack a walnut" between your shoulders blades.

**ASSESS:** CAN YOU SENSE WHEN YOUR HEAD IS SITTING FORWARD OF YOUR SPINE? ARE YOU AWARE OF THE BACK OF YOUR NECK BEING LONG OR SUCCUMBING TO THE WEIGHT OF YOUR HEAD? WHEN YOU BRING YOUR HEAD IN LINE WITH YOUR SPINE, CAN YOU SENSE THE MUSCLE WORK INVOLVED? IT'S HARD TO ALWAYS GET CONTROL OF THE BOBBLY BIT ON THE TOP OF OUR TOOTHPICK, BUT WHERE YOUR HEAD SITS IN RELATION TO YOUR SPINE IS A CRITICAL COMPONENT OF GETTING THE MAXIMUM YIELD FROM YOUR BODY.

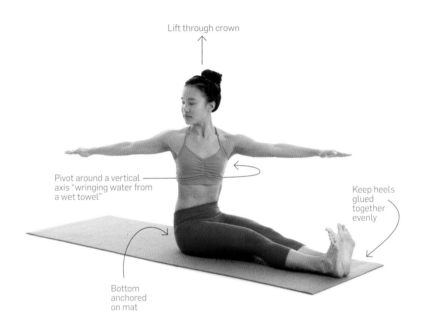

Lift through crown

Pivot around a vertical axis "wringing water from a wet towel"

Keep heels glued together evenly

Bottom anchored on mat

B

- Exhale slowly as you rotate your torso to the right, as far as you can without allowing the heels to separate or the hips to shift.
- From your farthest point of twist-i-tude, you now have two more chances to twist further, deepening your exhalation and trying to touch your chin to your right shoulder.
- Keep your arms pressing back and the blades stable on your back.
- Imagine you have tightened the coils of a spring and as you allow your inhale to happen, simply follow the uncoiling in your spine to return your torso to center.
- Repeat on the other side, working to stay long in your spine and lifted out through the crown of your head.

**REPS:** You get two or three chances to twist on each side, progressively deepening your exhalations (and therefore your inhalations) with each go.

VARIATIONS ON THE THEME:
## With a Pole
Sit tall with your legs straight out on the mat at a 90-degree angle to your body and squeezing together tightly. Place a long pole either across the backs of your shoulders with your hands wrapped around the ends 1 or behind your back, just above the base of your ribs, held in the crook of your elbows 2.

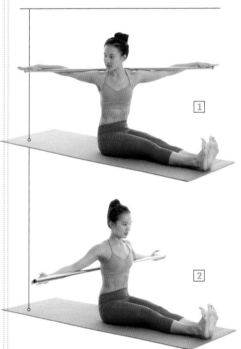

1

2

## Feet to the Wall (see photo on page 261)
Perform the Spine Twist with your heels butted up against a wall for stability and tactile feedback. As you twist, press your heels deeper into the wall, activating the movement from your hips.

# Side Kick Series

Body position—maintaining balance on the side edge of the body.

## SETUP POSITION:

- Lie on one side with your body in a straight line from the crown of your head through the spine, hips, and heels.
- Bring your legs forward until you have found an angle of stability (depending on your proportions, placing your feet on the front edge of the mat will usually do the trick). The more you wish to challenge your stability, the lesser the angle.
- Lift your head and layer your bottom hand behind the base of your head and your top hand on the mat.
- "Crack a walnut" between your shoulder blades and keep the elbows wide with the ribs drawn in.

## SIDE KICKS: SIDE BICYCLE

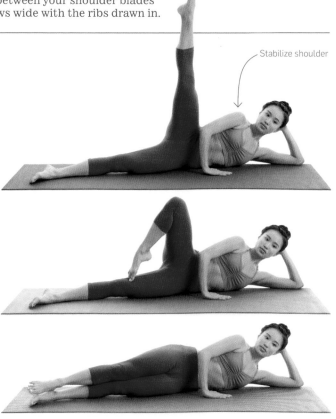

Light on hand

Stabilize shoulder

**A**

- Inhale with control as you kick your top leg straight to the ceiling and hold it at the topmost point.

**B** **C**

- Exhale slowly as you bend your knee and slide your toes along the inside of your bottom leg, past your foot, elongating your waist and stabilizing your upper body.
- Inhale with control as you kick the leg up again.

**REPS:** Repeat three side bicycles in one direction and three in the reverse, creating more imagined resistance from your "pedal" with each cycle.

# SIDE KICKS: SINGLE-LEG LIFTS

**A**

- With your body in a straight line from the crown of your head through the spine, hips, and heels, lay your head down on your arm—or a small pillow—and stretch your body in opposition from fingertips to toe tips.
- Cross your top foot in front of your bottom thigh or knee with your toes pointed toward the bottom foot.

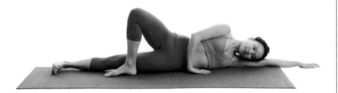

**B** **C**

- Inhale with control as you lift your bottom leg off of the mat, exhale slowly as you lower it.

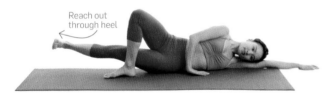

Reach out through heel

**NOTE:** *You can also draw circles with your leg from the hip socket.*

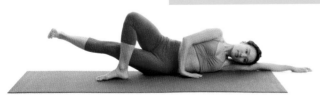

**REPS:** Lift and lower six times, lengthening the underside of your body more and more with each movement.

# SIDE KICKS: DOUBLE-LEG LIFTS

Press palm down firmly

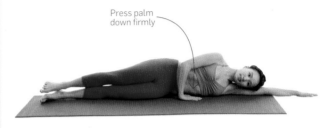

**A**

- With your body aligned in a straight line from head to heels, squeeze your legs together tightly, wrapping the backs of the upper inner thighs together, as if both legs were one.

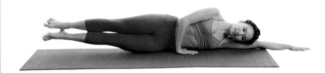

**NOTE:** *You can also keep your head propped up on your hand or hold your head up in line with your spine.*

Heels together

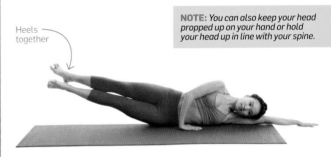

**B** **C**

- Inhale with control as you lift your legs off the mat, exhale slowly as your lower them.

**REPS:** Lift and lower your legs three times, staying long through the crown of your head and graduating the height of your legs with each opportunity.

# *Pilates on the Mat: Level II Mains*

## TEASER I

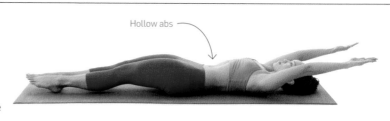

Hollow abs

- Lie back with your arms overhead, your biceps by your ears, and your lower legs in opposition to the fingertips, keeping your back flat and the legs squeezing together tightly.
- Your abs are scooped and your legs are wrapping from the backs of the upper inner thighs.

**NOTE:** *The Teaser was so named, the story goes, because Joe would stand by people's feet and "tease" that they couldn't reach him with their fingertips while staying in their powerhouse. But I know you can do this. Go get Joe!*

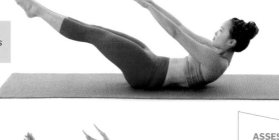

- Inhale with control as you bring your arms forward, shoulder-width apart, and begin lifting your legs.

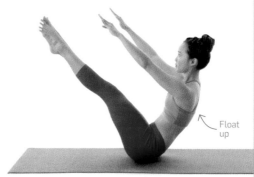

Float up

**ASSESS:** LIFT YOUR ARMS OVERHEAD AS IF SOMETHING WERE STOPPING THEM FROM LIFTING. CAN YOU FEEL THE ADDITIONAL MUSCLE WORK THAT MOVING WITH IMAGINED RESISTANCE CREATES? WHENEVER YOU'RE MOVING YOUR LIMBS, SEE IF YOU CAN CREATE SOME REASONABLE RESISTANCE TO KEEP MORE OF YOUR MUSCLES ALIVE AND ALERT.

- When your arms are parallel to your thighs, begin rolling up toward your feet, articulating one vertebra at a time and not allowing your pelvis to tip forward (stay balanced behind your tailbone).
- Exhale slowly as you descend, replacing each vertebra 1 inch behind where it was taken off.

**REPS:** You get three chances to count each vertebra on the way up and the way down.

## TEASER II

- Hold your topmost Teaser position and stabilize your torso.
- Lift your feet toward your hands, keeping your legs straight and your shoulders still.

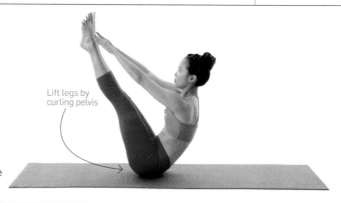

Lift legs by curling pelvis

**REPS:** Lift and lower your legs three times, seeking to move from the depth of your powerhouse muscles.

# HIP TWIST PREP

Like a propped-up corkscrew prep

- Lie back on the mat, propped up on your elbows, with your chest wide and your legs straight.
- Tightly wrap your legs together from the backs of the upper inner thighs and point your feet.

Lift through crown

- Inhale slowly, drawing the ribs in, and use your powerhouse muscles to bring your legs as one toward your head, without changing form in your upper body (your chest must remain lifted).

- Without moving anything above your waist, inhale slowly, swinging your legs to the right and then down toward the mat.

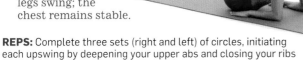

- Exhale slowly as you swing your legs to the left and back to center. (This breathing pattern can be reversed.)
- Only the hips and legs swing; the chest remains stable.

**REPS:** Complete three sets (right and left) of circles, initiating each upswing by deepening your upper abs and closing your ribs further with each subsequent circle.

# SWIMMING

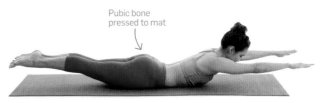

Pubic bone pressed to mat

- Lie on your stomach with your forehead down, the pubis anchored to the mat, and the inner thighs pressed tightly together.
- Your arms are stretched forward with the palms down, and your feet are pointed.
- Lift your arms, legs, chest, and head up on one count and hold.

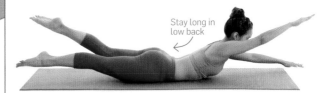

Stay long in low back

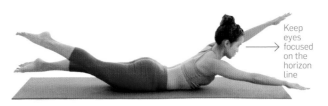

Keep eyes focused on the horizon line

- Inhale and exhale normally as you alternate lifting right arm/left leg and left arm/right leg without touching them down to the mat.
- Count slowly from 1 to 10 as you swim, lifting higher and reaching longer with each progressive count.
- Sit to Heels (page 96) for a counterstretch in your lower back, if needed.

# *Pilates on the Mat: Level II Mains*

## LEG PULL FRONT

**A**

- Stretch out into a plank position with your navel buttoned to your spine and a tight seat.

**B**

- Without allowing your hips to move, kick one leg up off the mat with a pulse at the top (like a double beat).
- Replace the foot on the mat and repeat with your other leg.

**REPS:** Complete two sets of kicks with the pulsing action, working to stabilize your pelvis more with each kick.

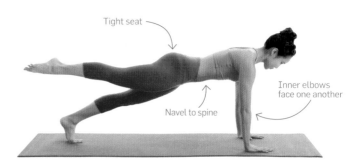

Tight seat

Inner elbows face one another

Navel to spine

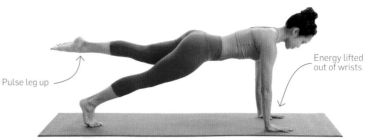

Pulse leg up

Energy lifted out of wrists

## SIDE BEND PREP II: SIDE PLANK

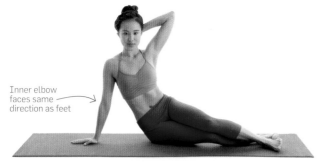

Inner elbow faces same direction as feet

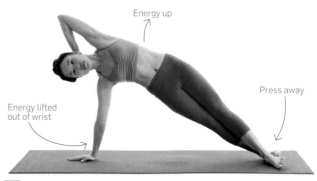

Energy up

Energy lifted out of wrist

Press away

**A**

- Sit on one hip, propped up on one hand, with your legs slightly bent to the side in line with your body.
- Place your top foot just in front of your bottom foot on the mat and your top hand behind the base of your head.

**REPS:** Do three on each side, seeking to gain more and more lift and elongation with each opportunity.

**B**

- Inhale with control as you lift your hip away from the mat, straightening your mat-side arm and elongating your legs.
- The top elbow is lifting to the ceiling, helping to create more length in your waist.
- Slowly exhale and return your hip to the mat with control.

# PILATES PUSHUP

Transitioning into any Pilates-style pushup from above is akin to the Roll-Up, only vertical!

**ASSESS:** WHEN IN PLANK POSITION, LOCK OUT HARD IN YOUR ELBOW AND FEEL THE SENSATION THAT CREATES IN THE JOINT. NOW "SOFTEN" (UNLOCK) YOUR ELBOW JOINT AND TURN THE INNER ELBOWS TO FACE EACH OTHER. CAN YOU FEEL THE MUSCLES IN THE BACKS OF YOUR ARMS TURN ON?

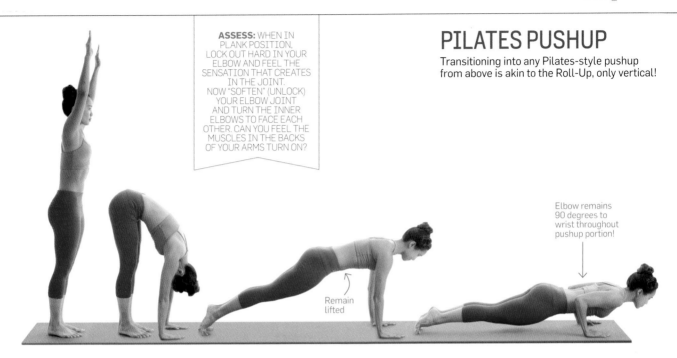

Elbow remains 90 degrees to wrist throughout pushup portion!

Remain lifted

**A**

- Stand tall, facing the mat at one end.
- Inhale with control as you bring your arms up, lengthening your waist and squeezing the backs of the upper inner thighs together tightly.

**B**

- Exhale slowly as you draw the ribs in, bring your head and arms forward, shoulder-width apart, and lower your hands to the mat by rolling through your spine (not folding at your hips); the abs remain scooped.
- Place your palms on the mat with your head on your knees (bending your knees as needed is perfectly acceptable).

**C**

- Walk your hands forward in 3½ giant steps until you are in a rigid plank position from head to heels with your upper-body weight just past your hands (your shoulders are past your wrists) and you are balanced on the tips of your toes.

**D**

- Inhale with control as you bend your elbows, keeping your upper arms pressed tightly to your sides, and lower your body, aiming your chin (not chest) to the front edge of the mat (stay forward on your toes and stretch your neck forward without allowing anything else to change in the body).
- Exhale slowly and push the mat away from you, bringing your body up in opposition to the push of your hands.
- Lift from your powerhouse muscles and draw the ribs in, folding your chest toward your thighs, like an upside-down Teaser.
- Lower your heels to the mat and push off your palms, walking your hands (with straight arms) back to your feet in 3½ giant steps. The legs remain as straight as possible until your forehead touches the knees.
- Roll back up to standing.

**REPS:** Complete three Pilates Pushups sequences, no matter how small the range of the actual pushup portion, with the intention of staying conscious of how your powerhouse muscles are working throughout each step.

# Mat Series

## LEVEL II
## > ENDERS

# ARM WEIGHTS: SIDE BENDS

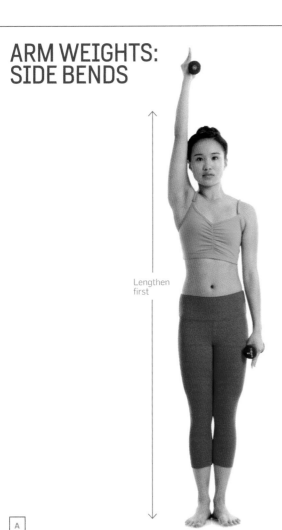

Lengthen first

A

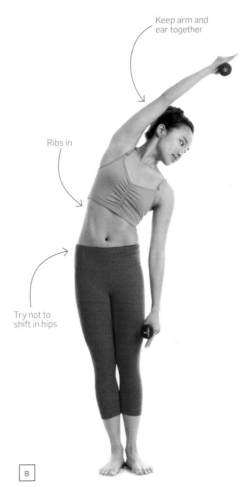

Keep arm and ear together

Ribs in

Try not to shift in hips

B

- Stand with your heels together and your toes fist-width apart, thighs wrapped.
- Make sure your body weight is evenly distributed between the balls of your feet and heels and draw the abs in and up.
- Lift your right arm overhead, your biceps by your right ear, and turn your head.

- Exhale with control as you bend to the left, reaching your right arm in opposition to your right foot and stretching your left hand toward your left foot. (Think of resisting gravity in your waist like in the Side Bend Prep II: Side Plank.)
- Inhale with control and reverse the movements, coming back to vertical and switching arms.

**REPS:** Repeat three bends to each side without allowing the hips to sway or the shoulders to roll in.

# *Pilates on the Mat: Level II Enders*

## ARM WEIGHTS: THE BUG

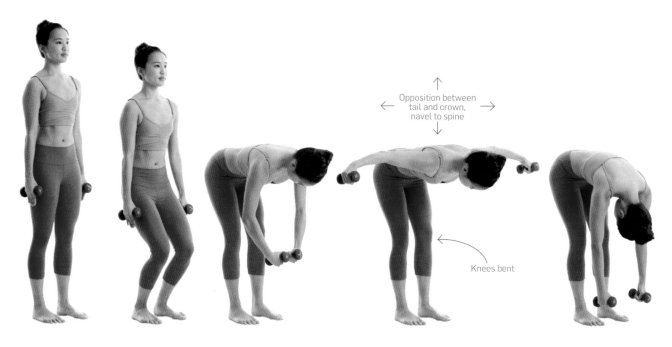

Opposition between tail and crown, navel to spine

Knees bent

**A**

- Stand tall with your feet hip-width apart and long, strong arms by your sides.

**B** **C**

- Bend your knees, break at the hips, and send your bottom back and your head forward until your back is in "table-top" position.

**D**

- Widen your elbows and face your knuckles toward one another, forming a circle with your arms.
- Inhale with control as you spread your bug wings and draw your shoulder blades together tightly.
- Exhale with control as you bring your knuckles together again without changing the size of your original circle.

**E**

- After five sets, let your arms and head hang and, with soft knees, roll up to standing, articulating your spine.

**REPS:** Complete five sets, deepening your exhalation and inhalation with each opportunity.

# ARM WEIGHTS: ZIP UP

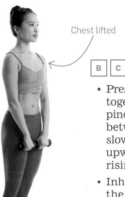

Chest lifted

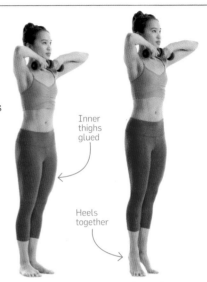

Inner thighs glued

Heels together

**A**

- Stand with your heels together and your toes fist-width apart, your thighs wrapped and squeezing toward the midline.
- Shift your entire body weight forward from the ankle so that it sits slightly over the balls of your feet, and draw the abs in and up.

**B** **C**

- Press the heads of your weights together in front of you, as if pinching the tab of a zipper between them, and exhale slowly as you draw the weights upward to your chin while rising up to your toes.
- Inhale with control and press the weights downward, "unzipping" your frontline and dropping your heels.

**REPS:** Do this three times and then reverse the breathing pattern (inhale up, exhale down), rising and lowering on the balls of your feet with each zip and unzip. Use each opportunity you get to improve your balance and strengthen from the ground up.

# ARM WEIGHTS: BOXING

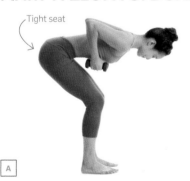

Tight seat

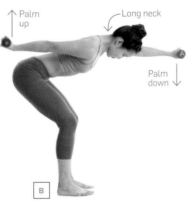

Palm up

Long neck

Palm down

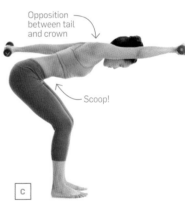

Opposition between tail and crown

Scoop!

**A**

- Stand tall with your feet hip-width apart and long, strong arms by your sides.
- Bend your knees, break at the hips, and send your bottom back and your head forward until your back is in "tabletop" position.
- Hold the weights outside of your shoulders, with your knuckles forward, palms down, and shoulder blades squeezing together.

**B**

- Inhale with control as you send one arm forward and one arm back, front palm down, back palm up.
- Exhale slowly as you return the weights to your shoulders.

**C**

- When finished, let your arms and head hang and, with soft knees, roll up to standing, articulating your spine.

**REPS:** Alternate sides and continue boxing until you've completed four sets, connecting the arms deeper and deeper to your back.

## WALL: FLUSH WITH CIRCLES

**NOTE:** *These can be done with or without light weights.*

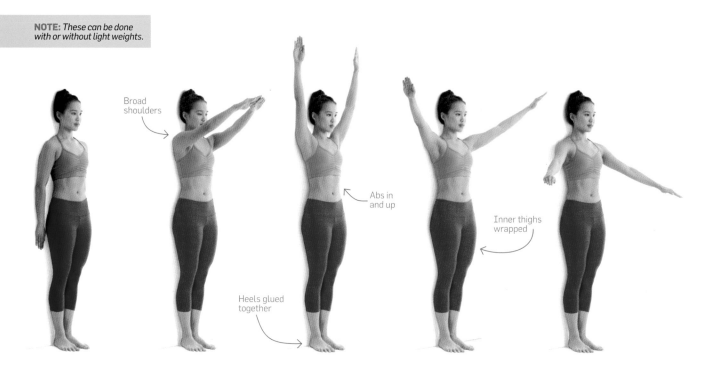

Broad shoulders

Abs in and up

Heels glued together

Inner thighs wrapped

A

- Stand with your back, head, and heels flush against the wall. Pin your pelvis, your shoulder blades, and the backs of your shoulders to the wall with strong powerhouse engagement. The heels are together, toes apart, thighs wrapped.

B C

- Inhale slowly as you circle your arms, lifting them as high as possible without losing the connection to the wall.

D E

- Exhale with control as you circle them to the sides as wide as possible without losing the connection to the wall.

**REPS:** Repeat the sequence, circling your arms five times forward and then reversing five circles. Use these ten chances to feel how deeply your arms connect to your back and waistline. With each lift and press of the arms, the waistline elongates.

# WALL: SQUATS WITH CIRCLES

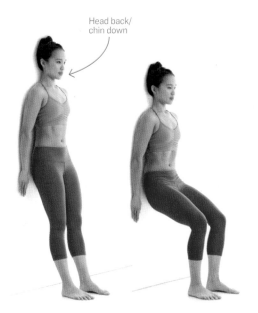

Head back/
chin down

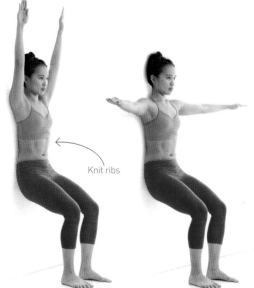

Knit ribs

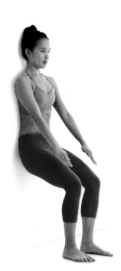

**A**
- Open your feet hip-width apart and walk them forward to where, when your hips and thighs are at right angles, your knees will be over your ankles (your shins are perpendicular to the floor).

**B**
- Breathe with control as you slide down the wall until your thighs are parallel to the floor. (If this is too great a strain in your knees, simply slide only halfway down to start and graduate each time you practice.)

**C**
- Inhale slowly as you lift your arms straight ahead, as high as possible without losing the connection to your back.

**D**
- Exhale with control as you circle your arms as wide to the sides as possible without losing the full connection between your back and the wall.

**E**
- Bring arms together in front of you and begin again.

**REPS:** Repeat the sequence, circling your arms five times forward and then reversing five circles. Use these ten chances to feel how deeply your arms connect to your back and waistline. With each lift and press of the arms, the waistline elongates.

# *Pilates on the Mat: Level II Enders*

## WALL: PUSHOFFS

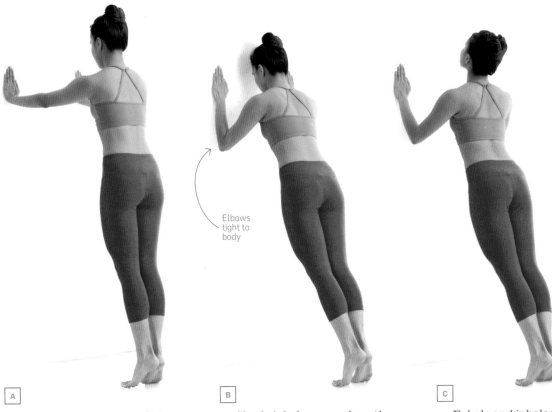

Elbows tight to body

**A**

- Stand with your palms flat against the wall at shoulder-height and -width and take a small step back until your body weight is supported on your straight arms.
- Bring your heels together and turn your toes apart, the inner thighs squeezing firmly toward your midline.

**B**

- Slowly inhale as you draw the abs in and up and rise to the balls of your feet, heels glued.

**C**

- Exhale and inhale with control as you do three consecutive Pushoffs, bending your elbows directly into your sides and not breaking anywhere in the body ("Steel from head to heel").
- Finish on an inhalation with your arms straight again, and lower your heels to the floor with control.

**REPS:** Complete three rounds, concentrating on stretching the chest forward and upward toward the wall more and more (like a vertical Pilates Pushup) with each opportunity.

# WALL: CORNER PUSHOFFS

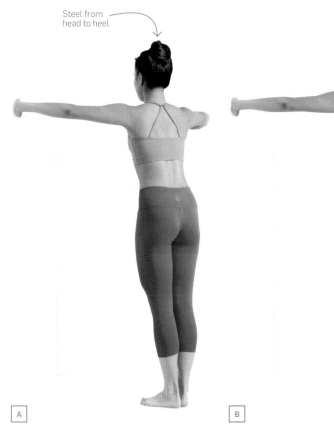

Steel from head to heel

"Crack a walnut" between blades

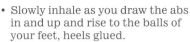

Squeeze backs of thighs together

**A**

- Stand facing a room corner and place your palms, the fingertips facing each other, one on each wall at shoulder-height or just below. When you look along each arm, your wrists should be in line with that shoulder.

- Take a small step back to shift your body weight toward the wall and bring your heels together and spread the toes apart. The inner thighs squeeze firmly toward your midline.

**B**

- Slowly inhale as you draw the abs in and up and rise to the balls of your feet, heels glued.

**C**

- Exhale and inhale with control as you do three consecutive Pushoffs, bending your elbows wide to the sides and not breaking anywhere in the body ("Steel from head to heel").

- Finish on an inhalation with your arms straight again, and lower your heels to the floor with control.

**REPS:** Complete three rounds, concentrating on stretching the chest forward and upward toward the wall more and more (like a vertical Pilates Pushup) with each opportunity.

# Mat Series: Level II

# Mat Sequence

**2** The Hundred (page 63)

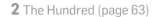

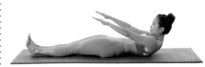

**3** Roll-Up (page 64)

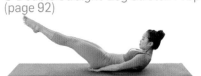

**4** Single-Leg Circles I (page 65)

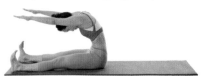

**8** Single Straight-Leg Stretch (page 92)

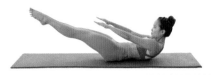

**9** Double Straight-Leg Stretch Prep (page 92)

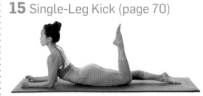

**10** Spine Stretch (page 68)

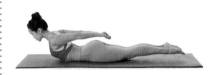

**14** Swan Dive Prep II (page 96)

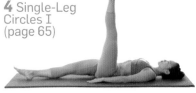

**15** Single-Leg Kick (page 70)

**16** Double-Leg Kicks (page 97)

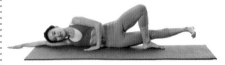

**20** Side Kicks: Front/Back (page 71)

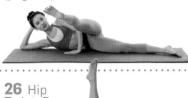

**21** Side Kicks: Side Bicycle (page 100)

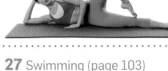

**22** Side Kicks: Single-Leg Lifts (page 101)

**26** Hip Twist Prep (page 103)

**27** Swimming (page 103)

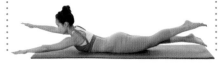

**28** Leg Pull Front (page 104)

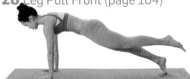

114

# >LEVEL II

**Start »**
Lowering Down to Mat
(page 93)

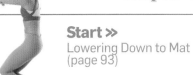

**5** Rolling Like a Ball
(page 91)

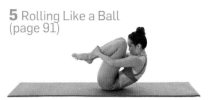

**6** Single-Leg Stretch (page 66)

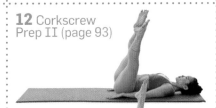

**7** Double-Leg Stretch (page 67)

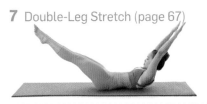

**11** Open-Leg Rocker Prep II
(page 94)

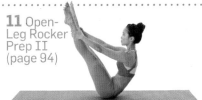

**12** Corkscrew Prep II (page 93)

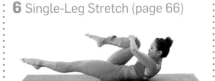

**13** Saw (page 95)

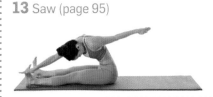

**17** Sit to Heels
(page 96) or
Jump through
to Seated
(page 97)

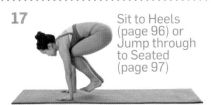
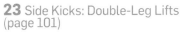

**18** Shoulder Bridge
(page 98)

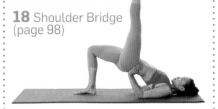

**19** Spine Twist
(page 98)

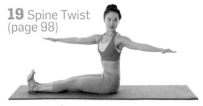

**23** Side Kicks: Double-Leg Lifts
(page 101)

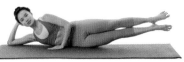

**24** Teaser I
(page 102)

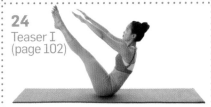

**25** Teaser II
(page 102)

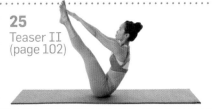

**29** Side Bend Prep II
(page 104)

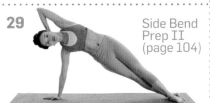

**30** Seal (page 76)

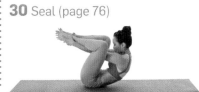

**End**
Pilates Pushup
(page 105)

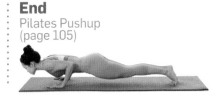

# Mat Series

## LEVEL III
> STARTERS

# KNEE-INS

**A**

- Stand tall at the end of the mat and inhale with control as you bring your arms up, wrapping your thighs together tightly and drawing the abs in and up.
- Exhale slowly and round forward with control, bringing your palms to the mat.
- Reach your forehead to your knees (bend your knees as needed).

**B** **C**

- Walk your hands forward with straight arms in 3½ giant steps until you are in a rigid plank position from head to heels with your upper-body weight just past your hands (your shoulders are past your wrists) and balanced on the tips of your toes.

**D**

- Holding a strong plank position with your arms, bring your right knee to your chest and your chest toward your knee (like an inverted Single-Leg Stretch).

**REPS:** Complete three sets.

**E**

- Draw the ribs in deeply and hold this position for a count of three, then return to your rigid plank position.
- Alternate legs a total of six times and increase the oppositional tension between the pull of the bent knee and the reach of the straight knee more and more with each chance you get.

**F**

- From your plank position, lift from your powerhouse muscles and fold your chest toward your thighs, like an upside-down Teaser.
- Lower your heels to the mat and push off your palms, walking your hands (with straight arms) back to your feet in 3½ giant steps.
- The legs remain as straight as possible until your forehead touches the knees.

**G**

- Reverse the movements of rolling down and roll your spine back up to standing tall with your arms and waist lifted.

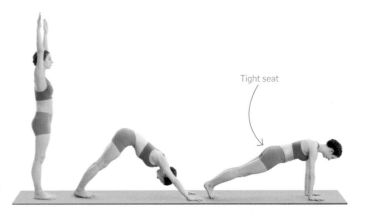

Tight seat

**NOTE:** *This move can also be done on your elbows.*

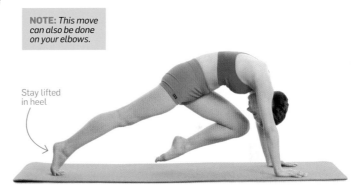

Stay lifted in heel

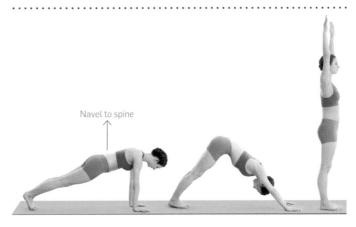

Navel to spine

# Pilates on the Mat: Level III Starters

## WAVE

**NOTE:** The Wave can also be done with your knees down, and you can play with the up/down combination possibilities: down right/up left or down right/up right, etc.

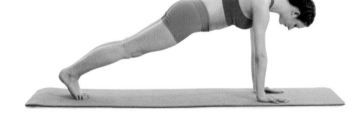

A

- Begin the same as Knee-Ins.
- Walk your hands forward with straight arms in 3½ giant steps until you are in a rigid plank position from head to heels with your upper-body weight just past your hands (your shoulders are past your wrists) and you are balanced on the tips of your toes.

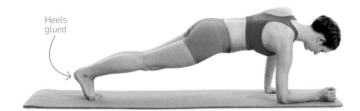

Heels glued

B  C

- Replace your right hand with your right elbow, palm, and forearm flat on the mat, then do the same with your left so that you are in a plank position on your elbows.

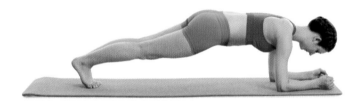

D  E

- Then reverse by replacing your right elbow with your right hand and do the same with your left so that you are back in an extended arm plank.

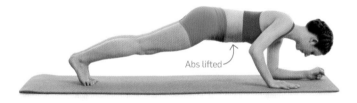

Abs lifted

**REPS:** Repeat the actions above, starting with your left side this time, and continue to alternate until you have been up and down evenly four times.

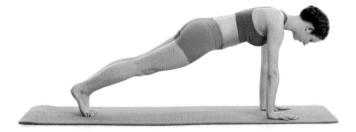

# UP-STRETCH COMBO

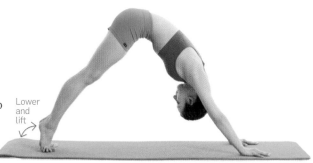

- Begin the same as Knee-Ins.
- Walk your hands forward with straight arms in 3½ giant steps, but instead of leveling out into plank position, keep your hips and heels high (like an inverted Teaser).
- Stabilize your upper body, with your head tucked toward your abs, as you lower and lift your heels three times, working from your deepest powerhouse muscles.

Lower and lift

- With your heels lifted, tuck your bottom under and begin curling your hips toward the floor.
- Create resistance by simultaneously curling your upper body deeper toward your abs.

Ribs up

*NOTE: This is taken from a combination of exercises on the Reformer in which the hips are working on mobility as the upper body is working on stability and then the pelvis becomes stable as the spine articulates. Try to find these opposing elements through the movements and see how they, in fact, spur one another on.*

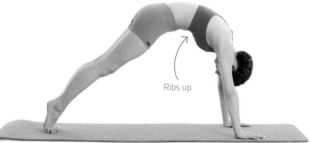

- Once your pelvis is level, stabilize your hips and waist and uncurl your upper spine, opening your shoulders and pressing your chest through (like an elevated Swan Dive).
- Your chest and chin are stretching upward, your hips remain perfectly still.
- Reverse the movement by bringing your head toward your chest, articulating one vertebra at a time and hollowing out your abs.
- The hips remain still as long as possible.

Push out through heels

Soften elbows

Lift abs

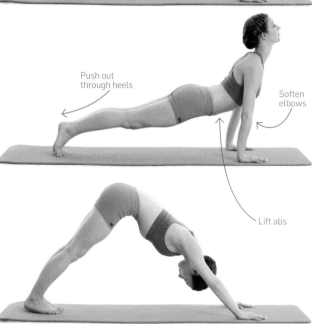

- When all spinal segments have been exhausted, allow the hips to lift with control, returning to the inverted Teaser position, and lower your heels.
- Repeat the Up-Stretch Combo three times, and then walk your hands back to your feet and roll up to standing.

**REPS:** Perform two full sets (of three Up-Stretch Combos), working on stabilizing what should be stable and when, while mobilizing what should be mobile and when.

# Mat Series

## LEVEL III
## >MAINS

# ROLLOVER I

Since this is a "rolling" exercise, we know that the movements are meant to facilitate, and be fueled by, the breath.

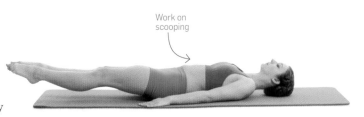

Work on scooping

**A**

- Lie flat with your legs squeezed together, your feet pointed, and long, sturdy arms held tightly to your sides. (The backs of your arms, palms, and shoulders are anchored to the mat.)

- Inhale with control as you lift both legs as one a few inches off the mat (like in the Hundred), using a strong squeeze of your buttocks and a deepening of your upper abs.

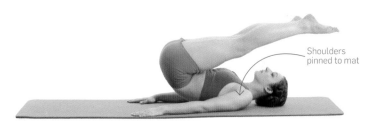

Shoulders pinned to mat

**B**

- Begin to bring your legs overhead, articulating your spine by removing one vertebra at a time from the mat beneath you.

- Use strong, stable arms to support your weight and balance evenly on your shoulder blades and the backs of your arms (the wrists are flat, the triceps are firing).

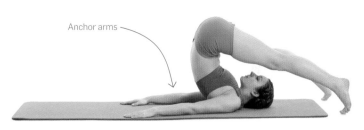

Anchor arms

**C**

- Exhale slowly as you open your legs to hip-width and begin to inhale as you reverse the movements slowly back down the mat.

**D**

- When your bottom reaches the mat, exhale slowly and lower your legs as close to the mat as possible while maintaining a flat lower back.

- Inhale slowly as you bring the legs together and repeat twice more before changing directions (i.e., bringing the legs over open and closing them overhead).

**REPS:** Perform six times.

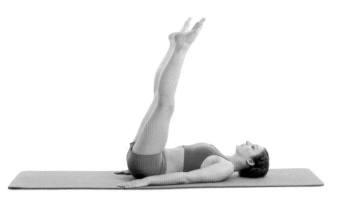

# Pilates on the Mat: Level III Mains

## SINGLE-LEG CIRCLES II

**A**

- Lie flat with your legs squeezed together and long, sturdy arms by your sides (the backs of your shoulders anchored to the mat).
- Stretch one leg up to the ceiling as straight and as close to perpendicular as possible.

**NOTE:** The size of the circle is completely dependent on your ability to control the movement.

**B** **C** **D**

- Draw circles in the air with your leg, beginning across your body, then down toward the ankle, out, around, and back up.

Keep chest stable

- Gradually increase the circumference of the circles to the degree that allows for your hip to lift off of the mat with control from your powerhouse muscles.

**REPS:** Complete five circles in each direction and then switch legs.

## DOUBLE STRAIGHT-LEG STRETCH II

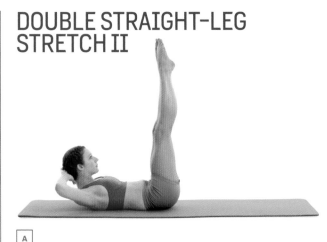

**A**

- Lie on your back with your hands layered, palm over palm, behind your lifted head and your legs held straight in the air perpendicular to your body.
- Open your elbows wide to the sides and wrap your thighs tightly together until both legs are one.

Keep tail curled under

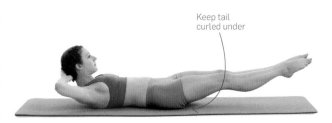

**B**

- Exhale slowly as you simultaneously pull the abs in and up and stretch your legs away to create oppositional pull.
- Lower your legs as far as possible while keeping your lower back firmly connected to the mat.
- Inhale with control as you bring your legs back to a 90-degree angle, making sure they remain resolutely straight.

**REPS:** Repeat six times, deepening your bottom ribs and opening your elbows wider with each opportunity.

# CRISSCROSS

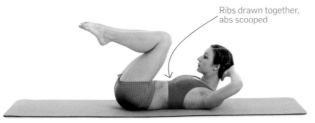

Ribs drawn together, abs scooped

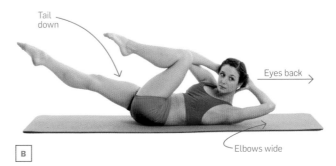

Tail down

Eyes back

Elbows wide

**A**

- Lie on your back with your hands layered, palm over palm, behind your lifted head and with your knees bent tightly into your chest.

**B**

- Inhale slowly and twist your torso to the left until your right elbow connects with your left knee, straightening your right leg forward and holding it a few inches above the mat.
- Exhale with control and twist right, connecting your left elbow to your right knee and extending your left leg.

**REPS:** Continue alternating sides, completing six sets of twists from a spinal rotation and not from rocking shoulders side to side. (Yes, I see you.)

# OPEN-LEG ROCKER (Legs Wide)

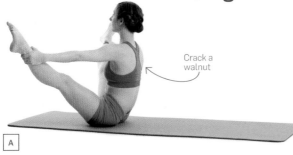

Crack a walnut

**BREATH FOR ROCKING AND ROLLING:** JOE RECOMMENDED INHALING IN THE STABLE POSITIONS AND EXHALING ON THE ROLLING PORTIONS IN ORDER TO "PRESS" THE AIR OUT. FIND THE PATTERN OF BREATH THAT BEST HELPS YOU STABILIZE AND MOBILIZE WHERE NEEDED.

Pull abs back

**A**

- Sit tall with your legs open mat-width and lengthen your spine up through the crown of your head.
- Hollow out your belly and round backward, lifting both legs up off the mat simultaneously and grabbing your ankles. Your abs lift your limbs.
- Balance there and inhale with control as you open your legs as wide as they'll go while still lengthening your waist.

**B**

- Look to your abs ("eyes on the prize") and exhale with control as you rock back, trying to touch your toes to the mat.
- Keep steady pressure between the legs and palms, without landing any weight on your neck.
- Control this movement so momentum doesn't!

**REPS:** Rock back and up six times, working to keep your chest lifting forward as you are rolling backward.

# Pilates on the Mat: Level III Mains

## CORKSCREW

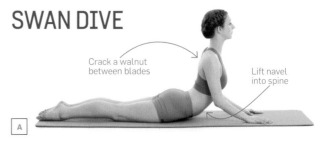

Squeeze as if both legs are one

**A**

- Lie flat on your back with long, sturdy arms by your sides.
- Squeeze your legs together tightly from the backs of the upper inner thighs.

- Inhale slowly as you lift your legs overhead, rolling back until you are balanced in the middle of your shoulder blades and the backs of your arms.

**B**

- Point your toes and exhale with control as you roll back down your spine, leaning your body slightly to the right.

Arms and shoulders anchored

**C** **D**

- When your right glute touches the mat, circle your legs to the left and inhale slowly, rolling up the left side of your body while scooping your abs and lifting your bottom.

**REPS:** Continue reversing the circle direction each time and complete three sets, deepening the scoop of your abs and seeking more articulation in your spine with each revolution.

## SWAN DIVE

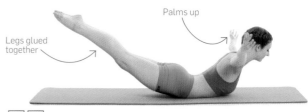

Crack a walnut between blades

Lift navel into spine

**A**

- Lie with your forehead down, pubic bone anchored to the mat, and inner thighs pressed tightly together.
- Place your palms down under your shoulders and press your elbows into your sides.
- Inhale with control as you lift your head and chest searching for a stretch from the pubic bone up through your chest and out from your chin.

Legs glued together

Palms up

**B** **C**

- Hold for one count, then lift both arms upward and out to your sides—palms faceup—as you begin to rock back and forth on your belly.
- Rocking forward "presses" the air from your lungs as an exhalation, while rocking back allows for a fuller expansion of your chest.

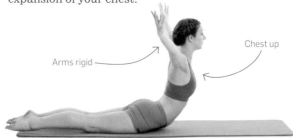

Arms rigid

Chest up

**REPS:** Rock six times, working on getting more and more lift from your dive.

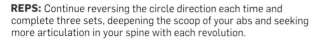

# NECKPULL

Since this is a "rolling" exercise, we know that the movements are meant to facilitate, and be fueled by, the breath.

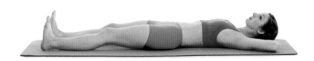

**A**

- Lie flat on your back with your legs narrowly open and in line with the hip bones, your feet flexed at the ankles and your palms layered behind the base of your head.
- The elbows are wide and your shoulders blades are drawn together.

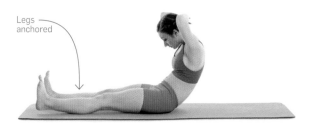

Legs anchored

**ASSESS:** SIT TALL AND INTERLACE YOUR HANDS BEHIND YOUR HEAD AND PRESS YOUR HEAD BACK INTO THEM. NOW LAYER YOUR HANDS, PALM OVER PALM, BEHIND YOUR HEAD AND DO THE SAME. CAN YOU FEEL THE DIFFERENCE? LAYERING YOUR HANDS BRINGS THE MUSCULAR WORK OUT OF YOUR SHOULDERS AND DOWN YOUR BACK TO YOUR BLADES.

*NOTE: When beginning, you may start this exercise from the tall, seated position and roll back into it, and you can leave out the hinging back portion. Practice the Roll-Back and the Roll-Up to get stronger at the Neckpull.*

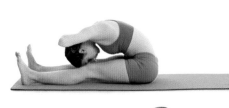

**B**

- Inhale slowly as you lift your head to your chest and round your upper back off of the mat with a deepening of your upper abs.

**C**

- Exhale slowly forward, trying to touch your forehead to your knees. The elbows remain wide.

**D**

- Inhale with control as you roll up to a tall seated posture, abs pulled in and up, walnut cracked between your blades.

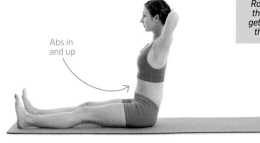

Abs in and up

**E**

- Ground the backs of your legs to the mat and lengthen your waist as you hinge backward 4 inches with a flat back.
- Suspend your torso in midair and exhale slowly as you curl your pelvis under, rolling your lower back down to the mat one vertebra at a time. Resist gravity's drag by "pulling" the neck in opposition to your heels.

**REPS:** Finish in the starting position and give yourself three more chances to increase the degree of spinal articulation you can muster in each step.

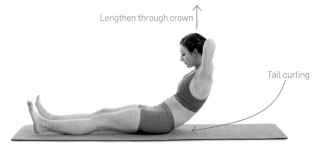

Lengthen through crown

Tail curling

# Pilates on the Mat: Level III Mains

## JACKKNIFE

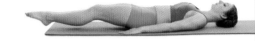

**A**

- Lie flat with your legs squeezed together, your feet pointed, and the backs of your arms anchored to the mat.
- Inhale with control as you lift legs a few inches off the mat (like in the Hundred), using a strong squeeze of your buttocks and a deepening of your upper abs.
- Exhale slowly as you bring your legs to a right angle with your body.

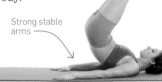

*Strong stable arms*

**B**

- While inhaling slowly, press your arms deeper into the mat and lift your bottom off until you are balancing on your shoulder blades.
- Hold for a count of two.

**C**

- Use your arms to support you as you "snap" your legs straight up (think of a jackknife). Pull your abs in opposition to your head.
- Hold for a count of two.

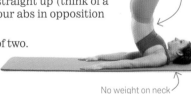

*Pull abs back*

*No weight on neck*

- Exhale slowly, break at the waist, and return to balance on your shoulder blades for a count of two.
- Inhale slowly and return your legs to a right angle.
- Exhale slowly and bring your legs to hover 2 inches from the mat.

**REPS:** Repeat three times, using each as a chance to create more steely strength in your knife blade.

## SIDE KICKS: BICYCLE

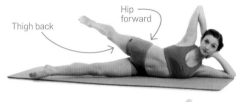

*Hip forward*

*Thigh back*

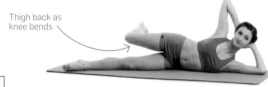

*Thigh back as knee bends*

**A** **B**

- From the backswing position of the Side Kicks: Front/Back (page 71), bring your heel to your bottom, creating a stretch over the front of your thigh and hip.

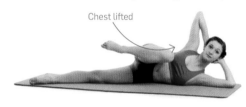

*Chest lifted*

**C**

- Keeping your heel and bottom connected, bring your knee forward to your chest and, keeping your thigh still, extend the leg toward your nose.
- Do not drop your foot below the height of your top shoulder.

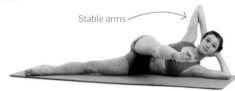

*Stable arms*

**D**

- Swing your leg back and pedal three times, elongating your waist and stabilizing your upper body more and more with each pass.

**REPS:** After three pedals backward, reverse the sequence and pedal forward three times, finding added length and oppositional forces at work.

# SIDE KICKS: GRAND LEG CIRCLES

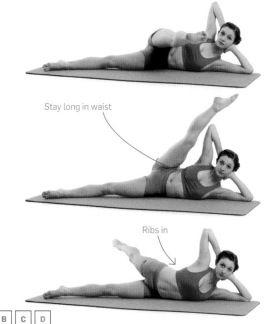

**A**

- Lift your top leg to the height of your hip, keeping it straight and connected to your abdominals.
- Imagine your leg is inside of a wide tunnel.

Stay long in waist

Ribs in

**B** **C** **D**

- Circle the leg with the intention of tracing the entire interior surface of the tunnel in both directions.
- The thigh can be turned out in the hip socket for more attention to the glutes or it can face forward for more inner/outer thigh work.

**REPS:** Perform three Grand Leg Circles forward and three Grand Leg Circles backward, working on stabilizing your upper body to target the hips and waistline

# SIDE KICKS: HOT POTATO

**A**

- Turn the top thigh out in the hip socket and kick your leg straight up to the ceiling with energy.

Lifted, stable upper body

**B**

- Bring it down straight, with your heel just forward of your bottom foot, and tap it on the mat sprightly three times, controlling the movement of the leg from your powerhouse muscles.

Light leg

**C** **D**

- Kick it up again and bring it down, this time tapping it three times just behind your bottom foot.

**REPS:** Repeat with two taps front and two taps back. And then one tap front and one tap back, keeping the energy of the movements alive.

# *Pilates on the Mat: Level III Mains*

## TEASER III

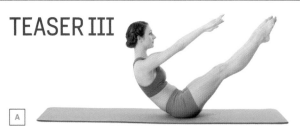

**A**

- Hold your topmost Teaser position (see Teaser I, page 102) and stabilize your torso.

**B**

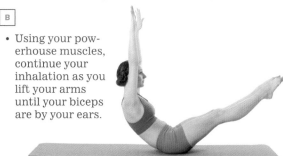

- Using your powerhouse muscles, continue your inhalation as you lift your arms until your biceps are by your ears.

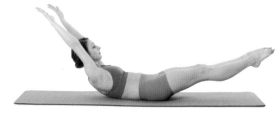

**C**

- As you exhale, slowly begin rolling down your spine one vertebra at a time, reaching your arms and legs far away from one another and lengthening like taffy through your waistline.

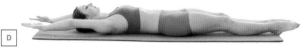

**D**

- The backs of your arms and legs should gently touch down on the mat simultaneously; then immediately reverse the sequence to fold your thighs and torso up to lifted Teaser again.

**REPS:** You get three chances to control this challenging movement, getting longer and stronger with each one.

## HIP TWIST

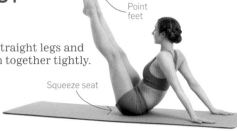

Point feet

**A**

- Sit tall with straight legs and squeeze them together tightly.

Squeeze seat

- Lift in your waist and place your hands, palms down, on the mat behind you for light support. Chest wide.
- Inhale with control as you bring your legs toward your head, without changing form.

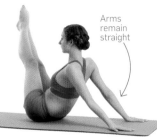

Arms remain straight

**B**

- Without moving anything above your waist, inhale slowly, swinging your legs to the right.

**C**

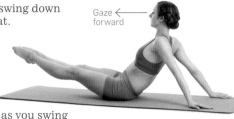

Gaze forward

- Continue the swing down toward the mat.

**D**

- Exhale slowly as you swing your legs to the left and back to center.

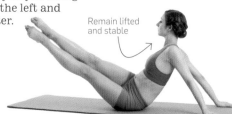

Remain lifted and stable

**REPS:** Complete three sets (right and left) of circles bringing the legs closer and closer to your head with each circle.

# LEG PULL

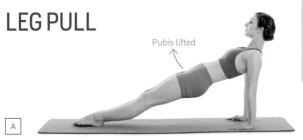

Pubis lifted

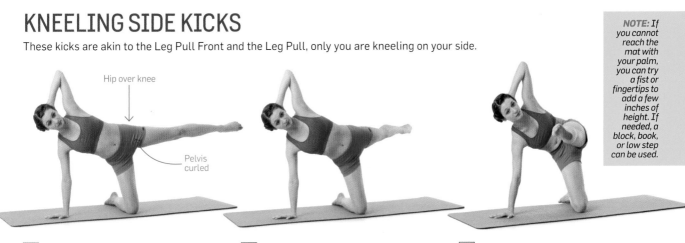

**A**

- Sit tall with straight legs extended and squeeze them together tightly. Your feet are pointed.
- Place your hands, palms down, on the edges of the mat behind you, with fingers pointed inward.
- Press into your hands and elevate your hips until your body is in a long diagonal line from head to heels.

**NOTE:** *For some of us, simply lifting into the Leg Pull position, holding for a count of three while broadening the chest and pointing the toes and feet and then lowering back down three times, will suffice.*

**B**

- Inhale slowly as you lift your right leg up as high as it will go without shifting from side to side or dropping your bottom.
- Exhale with control as you return your foot to the mat. Chest wide. Switch legs and repeat.

**REPS:** You get six chances to lift your legs and hips higher and higher with each round.

# KNEELING SIDE KICKS

These kicks are akin to the Leg Pull Front and the Leg Pull, only you are kneeling on your side.

Hip over knee

Pelvis curled

**NOTE:** *If you cannot reach the mat with your palm, you can try a fist or fingertips to add a few inches of height. If needed, a block, book, or low step can be used.*

**A**

- Kneel in the middle of the mat with a long waist.
- Put your right hand, palm down, on the mat while extending your left leg out to the side in line with your hip.
- The left hand is behind the head, the hip over the knee, and the shoulder over the wrist.

**B**

- On a swift inhale, swing your right leg back powerfully without shifting your hips forward of your knee or disturbing your upper-body position.

**C**

- Exhale forcibly as you kick your leg forward without shifting back in your hips or changing your chest and elbow.

**REPS:** Kick front and back six more times (eight kicks total) and then switch sides, using swinging back to open the front body, and all eight opportunities of kicking front to deepen your scoop.

# *Pilates on the Mat: Level III Mains*

## SIDE BEND

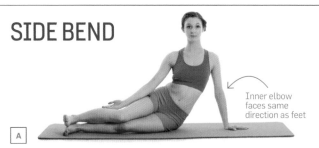

Inner elbow faces same direction as feet

**A**

- Sit on one hip, propped up on one hand, with your legs nearly extended (i.e., slightly bent) to the side and stacked ankle over ankle. The palm of the top hand is pressing onto your outer thigh.

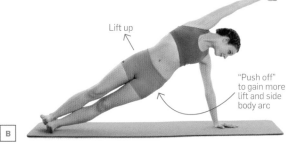

Lift up

"Push off" to gain more lift and side body arc

**B**

- Inhale with control as you lift your hip away from the mat and reach your arm overhead, creating a high, lifted arc in the torso.

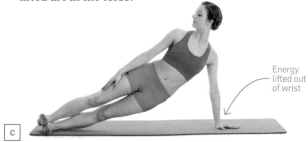

Energy lifted out of wrist

**C**

- Bring the hand from overhead back to your outer thigh and turn your chin to your outer shoulder.
- Exhale slowly as you lower the side of your calf to the mat.
- Inhale slowly as you return to your high arc.

**REPS:** Repeat three breath cycles, fueling the height and depth of your arc with each complete breath.

## CONTROL BALANCE PREP

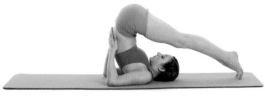

**A**

- Inhale with control as you roll your legs overhead, one vertebra at a time, until your toes touch the floor behind you.

**B**

- Use your strong, stable arms to support you as you raise your legs straight up and place your palms flat against the back of your lower back (your hands are above your hip bones, like a supported Jackknife).
- The legs are strong and your toes and feet are pointed.

Pull abs back into hands

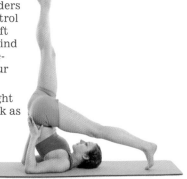

**C**

- Balance evenly on the backs of your shoulders and inhale with control as you reach your left foot to the floor behind you while simultaneously stabilizing your lifted right leg.
- Do not let your weight shift forward or back as your legs move.

**REPS:** Switch legs six times, using each rep as an opportunity to find more and more control of your torso.

# BOOMERANG

*Note:* The Boomerang combines the Teaser, the Roll-Up, and the Rollover into one beautiful flowing sequence.

**A**

- Sit tall with your legs straight out at a 90-degree angle to your body, your ankles crossed and the inner thighs squeezing together tightly.

Press down to lift up

**B**

- With your palms pressed to the mat at your sides, inhale with control as you lift your legs from the mat as one and roll back, bringing your legs overhead and balancing on your shoulder blades with long, strong arms pressed firmly to the mat (like the Rollover).

Scissor legs to switch ankles

**C**

- Holding this balanced position, switch ankles with a small, quick scissoring of the legs.

**D**

- Inhale with control as you roll up into the balanced Teaser position, reaching your forehead toward your knees and swooping your arms around your back, palms up, in opposition to your head.
- Do not allow your hands to touch the mat.
- Exhale with control as you lower the legs, your forehead to your knees, to the mat, lifting your arms even higher behind you.
- Roll up to the starting position with a steady inhalation and begin again.

**REPS:** Use each of six chances to further improve one element of the Boomerang.

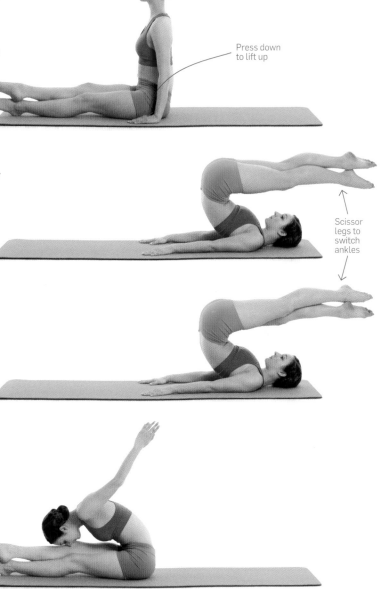

## HIGH BRIDGE PREP

**A**

- Lie back with your knees bent and your feet flat on the floor, with your ankles under your knees.

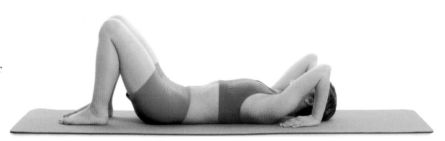

**B**

- Place the palms of your hands flat on the mat under your shoulders (or slightly wider) and inhale with control as you roll your bottom up until you feel weight on your palms.

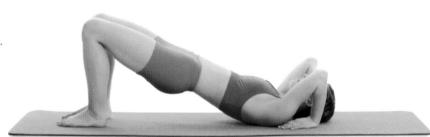

**C**

- Exhale with control as you press into your palms and lift your ribs in opposition to your hands. The arms are straight.
- Inhale slowly as you hold the position for a count of three.
- Exhale with control as you bend your elbows and gently lower your head to the mat; then roll slowly back down to the starting position.

**REPS:** Complete three bridges, paying close attention to your hands and feet: Do they press evenly into the mat as you raise and lower your body? Do they roll in or out when weighted? Can you control the articulation of your spine more and more with each opportunity?

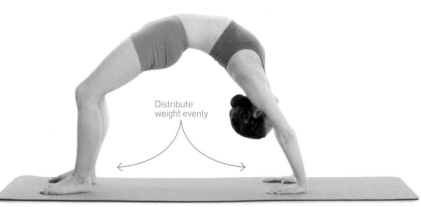

Distribute weight evenly

# SINGLE-LEG PUSHUP

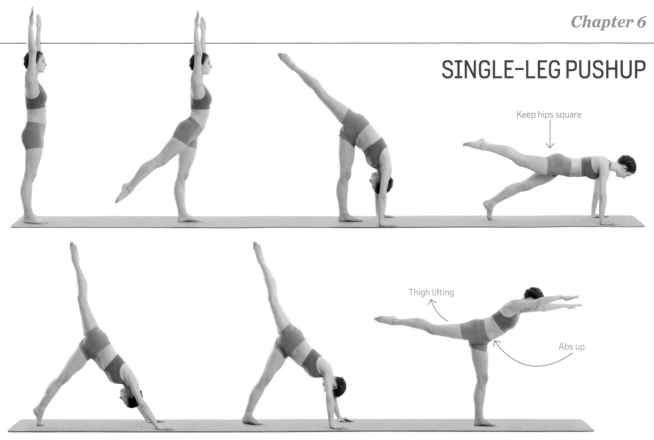

Keep hips square

Thigh lifting

Abs up

**A**
- Stand tall, facing the mat at one end.

**B**
- Inhale with control as you bring your arms up and lift one firm leg backward, stretching the front of your body on that side.

**C**
- Exhale slowly as you pivot in one piece around the head of your standing leg, bringing your arms and torso forward and your leg up simultaneously; the abs remain lifted in and up to control the movement.
- Place your palms on the mat with your forehead on your knee and your back leg lifted as high as is healthy for your body.

**D**
- Walk your hands forward to plank position with the hips square and back leg lifted (like the Leg Pull Front).

**E**
- Perform one Pilates Pushup with the leg lifted and initiate your fold by lifting your leg even higher (as if it were being pulled up and backward) as you press your palms away in opposition.

**F**
- Lower your standing heel and walk your hands (with straight arms) back to your feet in 3½ giant steps.

**G**
- Reverse the pivot to the mat and come back up to standing tall on both legs with your arms and waist lifted.

**REPS:** Complete one Single-Leg Pushup on each side, working for precision and balance with each opportunity.

# Mat
# Series

## LEVEL III
## > ENDERS

# ARM WEIGHTS: SHAVING THE HEAD

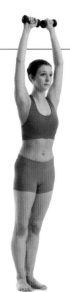

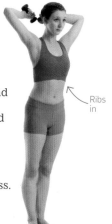

A

- Stand with your heels together and your toes fist-width apart, thighs wrapped and squeezing toward the midline.
- Shift your entire body weight forward from the ankle to sit slightly over the balls of your feet and draw the abs in and up.
- Press the heads of your weights together in front of your body and lift them up and overhead.

B

- Bend your elbows wide to the sides and bring the weights down behind your head—"shaving" the back of your head with the weights. Inhale with control and press the weights back up until your arms are straight.
- The elbows remain open as wide as possible throughout the shave and press.

Ribs in

**REPS:** Do this six times with the intention of lengthening your spine, vertebra by vertebra, with each arm movement.

# ARM WEIGHTS: TRICEPS EXTENSIONS

A

- Stand tall with your feet hip-width apart and long, strong arms by your sides.

B  C

- Bend your knees, break at the hips, and send your bottom backward and your head forward until your back is in a "tabletop" position.

D

- Hold the weights up by your shoulders, with your knuckles down, palms in, and shoulder blades "locked" together.

E

- Inhale with control as you straighten your arms back.
- Exhale slowly as you curl the weights back to your shoulders.
- After six sets, let your arms and head hang and roll up to standing.

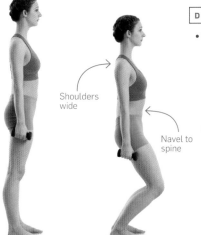

Shoulders wide

Navel to spine

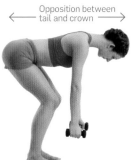

Opposition between tail and crown

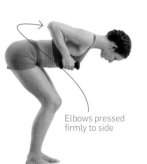

Elbows pressed firmly to side

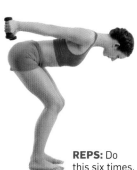

**REPS:** Do this six times.

# Pilates on the Mat: Level III Enders

## ARM WEIGHTS: SPARKLERS

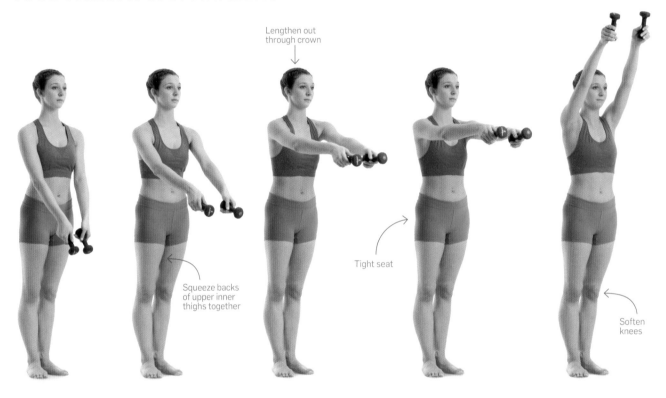

Lengthen out through crown

Squeeze backs of upper inner thighs together

Tight seat

Soften knees

A

- Stand with your heels pressed together and your toes apart, the backs of the upper inner thighs squeezing toward the midline.
- Shift your entire body weight forward from the ankle to sit slightly over the balls of your feet and draw the abs in and up.
- Hold the top ends of the weights in your hands and press the bottom ends of the weights together as if you were holding lit "sparklers."

**REPS:** Make eight circles up and eight circles down three times.

B C D E

- Inhale with control as you begin lifting the weights with tiny circles (8 to 10 circles should get you to the top), using the full length of your arms.
- Initiate the circles from all the way up at your shoulder blades! (Yes, they're connected back there.)
- Exhale with control as you reverse the circles, lowering your arms.

**NOTE:** These circles and the chest expansion can be done with or without weights, and you can add the coordination of raising and lowering of your heels as you bring your arms up and down.

# ARM WEIGHTS: CHEST EXPANSION

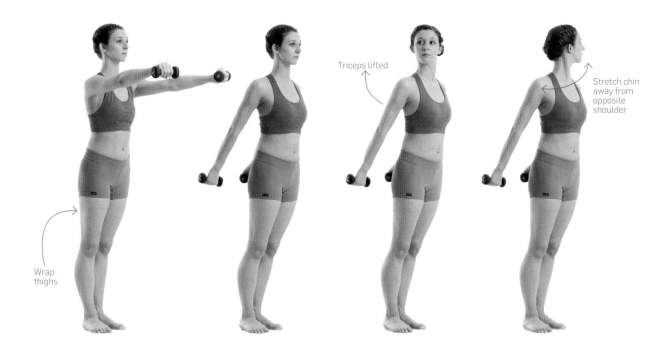

Wrap
thighs

Triceps lifted

Stretch chin
away from
opposite
shoulder

 **A**

- Stand with your heels together
  and your toes fist-width apart,
  thighs wrapped and squeezing
  toward the midline.
- Shift your entire body weight
  forward from the ankle to sit
  slightly over the balls of your feet
  and draw the abs in and up.
- Bring the weights up in front
  of you with straight arms at
  shoulder-height, palms down.

 **B**

- Inhale with control and press
  the weights down and back behind
  you as far as possible without
  breaking the line of your body
  ("steel from head to heels").
- Lift your chest in opposition to
  the weights.

 **C** **D**

- Hold your breath in this position
  and turn your head as far to the
  right as possible, and then as far to
  the left as possible.
- Return your head to center and
  exhale slowly as you lift the weights
  back to the starting position.

**REPS:** Do this four times, alternating which way you turn your head first. Reach your chest
higher and higher with each opportunity.

# *Pilates on the Mat: Level III Enders*

## ARM WEIGHTS: LONG LUNGE

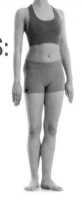

NOTE: These can be done with or without light weights.

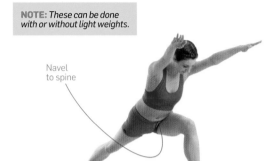

Navel to spine

Lengthen back body

**A**

- Stand with your heels together and your toes apart, then slide your left heel forward to the midpoint of your right arch.
- Turn your chest to face in the same direction that your left toes are pointing and pull the abs in and up.

**REPS:** Three on each side, lengthening the back body more and more.

**B**

- Inhale with control as you step your left foot out on the diagonal in a long lunge that lands you knee over ankle with your biceps by your ears. (Adjust if necessary to ensure your shin is perpendicular to the floor.)
- The chest is over your thigh, the back is flat, and the abs are scooped to the spine.

**C**

- Exhale slowly as you lower your arms and press back up to standing, sliding your lunging foot back to its starting position and engaging the inner thighs.
- On your third lunge, stay in the outstretched position and lower and lift your arms with control, then press up to standing and switch sides.

## WALL: SQUATS WITH WINGS

**A**

- From the squat position of Squats with Levers, opposite: Pin the backs of your hands to the wall.

NOTE: These squats can be done with or without light weights. They can also be done with your weights perpendicular to the wall, and you can alternate between parallel and perpendicular.

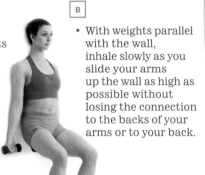

**B**

- With weights parallel with the wall, inhale slowly as you slide your arms up the wall as high as possible without losing the connection to the backs of your arms or to your back.

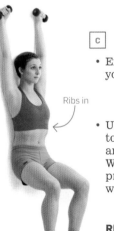

Ribs in

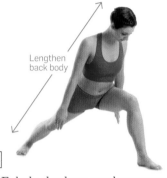

**C**

- Exhale with control as you lower them again.

- Use these five chances to deeply connect your arms to your back. With each lift and press of the arms, the waistline elongates.

Knees over ankles

**REPS:** Repeat the sequence five times and then slide back up to the starting position.

# WALL: SQUATS WITH LEVERS

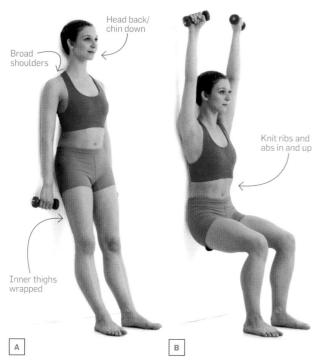

Broad shoulders

Head back/chin down

Knit ribs and abs in and up

Inner thighs wrapped

**A**

- Open your feet hip-width apart and walk them forward to where, when your hips and thighs are at right angles, your knees will be over your ankles (your shins are perpendicular to the floor).

**NOTE:** *These can be done with or without light weights.*

**B**

- Inhale with control as you slide down the wall while simultaneously lifting your arms as high as possible without losing the connection to your back.
- Exhale with control as you lower your arms and slide back up the wall.

**REPS:** Repeat the sequence five times. Use these five chances to feel how deeply each lift and press of the arms elongates the waistline.

# WALL: SINGLE-LEG SQUATS

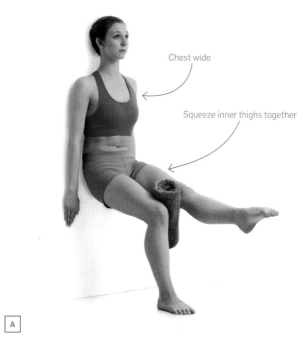

Chest wide

Squeeze inner thighs together

**A**

- Use a pillow or folded bath towel to squeeze between your knees with your feet together in parallel and move your feet forward to where, when your hips and thighs are at right angles, your shins will be perpendicular to the floor.
- Inhale with control as you slide down the wall until your thighs are parallel to the floor. (If this is too great a strain in your knees, simply slide only halfway down to start and graduate each time you practice.)
- Holding your breath in this position, the backs of your shoulders pinned to the wall, stretch one leg forward and hold for a count of three.
- Exhale slowly and replace your foot on the floor. Inhale with control and repeat with your other leg.
- Slide back up to the starting position.

**REPS:** Repeat the entire sequence three times, finding more control and stability with each opportunity.

# Mat Sequence
## >LEVEL III

**Start »**
Lowering Down to
the Mat (page 93)

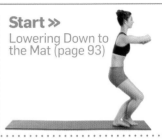

**6**
Rolling Like a Ball
(page 91)

**7**
Single-Leg Stretch
(page 66)

**8**
Double-Leg Stretch
(page 67)

**9**
Single Straight-Leg Stretch
(page 92)

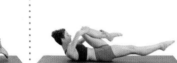

**14**
Corkscrew (page 124)

**15**
Saw (page 95)

**16**
Swan Dive (page 124)

**17**
Single-Leg Kicks
(page 70)

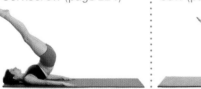
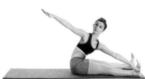
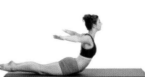
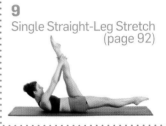

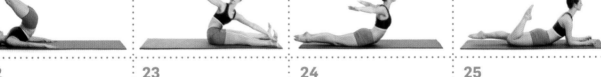

**22**
Side Kicks: Bicycle
(page 126)

**23**
Side Kicks: Grand Leg
Circles (page 127)

**24**
Side Kicks:
Hot Potato
(page 127)

**25**
Teaser III
(page 128)

**30**
Leg Pull
(page 129)

**31**
Kneeling Side
Kicks (page 129)

**32**
Side Bend
(page 130)

**33**
Boomerang
(page 131)

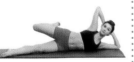
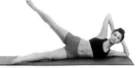
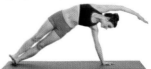
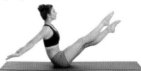
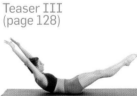

**2**
The Hundred
(page 63)

**3**
Roll-Up (page 64)

**4**
Rollover I (page 121)

**5**
Single-Leg Circles II
(page 122)

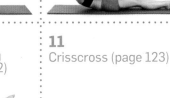

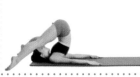

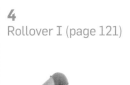

**10**
Double Straight-Leg
Stretch II (page 122)

**11**
Crisscross (page 123)

**12**
Spine Stretch
(page 68)

**13**
Open-Leg Rocker
(Legs Wide) (page 123)

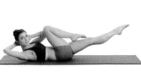

**18**
Double-Leg Kicks
(page 97)

**19**
Neckpull (page 125)

**20**
Spine Twist  (page 98)

**21**
Jackknife (page 126)

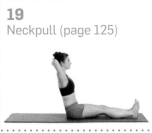

**26**
Hip Twist (page 128)

**27**
Swimming (page 103)

**28**
Leg Pull Front
(page 104)

**29**
Transition from
Leg Pull Front
to Leg Pull
(page 129)

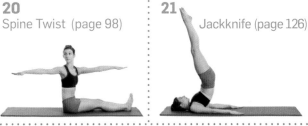

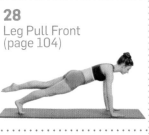

**34**
Seal
(page 76)

**35**
Control
Balance
Prep
(page 130)

**36**
High Bridge Prep
(page 132)

**End**
Single-Leg
Pushup
(page 133)

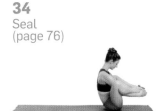

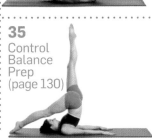

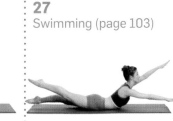

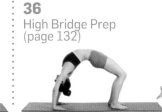

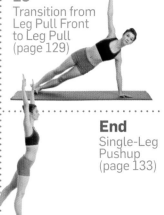

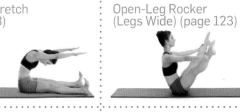

# Mat Series

## LEVEL IV
> STARTERS

# PLANK JACKS

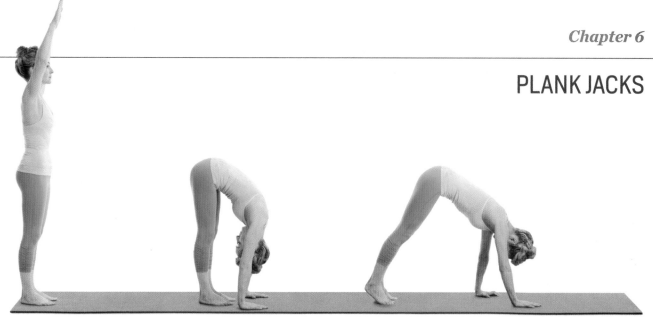

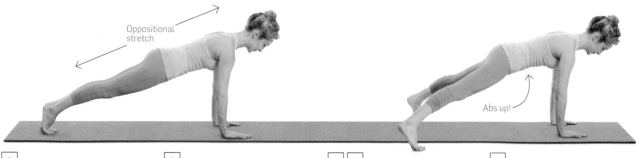

Oppositional stretch

Abs up!

| **A** | **B** | **C** **D** | **E** |

- Stand tall, facing the mat at one end.
- Inhale with control as you bring your arms up, lengthening your waist and squeezing the backs of the upper inner thighs together tightly.

- Exhale slowly as you bring your head and arms forward, shoulder-width apart, and lower your hands to the mat by rolling through your spine (not folding at your hips); the abs remain scooped.
- Place your palms on the mat with your head on your knees (bend your knees only as needed).

- Walk your hands forward in 3½ giant straight-armed steps until you are in a rigid plank position from head to heels, with your shoulders past your wrists, and you are balanced on the tips of your toes.

- Jump your legs open and closed six times, reinforcing your stable, shoulder-past-wrist position with each Jack.
- From your plank position, lift from your powerhouse muscles and fold your chest toward your thighs, like an upside-down Teaser.
- Walk your hands back to your feet with straight arms and roll up to standing.

**REPS:** Repeat the sequence three times total, finding a controlled rhythm.

# *Pilates on the Mat: Level IV Starters*

## SQUAT-THRUSTS

**A**

- Start by standing tall with your arms straight above your head.

**B**

- Squat and place your palms on the mat in front of you, slightly wider than shoulder-width apart.

**C** **D**

- While holding your upper body in place, jump ("thrust") your legs back and land on the balls of your feet with your body in a rigid plank position, your navel pulled firmly to your spine. (Do not let your hips drop.)
- Keeping your upper body in place, using a deep scoop of your abs, jump your feet forward to the original palms-down squat position and rise up to standing.

**REPS:** Try six to ten controlled Squat-Thrusts, emphasizing the balance element midjump when stable arms and strong abs rule the roost.

**NOTE:** *Squat-Thrusts (aka "burpees") are named after the physiologist who developed them in the 1940s as part of his fitness test. (For those Pilates practitioners familiar with the apparatus, the burpee is akin to our Third Knee Stretch on the Reformer). You can add so much to a burpee to progress: Jump up instead of stand up, add a pushup or Plank Jack while in plank position, etc.*

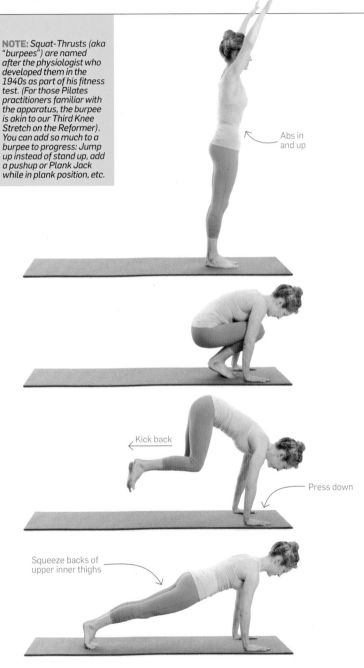

Abs in and up

Kick back

Press down

Squeeze backs of upper inner thighs

# TRANSITION: JUMP THROUGH TO THE HUNDRED

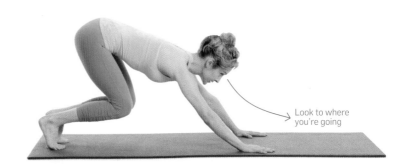

Look to where you're going

**A**

- From your plank position, lift from your powerhouse muscles and fold your chest toward your thighs, like an upside-down Teaser.
- Open your feet to parallel and stay high on your toes.
- Bend your knees, creasing at the hip, and crouch back like a tiger ready to pounce (chest open, eyes forward).

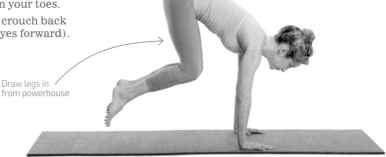

Draw legs in from powerhouse

**B** **C**

- Use the spring of your legs paired with the stability of your arms to smoothly jump your feet to the mat between your hands with bent knees and have a seat—or jump all the way through to a tall seated position with legs at a 90-degree angle to your torso. You can even try to land, or lift into, a balanced pike position. Have fun with your transitions.

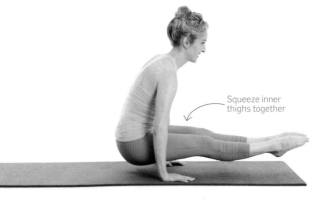

Squeeze inner thighs together

# Mat Series

LEVEL IV
> MAINS

# ROLLING LIKE A CANNONBALL

 **A**

- Sit on the mat with your knees bent to your chest and your hands wrapped tightly around the fronts of your ankles.
- Tuck your head down between your knees and pull your abs in and up away from the thighs.

**B** **C** **D** **E**

- Roll onto your upper back (never allowing the weight of your body to rest on your cervical vertebrae) and roll back up to balance on your tail—but this time, whenever you roll forward, press your knees and feet tightly together, release your hands, and jump up into the air.
- Land softly and reverse the movements back to the mat.

**REPS:** Roll back and cannonball up four to six times, finding full expansion in your cannon blast and full contraction in your ball.

**BREATH FOR ROCKING AND ROLLING:** JOE RECOMMENDED INHALING IN THE STABLE POSITIONS AND EXHALING ON THE ROLLING PORTIONS IN ORDER TO "PRESS" THE AIR OUT. FIND THE PATTERN OF BREATH THAT BEST HELPS YOU STABILIZE AND MOBILIZE WHERE NEEDED.

Keep legs together

Scoop!

**NOTE:** *For Cannonball Prep, do not jump up but stand up with control, squeezing your knees and feet together and lifting your arms.*

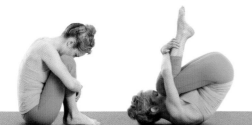
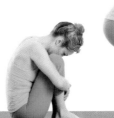
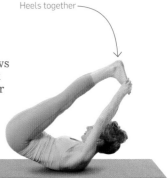

# CLOSED-LEG ROCKER

 **A**

- From the lifted, balanced Open-Leg Rocker Prep I position (page 69), sew your legs together as if they were one and take hold of your big toes, baby toes, or balls of your feet.

**B**

- Bring your head as close to your shins as possible with your elbows bent wide to the sides, then rock back to the base of your shoulder blades and back up.
- Control this movement so momentum doesn't!

Heels together

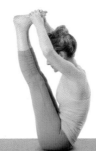

**REPS:** Give yourself four chances to find the muscular coordination and strength needed to achieve this version of Rocker.

# *Pilates on the Mat: Level IV Mains*

## TWISTED CORKSCREW

This is an exaggerated and complicated Corkscrew—
that is, a little twisted!

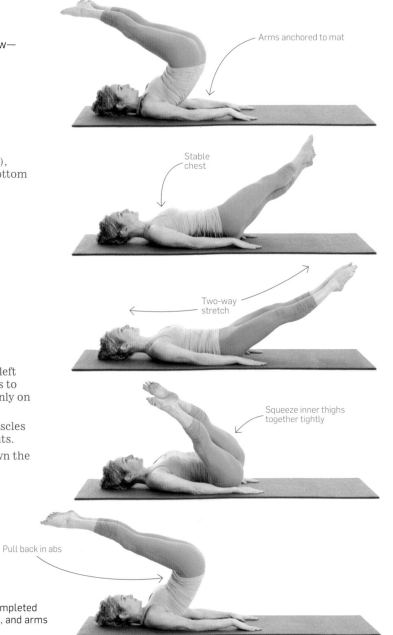

Arms anchored to mat

Stable chest

Two-way stretch

Squeeze inner thighs together tightly

Pull back in abs

A

- From the lifted Corkscrew position (page 124),
  keep your shoulders square and twist your bottom
  to the right (your legs will go left).

B C D E

- Roll down the left side of the body until your left
  buttock touches the mat, then circle your legs to
  the right(!) and come back up to balance evenly on
  your shoulder blades.
- The abs are scooped and the powerhouse muscles
  are working together to control the movements.
- Twist to the left and repeat the sequence down the
  right side of the body.

**REPS:** Continue alternating directions until you have completed
two or three sets, grounding your upper back, shoulders, and arms
more and more securely with each revolution.

# SCISSORS

- Lie flat with your legs squeezed together, your
  feet pointed, and long, sturdy arms held tightly to
  your sides. (The backs of your arms, palms, and
  shoulders are anchored to the mat.)

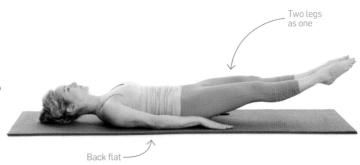

Two legs
as one

Back flat

B

- Inhale with control as you roll your legs overhead,
  one vertebra at a time, until you can place
  your palms flat against the back of your lower back
  (your hands are above your hip bones, like a
  supported Jackknife).

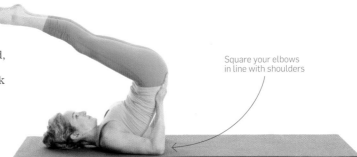

Square your elbows
in line with shoulders

C

- Balance evenly on the backs of your shoulders
  and inhale with control as you reach your right leg
  forward on a high diagonal and your left leg back
  in opposition.
- Split your legs as far as you are able while
  maintaining the lift in your hips (do not allow the
  weight of your body to fall into your wrists).
- Exhale with control as you switch legs, keeping
  the legs firm and the hips lifted.

**REPS:** Alternate legs six times, grounding your head and
upper body while seeking more lightness in your scissoring
legs at every opportunity.

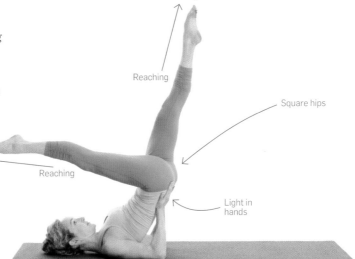

Reaching

Square hips

Reaching

Light in
hands

149

# *Pilates on the Mat: Level IV Mains*

## BICYCLE

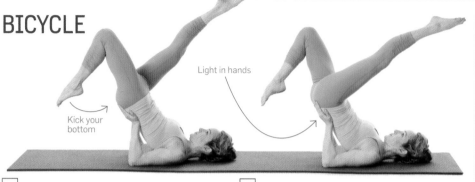

Kick your bottom

Light in hands

| A | B |

**A**

- From the lifted position of the Scissors, balanced evenly on the backs of your shoulders, inhale with control as you reach your left leg forward on a high diagonal and your right leg back in opposition.

**B**

- Stabilizing your left thigh, bend your left knee and exhale with control as you try to kick your bottom with your heel (like the Single-Leg Kick).
- Inhale slowly as you draw your bent knee toward you and then straighten it back on a high diagonal overhead as you simultaneously reach your right leg forward and repeat the sequence.

**REPS:** Bicycle six times, maintaining the lightness in your hips (do not allow the weight of your body to fall into your wrists) and trying with each opportunity to get your heel to your bottom.

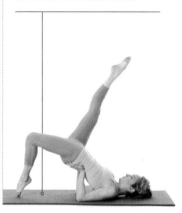

VARIATIONS ON THE THEME

For more of a hip opener, try to scrape the mat with your toes as you cycle forward and backward.

---

## SIDE KICKS: DOUBLE-LEG-LIFT SCISSORS

**A**

- With your body aligned in a straight line from head to heels, squeeze your legs together tightly, wrapping the backs of the upper inner thighs together, as if both legs were one.
- Inhale with control as you lift your legs off the mat and begin slowly scissoring the inner thighs past one another.

**B**

- Emphasize the lift and backswing of the legs and maintain a stable upper body throughout.

**REPS:** Scissor ten times, lifting the bottom leg higher with each effort.

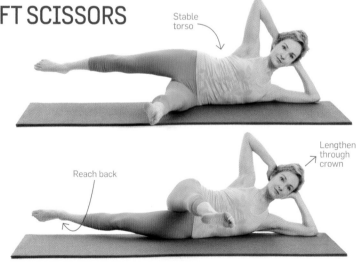

Stable torso

Lengthen through crown

Reach back

# TRANSITION: HIP-FLIP

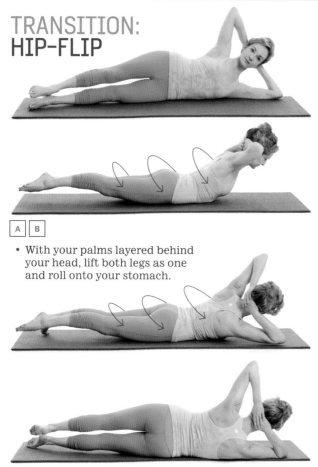

A  B

- With your palms layered behind your head, lift both legs as one and roll onto your stomach.

C  D

- Keep your head, chest, and thighs lifted off the mat as you twist your upper body (like a horizontal Spine Twist) in the direction you want to face and then, using strong employment of your powerhouse muscles, "flip" your hips to face the same way, curling your bottom under you.

**NOTE:** *This transition is meant to be fun. Remember, too, that there were no "sticky mats" in the early days of Pilates's popularity and so this would be much easier performed on slick studio Naugahyde.*

**REPS:** Practice until you are able to end in near-perfect alignment on your other side, ready to go right into the next exercise with a *minimum of motion.*

# TEASER IV: FIGURE 8s

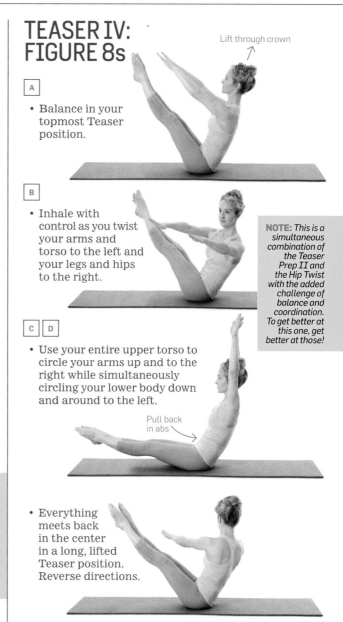

Lift through crown

A

- Balance in your topmost Teaser position.

B

- Inhale with control as you twist your arms and torso to the left and your legs and hips to the right.

**NOTE:** *This is a simultaneous combination of the Teaser Prep II and the Hip Twist with the added challenge of balance and coordination. To get better at this one, get better at those!*

C  D

- Use your entire upper torso to circle your arms up and to the right while simultaneously circling your lower body down and around to the left.

Pull back in abs

- Everything meets back in the center in a long, lifted Teaser position. Reverse directions.

**REPS:** Complete four Figure 8s (two sets), focusing on twisting from your waistline more than from your shoulders.

# *Pilates on the Mat: Level IV Mains*

## SIDE BEND: TWIST

**A**

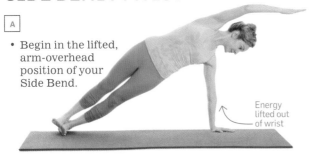

- Begin in the lifted, arm-overhead position of your Side Bend.

Energy lifted out of wrist

**B**

- Stabilize your hips and exhale slowly as you twist your upper body toward the mat, "threading" your arm and shoulder through the space between you and the mat.

Hips square to front

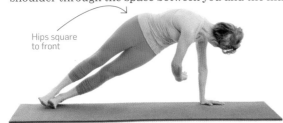

**C**

- Inhale with control as you unthread, opening your arm and chest to the back of the room while your pelvis remains facing front.
- Let your face follow the twist of your spine.
- Slowly exhale and return your hip to the mat with control.
- Switch sides.

Open from your chest

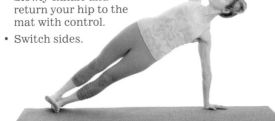

**REPS:** One smooth and steady twist on either side, if done well, should suffice—make it count!

## SIDE BEND: STAR

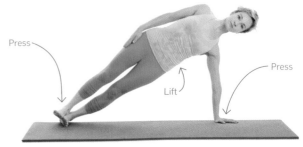

Press

Press

Lift

**A**

- From the lifted, palm-on-thigh position of your Side Bend, stabilize your hips.

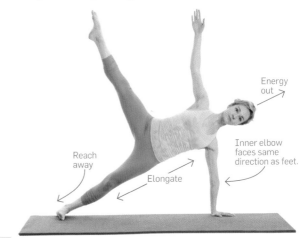

Energy out

Reach away

Elongate

Inner elbow faces same direction as feet.

**B**

- Inhale slowly as you raise your arm and top leg toward the ceiling.
- Exhale slowly as you return them to the starting position.
- Switch sides.

**NOTE:** You can choose which sidebend variations you want to do. The key is to keep energy lifted off your wrists.

**REPS:** Try two or three stars on each side, using the "press away" from the mat to energize the lift of your limbs.

# BOOMERANG ROWING

Press down

Lift up

Pull abs into back

Long, strong arms

Reach away

Lengthen

Abs lifted

**A**

- Sit tall with your legs straight out at a 90-degree angle to your body, your ankles crossed and the inner thighs squeezing together tightly.

**B** **C**

- With your palms pressed to the mat at your sides, inhale with control as you lift your legs as one from the mat and roll back, bringing your legs overhead and balancing on your shoulder blades with long, strong arms pressed firmly to the mat.

**D** **E** **F**

- Holding this balanced position, switch ankles with a small, quick scissoring of the legs.

**G**

- Inhale with control as you roll up into a balanced ankles-crossed Teaser position, reaching your fingertips for your toes.
- Flip your palms and bend your elbows into your sides.

**H**

- Slide your forearms back and clasp your hands behind you, stretching your arms long toward the mat.

**I**

- Exhale with control as you lower your legs, reaching your forehead to your knees, and lifting your arms straight up behind you in opposition.

**J** **K**

- Hold this position as you release your hands and circle them around to your feet.
- Roll up to a tall, seated position and begin again.

**REPS:** Complete four Boomerang Rowings (two sets of ankle crosses), getting higher and lighter in your limbs with each roll and row.

## CRAB

The rolling exercises in Pilates are meant as massages. Your back and organs are kneaded by the movements of the abdominal muscles pressing deeply toward the mat as you roll.

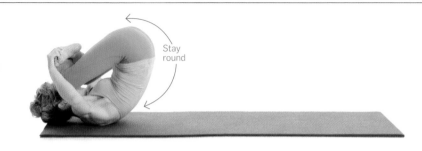

Stay round

**A**

- Sit on the mat with your knees bent into your chest and your legs crossed at the ankles.
- Take hold of your left foot's toes with your right hand and your right foot's toes with your left hand and pull your thighs as deep into the body as possible.
- Inhale with control and deepen your abs to initiate rolling back onto your upper back.

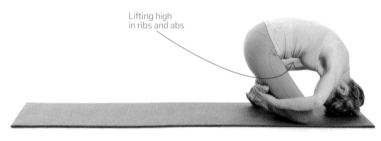

Lifting high in ribs and abs

**B**

- Exhale slowly as you roll up and forward until the crown of your head rests on the mat.
- The abs are strongly pulling in opposition to "put on the brakes" so momentum does not overtake you.
- Try three simple Crabs, staying centered on your mat and deepening your abs with each roll.
- When your head is on the mat, your abs are lifting up and back in opposition to keep the weight off your neck.

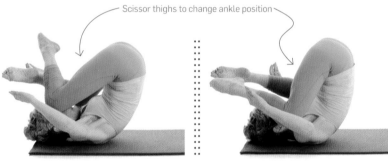

Scissor thighs to change ankle position

**C** **D** **E**

- Next, add your "pincers": When balanced on the back of your shoulders, switch the order of your ankles (if your right ankle had been on top of your left ankle, now it will be under) by scissoring your thighs away from one another and then back again from deep within your hip sockets.

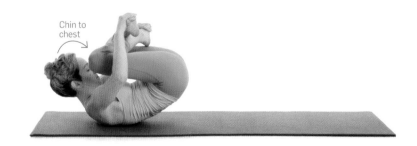

Chin to chest

**REPS:** Work your Crab claws six times, aiming to free your limbs more and more by using your abdominals to control the movements.

# ROCKING

After three flexed moves, it's time to open up the front of the body through an extension exercise.

- Lie on your stomach with your forehead down, the pubis anchored to the mat, and the inner thighs pressed tightly together.

- Bend your knees and reach both arms back evenly, taking hold of each foot with its corresponding hand and bringing your heels to your bottom for a stretch across your knees.

- Inhale with control as you lift your thighs and chest high off the mat (like you did for Swan Dive and Swimming).

- Exhale slowly as you press your feet back into your hands to create muscular tension (the good kind) from the tips of your toes, around the front of your body, up through the crown of your head, and back at your fingertips, effectively completing an energetic circle.

- Keep this muscular "lock" on the position throughout the Rocking movements.

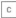

- Inhale slowly as you rock forward until your chest touches the mat.

- Exhale slowly as you rock back over your thighs, massaging the front of your body. (Lymph drainage, anyone?!)

**REPS:** Rock forward and back five times. contacting more and more front body surface to the mat.

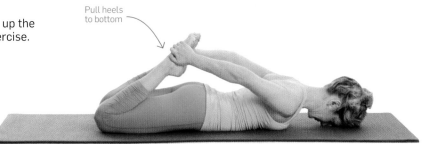

Pull heels to bottom

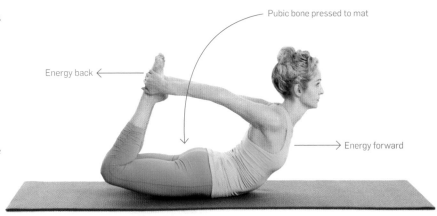

Pubic bone pressed to mat

Energy back ←

→ Energy forward

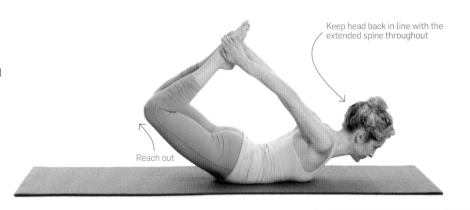

Keep head back in line with the extended spine throughout

Reach out

## CONTROL BALANCE

A

- Lie flat with your legs squeezed together, your feet pointed, and long, sturdy arms held tightly to your sides. (The backs of your arms, palms, and shoulders are anchored to the mat.)

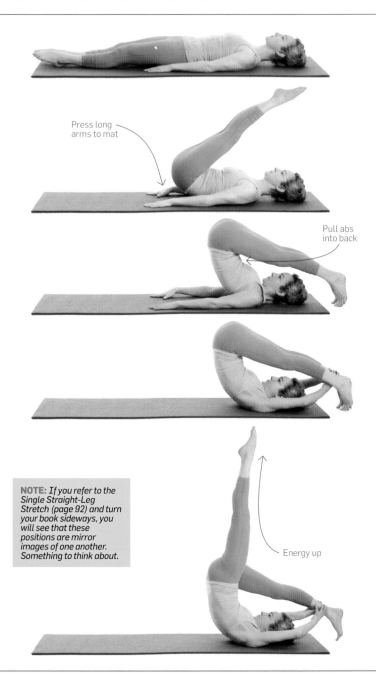

Press long arms to mat

Pull abs into back

B  C

- Inhale with control as you roll your legs and bottom overhead, one vertebra at a time, until your toes touch the floor behind you.

D  E

- Balance evenly on the backs of your shoulders and reach your arms around to take hold of your right ankle and lift the left leg as high in the air as possible. (Since you will no longer have the opposition of your arms to stop you from rolling onto your neck, it is critical to pull your upper abs as deeply away from your head and hands as possible.)

- Exhale with control as you bring the left leg back down and take hold of it with your hands, freeing your right leg.

- Inhale with control as you lift your right leg as high as possible without lifting weight onto your neck.

**NOTE:** *If you refer to the Single Straight-Leg Stretch (page 92) and turn your book sideways, you will see that these positions are mirror images of one another. Something to think about.*

Energy up

**REPS:** Switch legs six times, using each rep as an opportunity to find your inner core strength and balance.

# HIGH BRIDGE

This is a one-shot deal, so prepare to make the most out of the one repetition, on each leg, that you get.

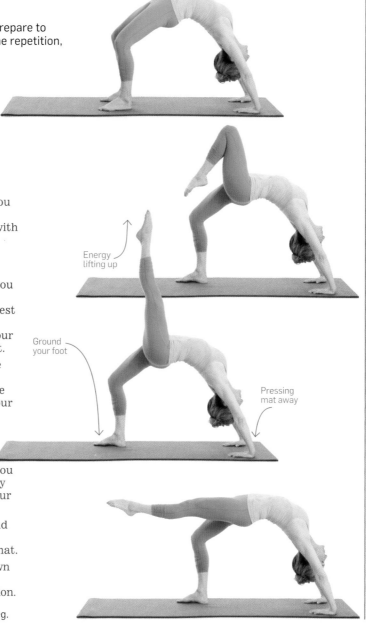

**A**

- Begin at the top of the High Bridge Prep (page 132) position.

**B** **C**

- Inhale with control as you straighten and lift your left leg to a right angle with the body.

**D**

- Exhale with control as you reach your left leg away from you, lifting your chest back in opposition and levering the weight of your hips away from your feet.

- Replace that foot on the mat and inhale with control as you repeat the lifted movement with your right leg.

- Exhale with control as you reach your right leg away from you and replace your foot on the mat.

- Inhale slowly as you bend your elbows and gently lower your head to the mat.

- Then roll slowly back down to the starting position on a slow, steady exhalation.

**REPS:** Perform once on each leg.

Energy lifting up

Ground your foot

Pressing mat away

## REVERSE YOUR MOVES FOR MAX EFFECT

Mastered your moves? Upped your tempo? Trumped your transitions? Still looking for a challenge? Perform your level matwork once forward and then reverse the order and perform the matwork once backward! The fun never ends.

# Mat Series

## LEVEL IV
> ENDERS

# ARM WEIGHTS: LUNGE BUTTERFLY

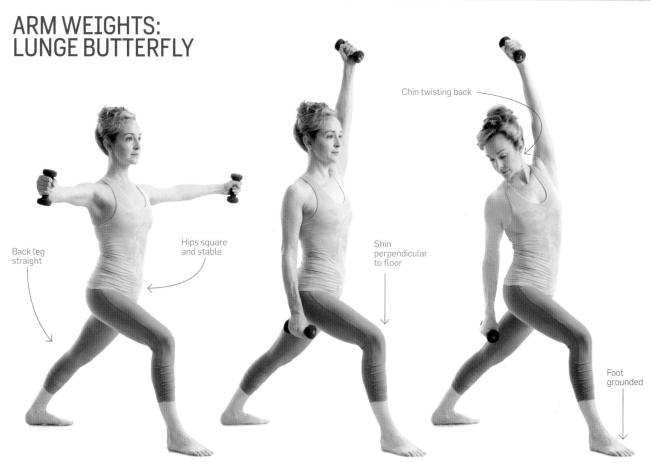

Back leg straight

Hips square and stable

Chin twisting back

Shin perpendicular to floor

Foot grounded

**A**

- Stand tall with your heels together and toes apart and step or slide your left foot back into a lunge with your arms long by your sides, your palms forward, and your shoulders back. Readjust your back foot as needed to keep the heel down.

- Keep your torso upright, stretching your chest upward in opposition to your weights, the abs pulled in and up.

- Inhale with control as you bring your arms out wide to your sides with your wings down and drawn together.

**B** **C**

- Exhale with control as you twist your head and torso to the right, lifting your left biceps by your ear and bringing your right arm down behind your right hip.

- Inhale with control as you return to center. Push off the front foot, bringing your feet back to the starting position.

- Step or slide the right foot backward into a lunge and repeat the entire sequence to the right.

**REPS:** Explore three chances on each side to distinguish the rotation of your spine from the rotation of your hips or shoulders, alternating sides with each go.

# Pilates on the Mat: Level IV Enders

## ARM WEIGHTS: LUNGE WITH WINGS

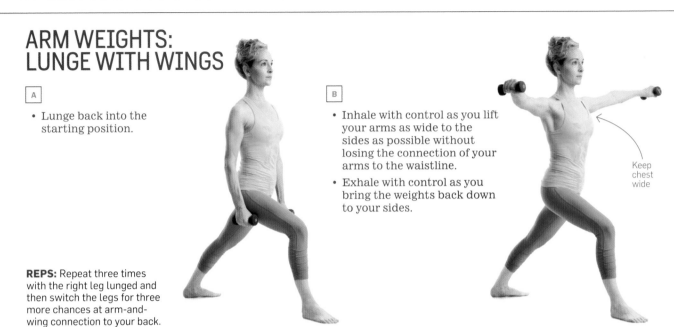

**A**

- Lunge back into the starting position.

**B**

- Inhale with control as you lift your arms as wide to the sides as possible without losing the connection of your arms to the waistline.
- Exhale with control as you bring the weights back down to your sides.

Keep chest wide

**REPS:** Repeat three times with the right leg lunged and then switch the legs for three more chances at arm-and-wing connection to your back.

## ARM WEIGHTS: LUNGE CHEST EXPANSION (Twisting Arms)

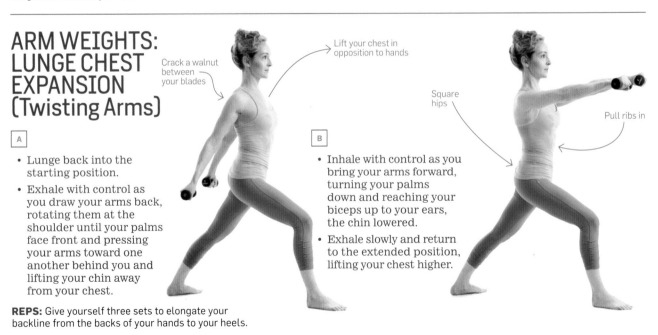

Crack a walnut between your blades

Lift your chest in opposition to hands

Square hips

Pull ribs in

**A**

- Lunge back into the starting position.
- Exhale with control as you draw your arms back, rotating them at the shoulder until your palms face front and pressing your arms toward one another behind you and lifting your chin away from your chest.

**B**

- Inhale with control as you bring your arms forward, turning your palms down and reaching your biceps up to your ears, the chin lowered.
- Exhale slowly and return to the extended position, lifting your chest higher.

**REPS:** Give yourself three sets to elongate your backline from the backs of your hands to your heels.

# ARM WEIGHTS: LUNGE SHAVING

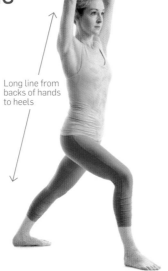

**A**

- Starting position same as Lunge Butterfly.
- Lift the weights up and overhead and pitch slightly forward over the lunging leg.

Long line from backs of hands to heels

**B**

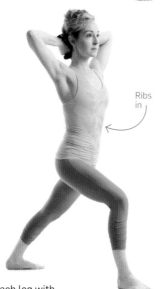

- Bend your elbows wide to the sides and bring the weights down behind your head—"shaving" the back of your head with the weights. Inhale with control and press the weights back up until your arms are straight.
- The elbows remain open as wide as possible throughout the shave and press.

Ribs in

**REPS:** Perform three times on each leg with the intention of lengthening your spine, vertebra by vertebra, with each arm movement.

# ARM WEIGHTS: LUNGE HUG

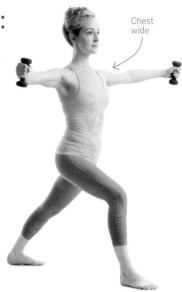

Chest wide

**A**

- Starting position same as Lunge Butterfly.
- Lift your arms forward to chest height and widen your elbows, facing your knuckles toward one another to form a circle with your arms.

Shoulders down your back

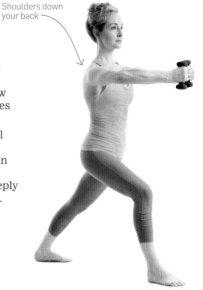

**B**

- Inhale with control as you spread your arms wide and draw your shoulder blades together tightly.
- Exhale with control as you bring your knuckles together in a giant bear hug. Draw the ribs in deeply to press the air out.

**REPS:** Give yourself three chances with your left leg back and three with your right leg back, changing the breathing pattern (exhale to open the arms, inhale to close them) and deepening your exhalation and inhalation with each opportunity.

# *Mat Series*

# Mat Sequence
## >LEVEL IV

**Start »**
Lowering Down
to Mat (page 93)

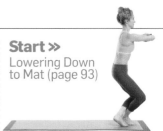

**6** Rolling Like a Cannonball (page 147)

**7** Single-Leg Stretch (page 66)

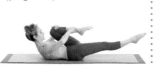

**8** Double-Leg Stretch (page 67)

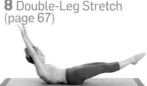

**9** Single Straight-Leg Stretch (page 92)

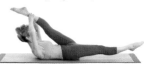

**14** Twisted Corkscrew (page 148)

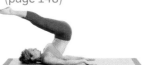

**15** Saw (page 95)

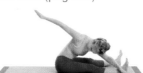

**16** Swan Dive (page 124)

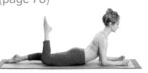

**17** Single-Leg Kicks (page 70)

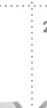

**22** Scissors (page 149)

**23** Bicycle (page 150)

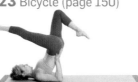

**24** Shoulder Bridge (page 98)

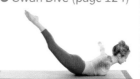

**25** Spine Twist (page 98)

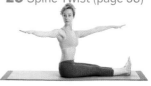

**30** Side Kicks: Double-Leg-Lift Scissors (page 150)

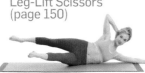

**31** Teaser IV-Figure 8s (page 151)

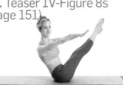

**32** Hip Twist (page 128)

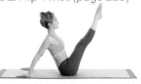

**33** Swimming (page 103)

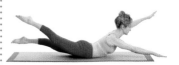

**38** Boomerang Rowing (page 153)

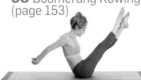

**39** Seal (page 76)

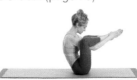

**40** Crab (page 154)

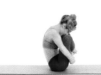

**41** Rocking (page 155)

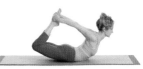

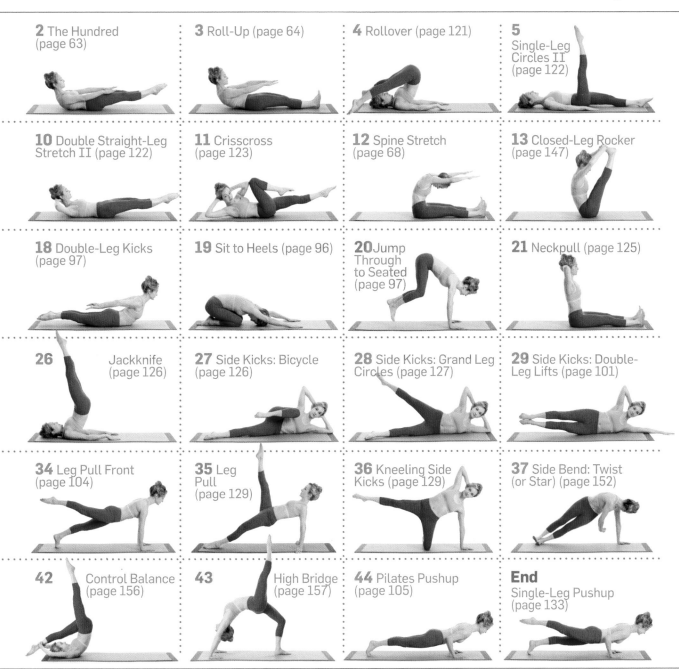

**2** The Hundred (page 63)

**3** Roll-Up (page 64)

**4** Rollover (page 121)

**5** Single-Leg Circles II (page 122)

**10** Double Straight-Leg Stretch II (page 122)

**11** Crisscross (page 123)

**12** Spine Stretch (page 68)

**13** Closed-Leg Rocker (page 147)

**18** Double-Leg Kicks (page 97)

**19** Sit to Heels (page 96)

**20** Jump Through to Seated (page 97)

**21** Neckpull (page 125)

**26** Jackknife (page 126)

**27** Side Kicks: Bicycle (page 126)

**28** Side Kicks: Grand Leg Circles (page 127)

**29** Side Kicks: Double-Leg Lifts (page 101)

**34** Leg Pull Front (page 104)

**35** Leg Pull (page 129)

**36** Kneeling Side Kicks (page 129)

**37** Side Bend: Twist (or Star) (page 152)

**42** Control Balance (page 156)

**43** High Bridge (page 157)

**44** Pilates Pushup (page 105)

**End** Single-Leg Pushup (page 133)

# Pushups and Planks

Pushups and planks work multiple parts of the body at the same time, engaging every muscle from head to toes. Considering you're supporting 70 percent of your body weight, a pushup is considered a resistance exercise, so you're also getting the similar bone-building effects you might see from weight lifting. Pilates Pushups bring even more benefits to the table by beginning and ending in an upright position, necessitating the addition of stretch, articulation, and control to master.

Pushups and plank variations are great to sprinkle into your workouts as Starters or Enders.

# PROPER POSITION

What do pushups and planks work? Well, everything, but especially your chest, triceps, abdominals, and back muscles. The serratus anterior (responsible for keeping your wings in place) gets direct stimuli during a pushup, keeping your posture strong. A Pilates Pushup is different from what you may be used to and has specific rules of engagement to get right in terms of form and intention. For example, in Pilates we do not simply lower to the ground; we aim forward for the front edges of our mats as if riding the springs of the Reformer carriage.

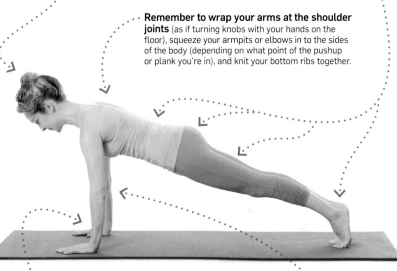

**Make sure your powerhouse muscles are active** by pulling your navel to your spine, tightening your seat, and pressing your inner thighs and heels together tightly throughout the pushup or plank sequence (unless otherwise indicated).

**Make sure your head remains in line with your spine** (a rod of steel from head to heel). You can place a pole or broomstick along your head and back and make sure you feel it contact the back of your head, your upper back (between your shoulder blades), and your sacrum.

**Remember to wrap your arms at the shoulder joints** (as if turning knobs with your hands on the floor), squeeze your armpits or elbows in to the sides of the body (depending on what point of the pushup or plank you're in), and knit your bottom ribs together.

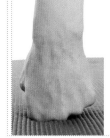

**DETAIL:** It takes practice to develop the strength in these often underused muscles. When bearing weight on the wrist, be sure to press through your first two knuckles and not allow any kink in the wrist. Start by keeping your knees bent and build up to a straight-body position.

**Wrist safety!** Since pushups and planks require so much weight to be placed on the wrists, and since wrists are not mechanically built to be weight bearers, it is critical for their health that you manage the damage. The less weight you can place on the heel of your hands the better. This means you will need to be conscious of distributing the weight evenly through the outer portion of your hands. Squeeze fingers tightly and cup the floor. If you are on a particularly thick mat, be careful of overflexing your wrist. Either move to a harder surface or try using fists (see detail).

**Your inner elbows should face one another without turning your hands or hiking your shoulders.** Assess this in plank position by locking out hard in your elbow and feeling the sensation that this creates in the joint. Now "soften" (unlock) your elbow joint and turn the inner elbows to face one another. Can you feel the muscles in the backs of your arms turn on?

# *Pushups and Planks*

**ASSESS:** WHEN LIFTING YOUR ARMS OVERHEAD, DO YOUR SHOULDERS AUTOMATICALLY FOLLOW THEM UP? TRY TO HOLD YOUR SHOULDERS DOWN, WHILE RAISING YOUR ARMS. CAN YOU FEEL YOUR ARM BONE MOVING WITHIN THE STABLE SHOULDER SOCKET?

## BEGIN

- Stand tall the end of the mat and inhale with control as you bring your arms up, wrapping your thighs together tightly and drawing the abs in and up.

- Exhale slowly and round forward with control, bringing your palms to the mat.

- Reach your forehead to your knees (bend your knees as needed).

**1**

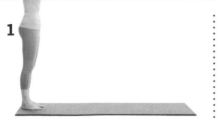

**2**

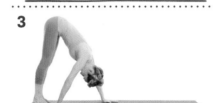

**3**

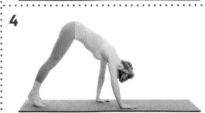

**4**

### PROGRESSIONS

- Planting your feet at a higher angle (such as up on a step) (see Incline Pushup and Planks, page 237)

- Placing your hands or feet on an unstable surface (like a stability ball or wobble cushion) (see Asymmetrical Pushups, page 237)

- Removing an arm or a leg from the equation (such as by lifting it off the mat) (see Superman Planks, page 171)

## 5 PILATES PUSHUP AND PLANK

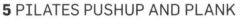

Lengthen in opposition

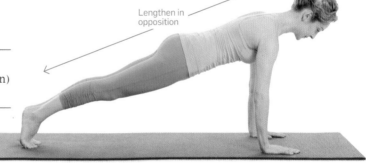

## END

- Lift from your powerhouse muscles and fold your chest toward your thighs, like an upside-down Teaser.

- Lower your heels to the mat and push off your palms, walking your hands (with straight arms) back to your feet in 3½ giant steps. The legs remain as straight as possible until your forehead touches your knees.

- Reverse the movements of rolling down and roll your spine back up to stand tall with your arms and waist lifted.

**6**

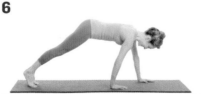

**7**

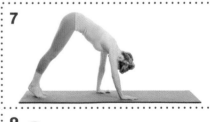

**8**

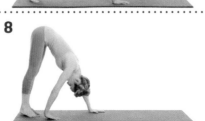

**9**

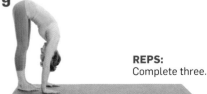

**REPS:**
Complete three.

# UP-STRETCH COMBO

**A**

- From the position of your Forward Fold: Walk your hands forward with straight arms in $3\frac{1}{2}$ giant steps, but instead of leveling out into plank position, keep your hips and heels high (like an inverted Teaser).

- Stabilize your upper body, with your head tucked toward your abs, as you lower and lift your heels three times, working from your deepest powerhouse muscles.

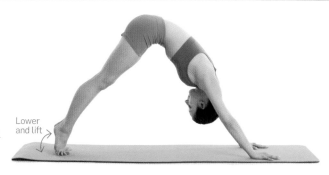

Lower and lift ↘

**C**

- With your heels lifted, tuck your bottom under and begin curling your hips toward the floor.

- Create resistance by simultaneously curling your upper body deeper toward your abs.

**NOTE:** *This is taken from a combo of exercises on the Reformer in which the hips are working on mobility as the upper body is working on stability and then the pelvis becomes stable as the spine articulates. Try to find these opposing elements through the movements and see how they, in fact, spur one another on.*

**D**

- Once your pelvis is level, stabilize your hips and waist and uncurl your upper spine,

Curl your bottom as much as possible

**E**

- Open your shoulders and press your chest through (like an elevated Swan Dive).

- Your chest and chin are stretching upward, the hips remain perfectly still.

- Reverse the movement by bringing your head toward your chest, articulating one vertebra at a time and hollowing out your abs.

- The hips remain still as long as possible.

- When all spinal segments have been exhausted, allow the hips to lift with control, returning to the inverted Teaser position, and lower your heels.

**REPS:** Repeat the Up-Stretch Combo three times and then walk your hands back to your feet and roll up to standing. Perform two full sets (of three Up-Stretch Combos), working on stabilizing what should be stable and when, while mobilizing what should be mobile and when.

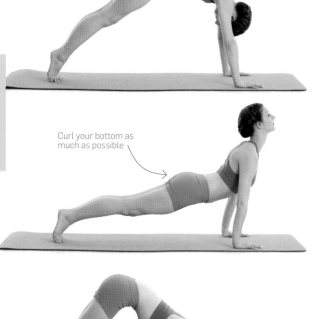

# *Pushups and Planks*

## WAVE

**A**

- From the position of your Forward Fold: Walk your hands forward with straight arms in 3½ giant steps until you are in a rigid plank position from head to heels with your upper-body weight just past your hands (your shoulders are past your wrists) and you are balanced on the tips of your toes.

> **NOTE:** *This movement can also be done in plank on your knees, and you can play with the up/down combination possibilities: down right/up left or down right/up right, etc.*

**B** **C**

- Replace your right hand with your right elbow, palm and forearm flat on the mat, then do the same with your left so that you are in a plank position on your elbows.

**D** **E**

- Then reverse by replacing your right elbow with your right hand and do the same with your left so that you are back in an extended arm plank.

**REPS:** Repeat the actions above, starting with your left side this time, and continue to alternate until you have been up and down evenly four times.

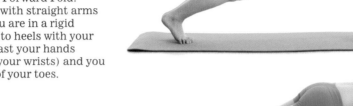
Tighten seat

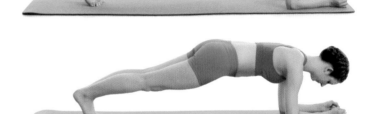
Scoop!

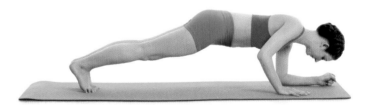

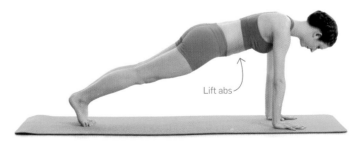
Lift abs

# SIDE-SWEEPER

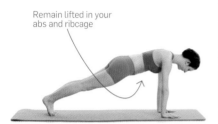

Remain lifted in your abs and ribcage

**A**

- Start in a rigid plank position with your arms straight, shoulders just past wrists, and light on toes.

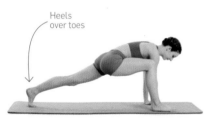

Heels over toes

**B**

- Swing your right leg around to the right and plant your right foot on the mat outside of your right hand, then swing it back to its starting position.

**REPS:** Repeat with your left leg. Continue to alternate sides and complete three sets before folding back up to starting position.

# KNEE-INS

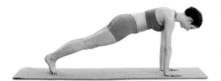

**A**

- Hold a rigid plank position with your arms pressing the mat away and abs lifted high into your back.

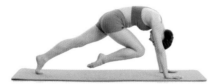

**B**

- Bring your right knee to your chest and your chest forward to your knee (like an inverted Single-Leg Stretch).
- Draw your ribs in deeply and hold this position for a count of three, then return to your rigid plank position.

**REPS:** Alternate legs a total of six times and increase oppositional tension between the pull of the bent knee and the reach of the straight knee more and more with each chance you get.

# MOUNTAIN CLIMBERS

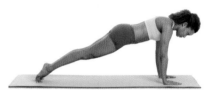

**A**

- These are like a sped-up version of the Knee-Ins. Take a strong plank positon with your body and draw one knee forward.

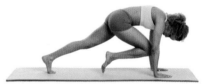

**B**

- Instead of holding your knee to your chest, keep your toes lightly on the floor and switch knees rapidly as if running, or climbing, in the horizontal plane.
- Keep your ribs knit and stay light on your feet and hands.

**REPS:** Complete eight to ten sets of Mountain Climbers before resetting your heels together and cycling through your pushup ending (that is, folding your chest to your thighs and walking back to your feet to roll up and stand).

# Pushups and Planks

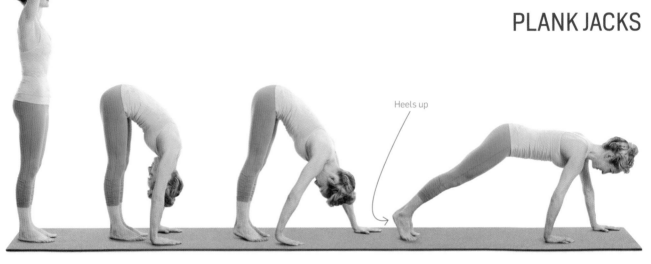

Heels up

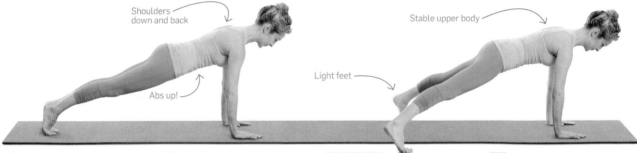

Shoulders down and back

Abs up!

Stable upper body

Light feet

**A**

- Stand tall, facing the mat at one end.
- Inhale with control as you bring your arms up, lengthening your waist and squeezing the backs of the upper inner thighs together tightly.

**B**

- Exhale slowly as you bring your head and arms forward, shoulder-width apart, and lower your hands to the mat by rolling through your spine (not folding at your hips); the abs remain scooped.
- Place your palms on the mat with your head on your knees (bend your knees only as needed).

**C** **D** **E**

- Walk your hands forward in 3½ giant straight-armed steps until you are in a rigid plank position from head to heels with your shoulders past your wrists and you are balanced on the tips of your toes.

**F**

- Jump your legs open and closed six times, reinforcing your stable, shoulder-past-wrist position with each Jack.
- From your plank position, lift from your powerhouse muscles and fold your chest toward your thighs, like an upside-down Teaser.
- Walk your hands back to your feet with straight arms and roll up to standing.

**REPS:** Repeat the sequence three times, total, finding a controlled rhythm with impeccable form.

# SPIDER PLANKS

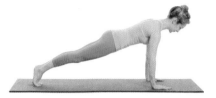

**A**

- Start in a rigid plank position and lift abs until feet are light and hips are floating.

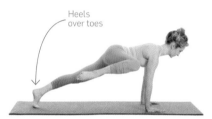

Heels over toes

**B**

- Bring your right knee up and around your right armpit and then replace it down on the mat.

> **NOTE:** *This move can also be executed while performing a slight pushup: As your knee comes toward your shoulder, lean forward and allow your elbows to bend, then press up and back as you return your foot to the mat.*

**REPS:** Repeat with your left knee. Continue to alternate sides, remaining light in the legs and hips and lifted in your abs and ribcage.

# SUPERMAN PLANK

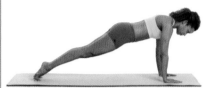

**A**

- Start in your rigid plank position (can also be done on elbows or on knees).

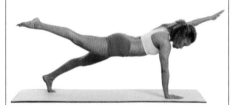

**B**

- Open your feet at least hip-width but keep your hands or elbows directly beneath the shoulders.
- Make sure your abs are lifted toward your back and your seat is tight as you reach your left arm forward with your biceps next to your left ear.
- Replace that arm and repeat with your right arm.

**REPS:** After two sets, see if you can lift your left arm and right leg in opposing directions without losing form. Then switch and try lifting your right arm and left leg. Two times is plenty before heading into your pushup ending.

# SIDE PLANKS

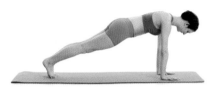

**A**

- Start in your rigid plank position with heels together and tail curled under.

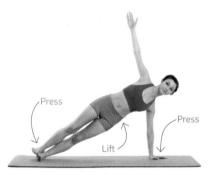

Press

Press

Lift

**B**

- Inhale with control as you rotate right, lifting your right arm off the mat and up to the ceiling.
- Allow your feet to either stack on top of one another or position your front foot to just sit in front of your bottom foot.
- Hold for a count of three and then return to plank before repeating the sequence to the left.

**REPS:** Complete only one set before coming back up to standing so as not to remain on your wrists for too long. You may always go back down and perform another set should you feel so inclined.

# *Pushups and Planks*

## SQUAT-THRUSTS

**A**

- Start by standing tall with your arms in the air.

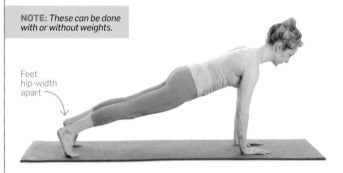

Energy up

Lengthen

**B**

- Squat and place your palms on the mat in front of you, slightly wider than shoulder-width apart.

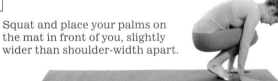

**C** **D**

- While holding your upper body in place, thrust your legs back and land on the balls of your feet in a rigid plank, your navel pulled firmly to your spine. (Do not let your hips drop.)

Press down to lift up

Energy up

- Keeping your upper body in place, using a deep scoop of your abs, jump your feet forward to the original squat position and rise up to standing.

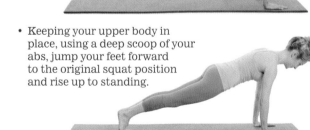

**REPS:** Try six to ten controlled Squat-Thrusts, emphasizing the balance element midjump when stable arms and strong abs rule the roost.

## PUSHUP WITH A DUMBBELL ROW

> **NOTE:** *These can be done with or without weights.*

Feet hip-width apart

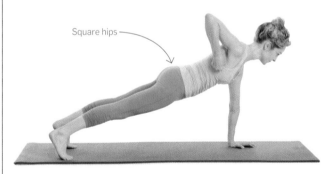

**A**

- If performing the row with weights, leave a set of weights at the far end of the mat where you will end up in your plank position. (You can also create imagined resistance.)

Square hips

**B**

- Once there, take hold of one weight in each hand and, holding a strong plank position, row the dumbbell in your right hand to the side of your chest by bending your arm and pulling it upward.
- Then lower the dumbbell and repeat the same

**REPS:** Complete three sets before walking your hands, weight free, back to your feet for your pushup ending.

# INVERTED TEASER PUSHUPS
## (aka Pike Pushups)

These target your shoulders and triceps from a new angle.

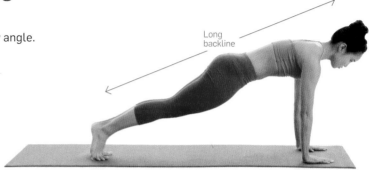

Long backline

**A**

- Squeeze your heels together or open your feet hip-width apart and walk your hands forward with straight arms in 3½ giant steps with hips high.

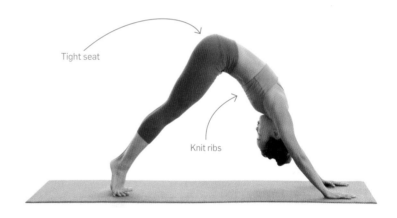

Tight seat

Knit ribs

**B**

- Instead of leveling out into plank position, keep your hips and heels high (like an inverted Teaser).

**C**

- Keeping your head between your arms, bend your elbows with control, allowing them to open only slightly away from your body, as you lower the crown of your head to the mat between your hands.

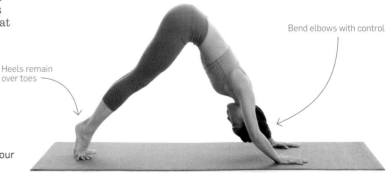

Bend elbows with control

Heels remain over toes

**REPS:** Complete three inverted pushups and walk your hands back in to your feet for your pushup ending.

# *Pushups and Planks*

## ASYMMETRICAL PUSHUP/PLANK

**NOTE:** *This exercise is akin to one-arm pushups on the wunda chair.*

**A**

- This is a great way to work a weaker side or to add a challenge to a regular pushup.
- Leave a yoga block or low step at the far end of the mat where you will end up in your plank position.
- Once there, place one hand up on the block while the other remains directly under the shoulder.
- The feet and inner thighs are squeezing together tightly.

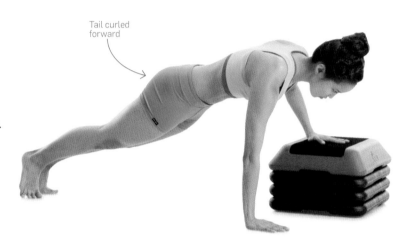

Tail curled forward

**B**

- Perform three pushups and then fold your chest to your thighs and walk your hands back to your feet before rolling up one vertebra at a time.

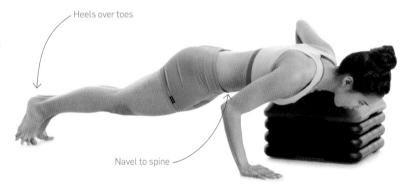

Heels over toes

Navel to spine

**REPS:** Complete two rounds on your right side, and then move the block to the other side and complete two more. If you are working a weaker side, you can do an extra round on the weaker side.

# ELEPHANT PLANKS

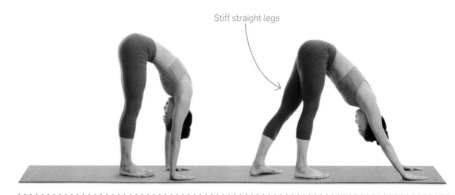

Stiff straight legs

 A B

- From the position of your forehead on your knees: With stiff legs and feet, march your heels backward using just $3\frac{1}{2}$ strides to get you down to a rigid plank position ("steel from head to heels").

C

- Hold your plank for a count of three, using the time to broaden the chest and press the mat away.

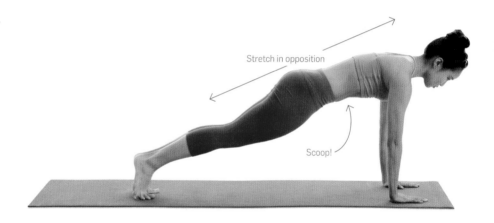

Stretch in opposition

Scoop!

D

- Lift from your powerhouse muscles, draw the ribs in and fold your chest toward your thighs, like an upside-down Teaser.

E

- Lower your heels to the mat and, keeping your knees dead-straight and your feet flexed, walk your feet as far between your hands as possible, scooping your abs to make room for the length of your legs.

**REPS:** Complete three Elephant Planks, alternating between walking your feet to your hands and your hands to your feet.

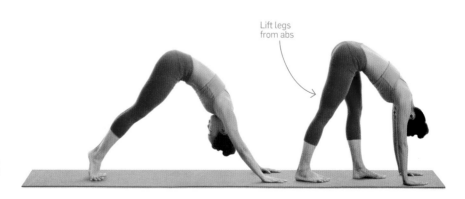

Lift legs from abs

# Archival Starters and Enders

Over the years, as Pilates has gained popularity, more and more footage of Joe's original work has emerged. While some may argue that "archival" means outdated or unevolved, many of us know the value and joy in these upbeat Starters and Enders often given to us by Romana to start or cap off our athletic Pilates sessions. See if, where, and how they feel best for you.

# KNEES TO ELBOWS FRONT

**A**

- Fold your arms like a genie and hold them up at shoulder-height. Beginning with your heels together and toes apart, push off your right foot with energy and lift your right knee up to touch the outer edge of your right elbow.

- Swiftly return the right foot to its starting position and press through your left foot to repeat on the left side.

Chest lifted

Legs light

**REPS:** Continue alternating sides until you've completed four sets on each side without allowing your elbows to drop.

# KNEES TO ELBOWS SIDE

Reach            Reach

**A**

- Transitioning seamlessly from Knees to Elbows Front, open your arms wide to the sides and bring your right knee up to the side toward your right elbow.

- Replace it deftly to the floor and repeat on the left side. Your chest should remain lifted and your palms down.

**REPS:** Continue alternating lifts until you've completed four on each side.

# STANDING BICYCLE

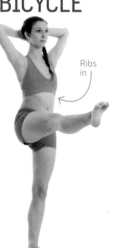

Ribs in

**A**

- Standing tall with your arms wide to the sides or layered behind your head, slowly and with control bring one leg straight up in front of your body as high as you are able to manage without sinking in your waist or bending your standing leg.

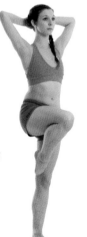

**B**

- At the leg's peak, bend your knee and pass it alongside your standing knee, lifting it back behind you without twisting in your hips.

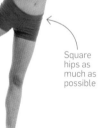

**C**

- Straighten your leg behind you and sweep it through to begin again.

Square hips as much as possible

**REPS:** Complete two forward bicycles and then reverse the movements for two backward bicycles. Repeat with your left leg.

# *Archival Starters and Enders*

## SINGLE-LEG BALANCES TO FRONT/SIDE/BACK

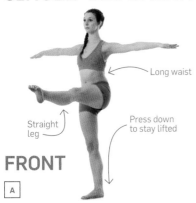

Long waist

Straight leg

Press down to stay lifted

### FRONT

A

- Standing tall with your arms wide, slowly bring one leg straight up as high as you can, pressing the floor away with your standing leg.

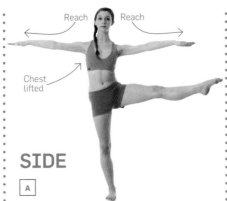

Reach    Reach

Chest lifted

### SIDE

A

- Bring your right leg straight up to the side as high as you are able without side bending or losing your balance.

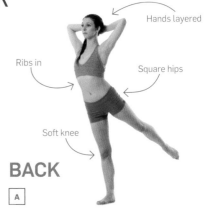

Hands layered

Ribs in

Square hips

Soft knee

### BACK

A

- Lift a leg to the back without twisting your hips or leaning forward.

**REPS:** Once on each leg is enough, so make them count.

## BUTTERFLY TWIST

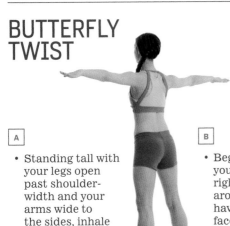

A

- Standing tall with your legs open past shoulder-width and your arms wide to the sides, inhale and lengthen your waist as you rise to your toes and balance.

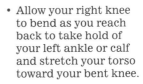

B

- Begin twisting your torso to the right and continue around until you have turned to face the other way.

C

- Allow your right knee to bend as you reach back to take hold of your left ankle or calf and stretch your torso toward your bent knee.

- To come up, reverse the movements of the twist, unwinding yourself and coming back to face front, balancing on your toes.

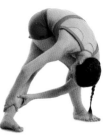

**REPS:** Repeat the twist to the other side. One time on each side is plenty to wring the tension out of your body.

# JOGGING KNEES UP, HEELS UP

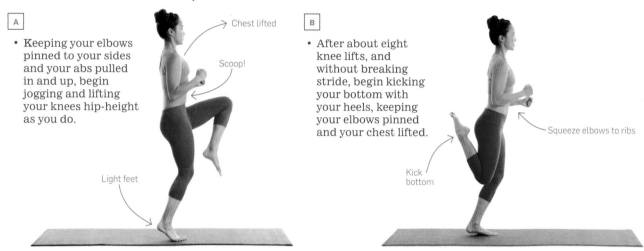

**A**
- Keeping your elbows pinned to your sides and your abs pulled in and up, begin jogging and lifting your knees hip-height as you do.

Chest lifted

Scoop!

Light feet

**B**
- After about eight knee lifts, and without breaking stride, begin kicking your bottom with your heels, keeping your elbows pinned and your chest lifted.

Squeeze elbows to ribs

Kick bottom

**REPS:** After eight bottom kicks, either move on to the next exercise or complete another set, this time reducing your lifts and kicks to six, then four, then two.

# STANDING SAW

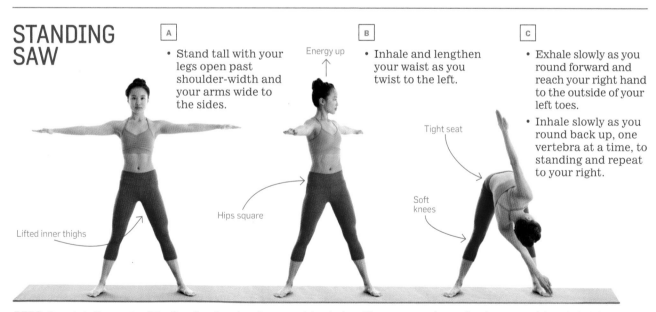

**A**
- Stand tall with your legs open past shoulder-width and your arms wide to the sides.

Hips square

Lifted inner thighs

**B**

Energy up

- Inhale and lengthen your waist as you twist to the left.

**C**
- Exhale slowly as you round forward and reach your right hand to the outside of your left toes.
- Inhale slowly as you round back up, one vertebra at a time, to standing and repeat to your right.

Tight seat

Soft knees

**REPS:** Complete three sets of the Standing Saw, keeping your abdominals pulling up as you descend and your seat tight to help bring you up.

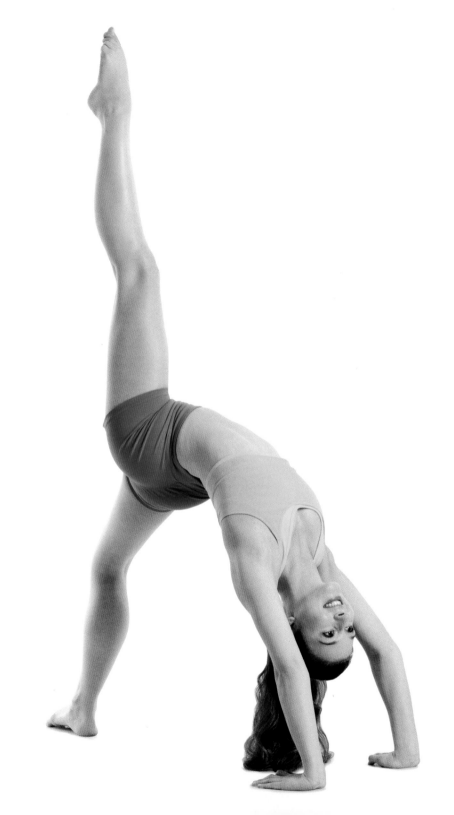

# CHAPTER 7
# *Pilates Props*

# Creating Your Home Studio

Props are great tools for using your creativity and imagination to inspire new ways to feel the Pilates movements. Use these accessories and moves wisely to complement your workouts. Props don't make the work easier. They help create tactile awareness, resistance, stability, or instability so you can work in a more focused manner (which is usually hard in a whole new way).

Joe's apparatus were originally designed to support those not strong enough to use their own bodies in coordinated, weight-bearing ways and also to challenge the body with weighted resistance, range of motion, and coordination. Using Joe's apparatus, you are able to take your body to places it may not be able to reach on its own. For the purposes of this book, though, I assume you don't have a Cadillac or Reformer in your living room! So I've designed a series of exercises that use props and help you get many of the benefits you'd experience in a fully equipped Pilates studio. (For those of you familiar with Pilates apparatus exercises, I've indicated when the prop variations are similar to those done in the studio.)

Over the years, as fitness trends expanded and Pilates made its way into gyms and weekend workshops, the demand grew for more challenging matwork. Many practitioners chose to adapt the exercises of the apparatus into floorwork (matwork) exercises. While this is fun and challenging, there are many reasons why mat exercises should be performed on the mat and apparatus exercises should be performed on the apparatus—mostly due to angles and support. That said, I have chosen a few exercises from the apparatus that add new direction and orientation to the classic mat series. With a strong sense of imagination and awareness, you may be able to envision the resistance of the apparatus as you move, thus adding a new element to your workout.

Remember, your body doesn't know whether you are holding a resistance spring or not; simply work as if you were using it, and your muscles will react accordingly.

The Pilates Body - Brooke Siler

✓ Spine stretch forward
Single leg stretch
Double stretch
Double straight leg
Single straight leg

✗ Breathing - contract power house
breathe from diaphragm
Deep down by belly button

**NOTE:** *Sources for these props can be found in the Resources section at the end of the book.*

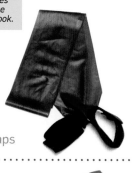

Bands/
Ankle straps

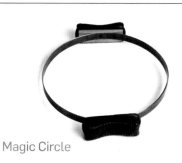

Magic Circle

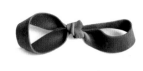 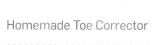

Homemade Toe Corrector

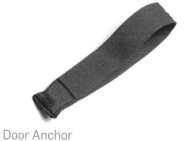

Door Anchor

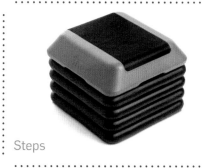

Steps

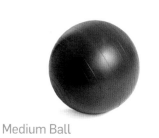

Medium Ball

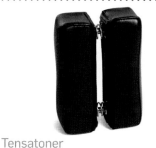

Tensatoner

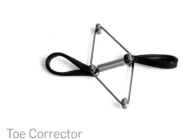

Toe Corrector

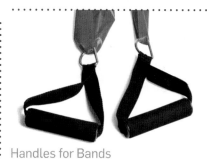

Handles for Bands

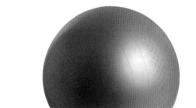

Big Ball

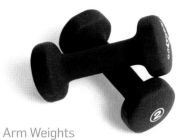

Arm Weights

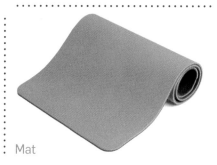

Mat

# Bands

The Pilates system derives much of its power from spring resistance. Using apparatus and props with springs is ideal for building strength and stability. Unfortunately, the spring setup is not an easy one, nor are springs travel friendly, since you would need to drill holes into walls to secure them to a stable surface. A nice alternative to springs is the resistance band. Bands allow for constant tension on the muscles, which makes exercises feel distinctly harder than simply lifting and lowering a weight. You also use more of the stabilizing muscles needed to keep the oppositional pull on the band, thus doubling up on the efficiency of the exercise and improving coordination (doing two things at once). And for those counting calories, you'll remember that using more muscles burns more calories.

Bands are inexpensive and easy to take anywhere. You'll just need to figure out which resistance level works best for your body.

If the bands' resistance is too light or loose, you

won't receive the necessary support you may be looking for, and if it's too tight or heavy, you'll strain yourself trying to use it. Remember, too, that the farther a band is pulled, the greater the resistance. When trying out different bands, make sure to pull each one from the floor to gauge its tension at different lengths.

Throughout the following exercises, commit to the idea that the band is an extension of your muscle: If you let the band go slack, then it means you have let go with your muscles. If slack muscle is what you're after, then make that a conscious choice. Otherwise, maintain tension on the bands throughout the movements, flowing from one move to the next within each exercise.

# Door Anchor Setup

### Hinge setup

Use this setup if you have an anchor with a loop on each end. Open your door and thread one end of the nylon loop through the crack over the selected hinge, feed it back through the crack underneath the hinge, and thread it through itself, pulling it tightly until one end cinches around the hinge. Then simply thread one end of your band through the open loop of nylon anchor and you're ready to go. You can use any of the three heights of hinges on your door to create varying resistance and to take your workouts from the ground on up.

### Stopper setup

Use this setup if you have an anchor loop with one large end that acts as a stopper in your doorjamb. Simply mark the height you will be working at and close the strap in the door, keeping the stopper on the outside of the door and the loop on the inside with you.

When you use bands there are no poles to push off from or hold, as there would be on the apparatus, so finding a healthy hand position on the wall will be important. I offer some suggestions ahead, but you'll have to stay conscious of how your wrists feel.

Also, consider investing in ankle straps and handles, if you do not already have them. Bands generally roll up into thin lines when pulled and can be painful on your hands and feet.

# Pilates Props: Bands

The most important thing is to make sure that you are working evenly! Since we are creating faux apparatus, we must bear in mind that the pieces are not originally made to be Pilates equipment. On the actual apparatus, springs are hooked to stable metal poles set at specific distances, whereas your bands will be coming from the single center point of your anchor. Therefore, the line of pull changes. This isn't a bad thing, but allow for adaptability and stay focused on the intent instead.

To receive maximum reward and minimum risk, we must work to align everything just right.

Make sure your mat is placed so that the door anchor exactly bisects the centerline of your mat (you can measure and put a tape line down the middle of your mat) so that your pull on the bands is always even in your body.

## Stopper heights

I tested *a lot* of band, tube, and anchor combinations for this book, and the following anchor heights and band resistances are what I came up with as being the closest in feeling to the tension and movement of the apparatus springs without having to drill holes in walls (which I've been very tempted to do!).

These are the anchor settings referenced in this chapter's band exercises.

**Lowest:** Anchor 3 to 5 inches from the floor.

**Low:** Anchor 23 to 25 inches from the floor.

**Mid:** Anchor 33 to 35 inches from the floor.

**High:** Anchor 53 to 55 inches from the floor, or simply anchor at shoulder-height for many of the standing exercises.

In the studio, we rotate between the arm springs and the leg springs so we're never stuck in any one position very long. It will behoove you to have both setups in place so that you can jump around as needed. Read through your chosen routine. If both heavy and medium-weight bands are called for, or handles and then ankle straps are needed, have them set up and ready to go.

# Band Needs

## THESE ARE THE TOOLS YOU'LL NEED FOR THE BAND EXERCISES:

- **1 OR 2 BANDS** ($10 to $20); I recommend buying both a heavy resistance band and a medium band
- **1 DOOR ANCHOR** ($6)
- **1 SET OF HANDLES** ($8)
- **1 SET OF FOOT/ANKLE STRAPS** ($6)

TOTAL = $40 (That's much less than a pair of sneakers!)

# Bands
## >LYING DOWN

## Arm "Spring" Series

**ANCHOR SETTING**
LOW

**BAND RESISTANCE**
MEDIUM

These exercises are derived from the Arm Spring Series on the Cadillac. Don't be fooled by the name: Like all Pilates exercises, they work more than one area of the body at a time.

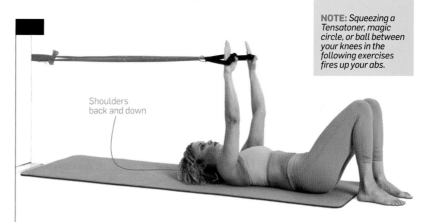

**NOTE:** *Squeezing a Tensatoner, magic circle, or ball between your knees in the following exercises fires up your abs.*

Shoulders back and down

### UPPER BODYWORK SETUP POSITION

- Lie on your back and slide your bottom to the front edge of the mat.
- Lift your arms so your wrists are over your shoulders, bend your knees, and plant your feet flat on the floor with your heels under hip-width knees. (It is correct to end up on the bottom edge of the mat with your legs off.)
- Begin with tension on the bands and use this series to establish a broad, open chest by pinning the backs of your shoulders to the mat without releasing your powerhouse muscles.

187

# *Pilates Props: Bands*

## SUPINE: CHEST EXPANSION

A

- Inhale slowly as you curl your bottom off the mat against the tension of the bands and then press your hands past your hips—the backs of your arms and shoulders press to the mat but your hands and forearms reach forward 1 inch above the mat.
- Press into the balls of the big toes.

B  C

- Hold your breath in this lifted position for 5 to 10 counts and then exhale with control as you roll your spine to the mat one vertebra at a time, returning your arms to the starting position without letting go of the tension on the bands.

**REPS:** Give yourself three to five opportunities to increase the expansion of your ribcage with each inhalation and to press all the air from your lungs with each exhalation. (There are no head turns in this position as there are with chest expansions elsewhere.)

**NOTE:** The closer you can squeeze your heels to your backside, the more hamstring is activated. The more hamstring, the less hip flexor; the less hip flexor, the more low abs. Therefore squeeze those heels in tight to make this supine series ab-tastic.

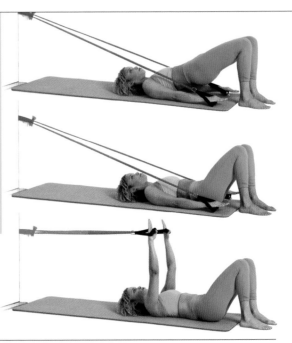

## SUPINE: ARMS UP/DOWN

A

- Start in the proper upper-body position and press your knees and feet together or hip-width apart, with your heels close to your bottom.
- Glue your inner thighs together tightly.

B

- Inhale and press your arms straight down to your sides, trying to touch the backs of your upper arms to the mat.
- Hold there for a count of three and then slowly resist the pull of the band as you return your arms to the starting position.

**REPS:** Give yourself five chances to deepen the work of the powerhouse and reach farther and farther past your bottom with your wrists.

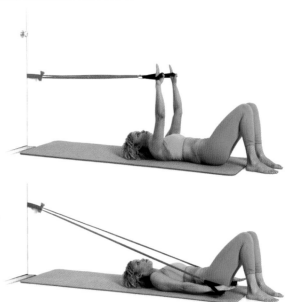

# SUPINE: ARM CIRCLES

- As in Supine: Arms Up/Down, press your knees and feet together or hip-width apart, with your heels pressed as close to your bottom as possible.
- Glue your inner thighs together tightly.

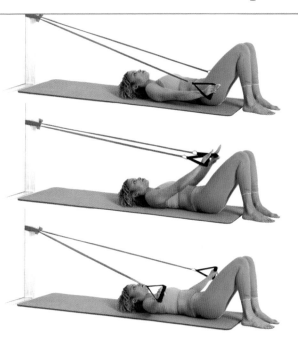

B  C

- When your arms are hovering just above the mat, initiate small circles with long arms by your sides, sweeping the backs of your arms on the mat.

**REPS:** Complete six circles in one direction and then reverse for six circles, continuing to reach your wrists past your bottom.

# SUPINE: TRICEPS EXTENSIONS

- As in Supine: Arm Circles, press your knees and feet together or hip-width apart, with your heels pressed as close to your bottom as possible.
- Glue your inner thighs together tightly, or squeeze a Tensa-toner, magic circle, or ball between your knees or between your heels and your backside.
- Inhale and press your arms straight down to your sides, trying to touch the backs of your upper arms to the mat.

- Hold there and bend your arms, keeping the backs of the arms and shoulders pinned to the mat.
- Exhale slowly as you allow your wrists to come to a 90-degree angle with the upper arm *only* (do not give in to the pull of the band) and then press your palm down to the mat again.

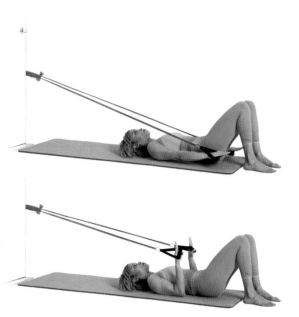

**REPS:** Give yourself five chances to feel the burn of your triceps as you work to maintain a stable upper arm throughout.

# *Pilates Props: Bands*

## SUPINE: WINGS

A

- As in Supine: Triceps Extensions, press your knees and feet together or hip-width apart, with your heels pressed as close to your bottom as possible.
- Glue your inner thighs together tightly, or squeeze a Tensatoner, magic circle, or ball between your knees or between your heels and your backside.
- Inhale and press your arms straight down to your sides, trying to touch the backs of your upper arms to the mat.

B

- Exhale slowly as you allow your arms to open to the sides, keeping your upper arms on the floor.
- Inhale with control as you press your arms back toward your sides, making a motion like you would to create a snow angel.

**REPS:** Open and close your arms six times, reaching farther and farther away. with each flap of your snow-angel wings.

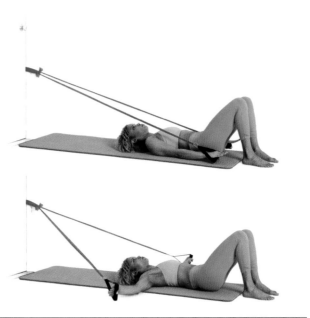

## PRONE: PULLING STRAPS

A

- Lie facedown. Hold the bands (not handles) in a "T" shape formed between your arms and body.

B

- Begin with your arms lifted to shoulder-height with tension on the bands.

C

- Inhale and draw your hands back toward your hips as you lift your chest off the mat (the bustline remains down).
- Hold for a count of three and then slowly release your breath and some tension in the bands as you return to the starting position.
- Your navel remains firmly lifted throughout.

**REPS:** Give yourself five chances to find the opposition between your hands pulling back and your chest reaching forward, then sit to heels to release your back.

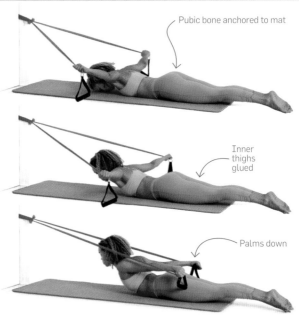

Pubic bone anchored to mat

Inner thighs glued

Palms down

# Leg "Spring" Series

### ANCHOR SETTING
`MID`

### BAND RESISTANCE
`MEDIUM TO HEAVY`

These exercises are derived from the Leg Spring Series on the Cadillac. They are excellent for shaping and toning your legs as well as offering new ways to access your powerhouse muscles. Maintain a softness in the back of your knee so that you are working from the correct muscles and not placing tension into your joints.

Make it your intent to focus not simply on the movements of your legs but on the stability of your torso that is maintained through proper powerhouse engagement.

**NOTE:** *By working all muscle in concert, you achieve a greater goal than any one grouping might accomplish alone.*

Heels glued

Ribs down

Tight seat

Long, strong arms pinned to the mat

## LOWER BODYWORK SETUP POSITION

- Lie on your back with the crown of your head toward the wall and your hands either long by your sides, with the entire length of the arm pressed firmly to the mat, or reaching overhead with your hands pressing flat against the wall or in fists to spare your wrists.
- To simulate the Cadillac poles, you can use two blocks pressed together against the wall and squeeze the edges of the blocks with your hands.
- Experiment a little to find what position allows you to gain the most stability in your torso and the most ability to work oppositionally.

# *Pilates Props: Bands*

## FROGS

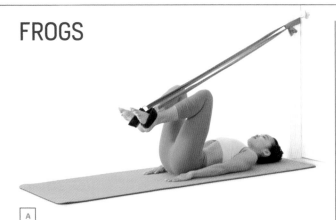

**A**

- Start in the proper bodywork position and bring your heels together at your bottom with your knees shoulder-width apart.

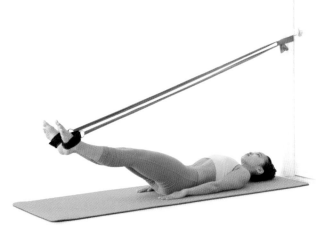

**B**

- Inhale with control as you press your heels away from you on a 45-degree angle, keeping them glued together; continue pushing until your inner thighs touch.
- Exhale slowly as you resist the pull of the band and bring your heels back to the starting position.

**REPS:** Give yourself five to eight chances to increase the length from the base of your ribs to the tips of your toes.

## CIRCLES

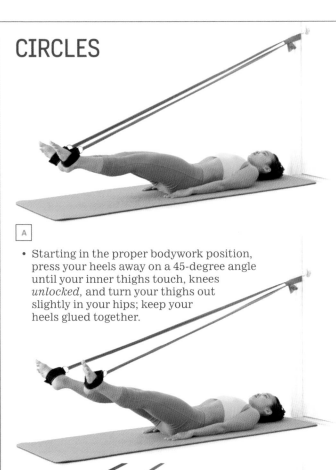

**A**

- Starting in the proper bodywork position, press your heels away on a 45-degree angle until your inner thighs touch, knees *unlocked*, and turn your thighs out slightly in your hips; keep your heels glued together.

**B** **C**

- Circle your thigh bones in their hip sockets to the rhythm of: open, down, together, lift.

**REPS:** Complete five circles in one direction and five in the other, working from your knee up to your pelvis and stabilizing the action more and more with your powerhouse and torso.

# WALKING

- Starting in the proper bodywork position, press your heels away on a 45-degree angle until your inner thighs touch, knees *unlocked,* and turn your thighs parallel, with your feet slightly flexed.

- Press your right thigh down an inch past your left thigh without moving in your hips.
- Then bring your left thigh an inch below your right thigh.
- Continue "walking" until the backs of your thighs approach the mat and then reverse the steps to walk back up.

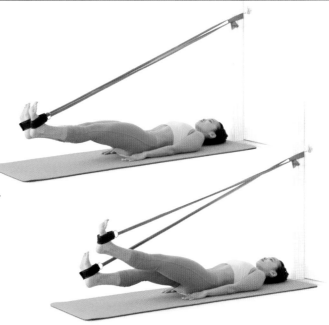

**REPS:** Inhale for six steps down and exhale for six steps up. Allow yourself three rounds of walking to improve stabilizing one leg as the other moves.

# HAMSTRING CURLS

- Lie with the crown of your head facing away from the wall and your forehead resting on the backs of your hands.
- Slip the bands or straps around the arches of your feet and move away from the anchor until there is tension on your bands when your legs are bent to a 90-degree angle.

Pubic bone anchored to mat

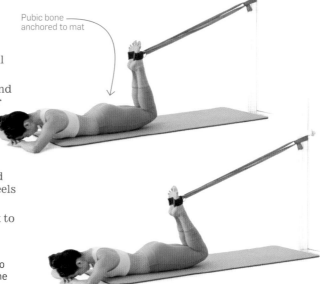

- With your inner thighs squeezing together, abs lifted, and pubic bone anchored to the mat, inhale and bring your heels to your bottom, holding them there for a count of three.
- Exhale with control as you slowly release your heels back to the starting position.

**REPS:** Continue curling your heels to your bottom five times, trying to gradually reach the point where you can lift your knees together off the mat and still get your heels to your bottom.

# Bands
## >SITTING UP

## ROLL-BACK

ANCHOR SETTING **HIGH**
BAND RESISTANCE **HEAVY**

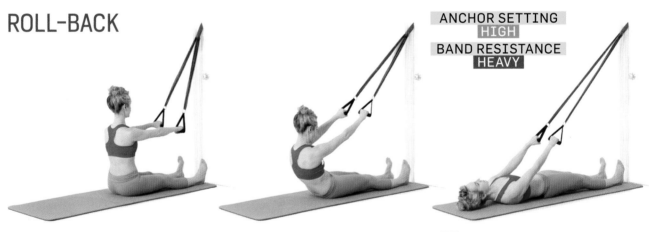

**A**

- Sit tall with your heels against the wall with your feet open shoulder-width.
- Take hold of one band in each hand. Your arms are straight and also open shoulder-width.

**B**

- Inhale slowly, expanding your rib-cage in all directions, and exhale with control as you roll your back to the mat from the bottom to the top, one vertebra at a time, pressing all the air from deep within your lungs.

**C**

- Inhale with control as you roll back to the starting position, "peeling" one vertebra off the mat at a time.

**REPS:** Give yourself five chances to best articulate your spine, opening the back body and coordinating movement with breath.

# SINGLE-ARM ROLL-BACK

**A**

- Hold both bands in your left hand, with your right arm folded across the front of your hips. (Your box is square.)

**B**

- Roll back.

Articulate each bone of your spine

Push heels away

**C**

- Once your entire back is on the mat, take your arm from across your hips and reach it back away from your left leg on a long diagonal cross.
- There is opposition at work from your fingertips to your heels.
- Bring your arm back across your hips, squaring your shoulders and hips on the mat, and roll up evenly.

**REPS:** Switch hands and repeat the sequence, staying conscious of articulating your spine and squaring your box.

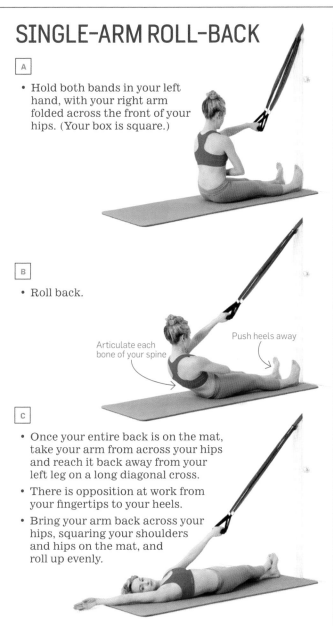

# ROWING SHAVE

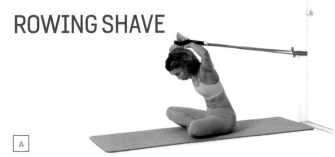

**A**

- Sit cross-legged (or with legs straight) and check that there is enough starting tension.
- Bring your hands up behind the base of your head with your fingertips pressed together in a triangle and your elbows wide.

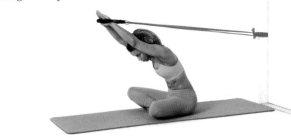

**B**

- Inhale as you press the handles up and away from the base of your spine and exhale as you bring them behind your head with control.

**REPS:** Complete six shaves, working to lengthen your waistline with each lift and lower of the hands.

VARIATIONS ON THE THEME
## Single-Arm Rowing Shave

Leave one hand behind your head and only straighten and bend the weaker arm or side. Notice torso torque and minimize as much as possible.

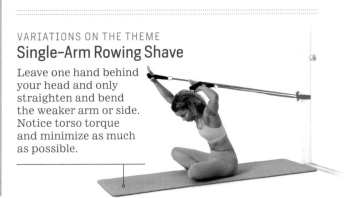

# *Pilates Props: Bands*

## ROWING HUG

**ANCHOR SETTING**
**LOW**

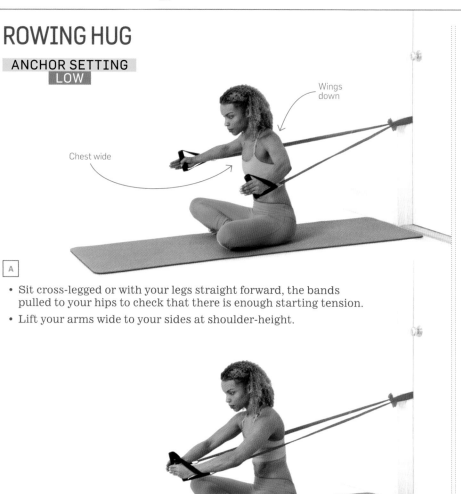

Chest wide

Wings down

A

- Sit cross-legged or with your legs straight forward, the bands pulled to your hips to check that there is enough starting tension.
- Lift your arms wide to your sides at shoulder-height.

B

- Inhale as you close your arms, bringing your fingers to touch in front of you.
- Exhale with control as you open your arms, resisting the pull of the bands.

**REPS:** Complete five hugs, inhaling on the hug and exhaling on the release, and then reverse your breathing pattern for five more hugs.

**NOTE:** *Pilates works best when what is meant to be stable does not move and what is meant to be mobile does! Concentrate on these principles of contrology throughout this band series (and beyond).*

VARIATIONS ON THE THEME
### Single-Arm Rowing Hug

Sit cross-legged or with your legs straight forward, but when your fingers are together in front of you, leave your strong arm in front and open the arm of the weaker side. Notice if one arm opening pulls your torso to that side. Can you inhibit that?

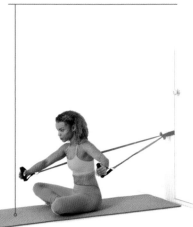

**REPS:** Give yourself five times to try to stabilize your torso as one arm opens.

# DOOR OPENERS: EXTERNAL ROTATORS

ANCHOR SETTING
LOW OR LOWEST

**A**

- Sit cross-legged in the middle of your mat, with your left shoulder toward the door.
- Slide your right arm through the back band behind you until it is past your elbow, and hold the front band in your right hand.
- Move away from the door to where there is starting tension on the front band.
- The back band is helping to pin your right arm to your side body.
- Sit tall and place your left hand behind your head.

**B**

- Inhale as you draw your right forearm away from your body as if opening a door.
- Exhale with control as you bring your forearm back in line with your body.

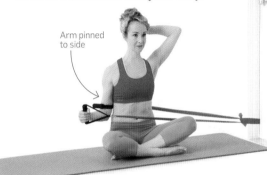

Arm pinned to side

**REPS:** Give yourself five chances to stabilize your torso as you externally rotate your arm in the shoulder socket.

# DOOR CLOSERS: INTERNAL ROTATORS

ANCHOR SETTING
LOW OR LOWEST

**A**

- Remain in your Door Openers: External Rotators position.
- Slide your left arm through the back band until it is past your elbow, and hold the front band in your left hand.
- Move away from the door to where there is starting tension on the front band.
- You are pulling the back band to your left side body.
- Sit tall and place your right hand behind your head.

**B**

- Inhale as you draw your left forearm toward your body as if closing a door.
- Exhale with control as you bring your forearm back in line with your body.

Arm pinned to side

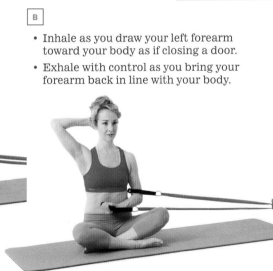

**REPS:** Give yourself five chances to stabilize your torso as you internally rotate your arm in the shoulder socket.

# Bands

**NOTE:** *Make sure your kneecaps are well cushioned! If your mat is not thick, then double or triple it. Or place a folded towel under your knees. Any way you do it, make sure the kneecaps are protected. Bands are at Arm Spring height—or Leg Spring height, if more tension is needed.*

## >KNEELING DOWN

### KNEELING ARM SPRINGS: CHEST EXPANSION

**ANCHOR SETTING**
**HIGH**

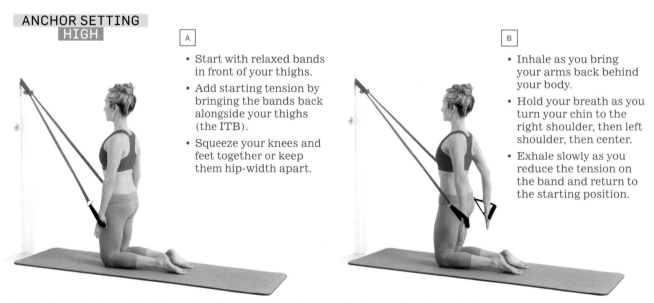

**A**
- Start with relaxed bands in front of your thighs.
- Add starting tension by bringing the bands back alongside your thighs (the ITB).
- Squeeze your knees and feet together or keep them hip-width apart.

**B**
- Inhale as you bring your arms back behind your body.
- Hold your breath as you turn your chin to the right shoulder, then left shoulder, then center.
- Exhale slowly as you reduce the tension on the band and return to the starting position.

**REPS:** Do this four times, alternating your head turns and broadening your collar bones with each opportunity.

# KNEELING ARM SPRINGS: REVERSE CHEST EXPANSION

**ANCHOR SETTING**
**HIGH**

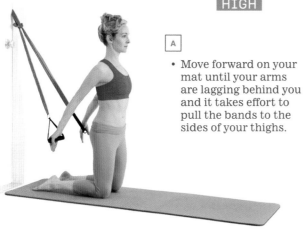

**A**

- Move forward on your mat until your arms are lagging behind you and it takes effort to pull the bands to the sides of your thighs.

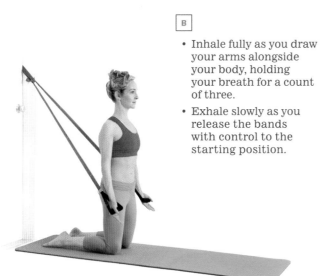

**B**

- Inhale fully as you draw your arms alongside your body, holding your breath for a count of three.
- Exhale slowly as you release the bands with control to the starting position.

**REPS:** Give yourself five chances to challenge your lungs on the inhalation and open your chest and shoulders more with each exhalation.

# KNEELING ARM SPRINGS: LONG BACK STRETCH

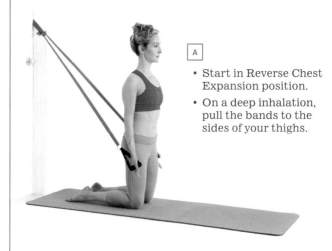

**A**

- Start in Reverse Chest Expansion position.
- On a deep inhalation, pull the bands to the sides of your thighs.

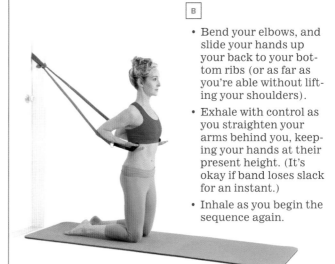

**B**

- Bend your elbows, and slide your hands up your back to your bottom ribs (or as far as you're able without lifting your shoulders).
- Exhale with control as you straighten your arms behind you, keeping your hands at their present height. (It's okay if band loses slack for an instant.)
- Inhale as you begin the sequence again.

**REPS:** Repeat four times in one direction and then switch the direction of the arms for four more chances.

# Pilates Props: Bands

## KNEELING ARM SPRINGS: BUTTERFLY

A

**ANCHOR SETTING**
**HIGH**

- Kneel in the middle of your mat, facing away from the anchor with your knees and feet squeezing together or open hip width.

- Hold your arms open to the sides of the room at shoulder-height and pitch your body forward in one piece as if leaning into the wind. (If there is not enough tension to hold your weight, then simply move farther away from the anchor.)

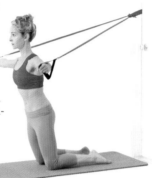

B

- Inhale with control as you twist your torso to the left, bringing your right arm overhead (biceps to your ear) and your left arm just behind you (hand by your bottom).

- Maintain equal tension on both bands as you twist.

- Exhale slowly as you return to the starting position and repeat the twist to the other side.

- Make sure you are exhaling completely as you twist.

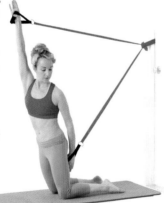

**REPS:** Complete two sets of Butterfly twists with inhalation on the twist, and then switch the breathing pattern and perform two sets exhaling on the twists. Notice: Which breathing pattern feels more supportive?

## KNEELING ARM SPRINGS: THIGH STRETCH

A

- Kneel in the middle of your mat, facing the anchor with your knees and feet squeezing together or open and aligned hip-width apart.

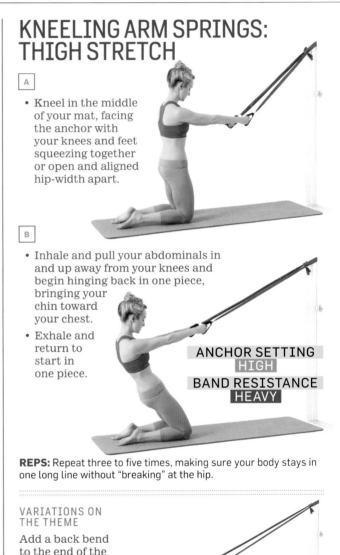

B

- Inhale and pull your abdominals in and up away from your knees and begin hinging back in one piece, bringing your chin toward your chest.

- Exhale and return to start in one piece.

**ANCHOR SETTING**
**HIGH**
**BAND RESISTANCE**
**HEAVY**

**REPS:** Repeat three to five times, making sure your body stays in one long line without "breaking" at the hip.

### VARIATIONS ON THE THEME

Add a back bend to the end of the thigh stretch and then return to the starting position in one piece.

# Swakate Series

**ANCHOR SETTING**
**LOW OR MID**

This series of four moves is adapted from the Reformer Sequence, where we were warned "This is only for men." We've come a long way, ladies!

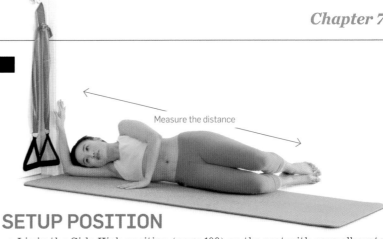

Measure the distance

## SETUP POSITION

- Lie in the Side Kick position (page 100) on the mat with your elbow to the wall and your body straight.
- Mark the spot where your knees are on the mat and come up to kneel sideways on your mat on that spot.
- Depending on your bands, that should be a good measurement for where to begin the Swakate Series.

**REPS:** Complete the entire series on one side before turning around to better it on the other side.

## OOPAH

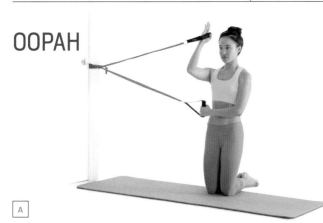

A

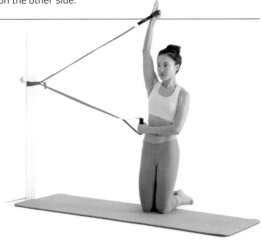

B

- Take the Swakate setup position, with your knees and feet squeezing together or open and aligned hip-width apart.
- Hold one band across your belly with the outside hand (the farthest from the anchor) while the inside hand holds the band close to your head with your elbow bent.

- Inhale and straighten the inside arm to the ceiling, keeping it as close to in line with the shoulder as possible (don't let it drift toward the door).
- Exhale with control as you return to the starting position.

**REPS:** Repeat four times, securing your torso more and more with each opportunity.

# *Pilates Props: Bands*

## SWAKATE

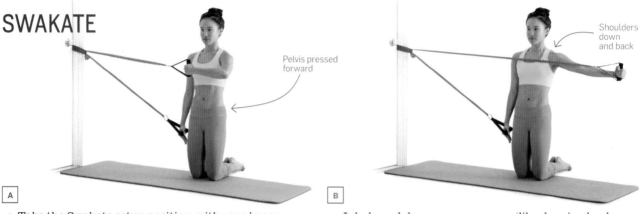

Pelvis pressed forward

Shoulders down and back

**A**

- Take the Swakate setup position, with your knees and feet squeezing together or open and aligned hip-width apart.
- Hold the inside band tight to your thigh with your inside arm, while your outside hand holds the outside band up in front of your chest, your elbow bent and tension on the band.

**B**

- Inhale and draw your arm open (like drawing back curtains), pulling the band across your chest to its full extension.
- Exhale with control as you bend your arm back to the starting position.

**REPS:** Repeat four times, securing your torso against the temptation to rotate each chance you get.

## LOTUS

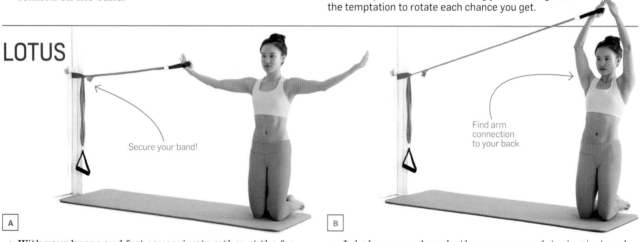

Secure your band!

Find arm connection to your back

**A**

- With your knees and feet squeezing together at the far end of your mat, release the outside band (making sure the band is secured around the anchor and won't slip out) and open both arms wide to the sides of the room at shoulder-height.
- The inside hand has the inside band, and the outside hand is acting.

**B**

- Inhale as you draw both arms upward, trying to touch your hands above your head like the petals of a lotus flower closing.
- Exhale with control as you slowly open your arms, resisting the band's pull.

**REPS:** Open and close your lotus four times, keeping your shoulders down and chest up.

# SIDE BEND
# ARM CIRCLES

**NOTE:** *Work on finding your arms' connection to your back. Keep the muscular action below the shoulders and under your armpits in order to access more powerhouse!*

- Walk your knees farther away from the anchor for more tension and squeeze your knees and feet together.
- Side bend toward the anchor and prop yourself up on your inside fist.
- Extend your top leg away from you and bring the band up overhead to where there is starting tension.
- Keep your hip over your knee, pubic bone pressed forward, and shoulders square like your kneeling side kick position (page 129).

**B**

- Inhale and draw your arm over to your top hip, allowing your palm to turn in as needed.

**C**

- Exhale with control as you circle the band around and return overhead.

**REPS:** Repeat three times and then allow your arm to complete three full circles in one direction and three in the other. (It's okay for the tension to lessen momentarily as the circling hand nears the door.) Want an added challenge? Keep your extended leg lifted off the mat throughout!

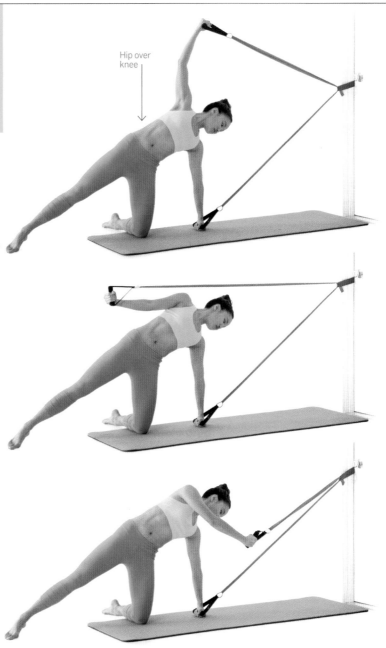

Hip over knee

# Bands
## >STANDING UP

Any of the following exercises (and then some) can be performed in either Standing Arm Spring position or Lunging Arm Spring position. When choosing a lunging position, make sure to switch legs every three or four movements to work both sides of the body evenly.

# Standing Arm "Spring" Series

ANCHOR SETTING
SHOULDER

## SETUP POSITION

- Face away from the anchor and open your arms wide to the sides of the room.
- Step to where there is sufficient tension on your bands to hold you when you lean your body into the wind. (Your arms are in line with your shoulders, not behind them).
- Your heels are together and your toes are apart, and the inner thighs are zipped together tightly.
- Abs in and up—as always.

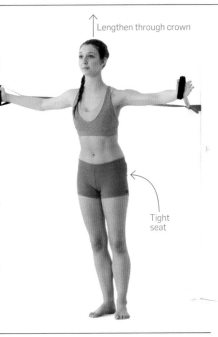

Lengthen through crown

Tight seat

# Lunging Arm "Spring" Series

ANCHOR SETTING
HIGH

## SETUP POSITION

- Face away from the anchor, starting on the centerline of your mat, and take a deep lunge forward with one leg, finding a place where there is sufficient tension to challenge you without being too heavy to bring bands together.
- Your front foot is to one side of the centerline of the mat, and your knee is directly over the front ankle. Do not allow your knee to roll in.
- Your back leg is slightly turned out and can be moved out toward the edge of the mat for more stability.

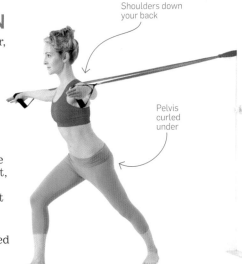

Shoulders down your back

Pelvis curled under

# *Pilates Props: Bands*

## HUG

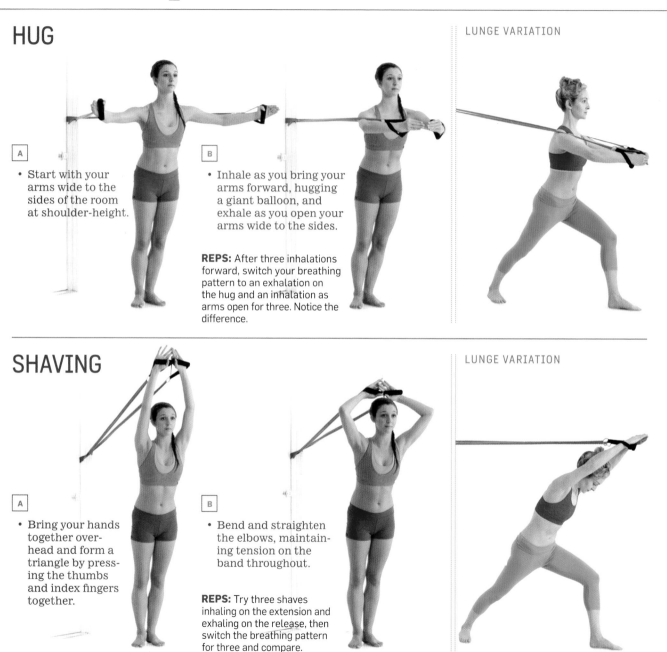

**A**
- Start with your arms wide to the sides of the room at shoulder-height.

**B**
- Inhale as you bring your arms forward, hugging a giant balloon, and exhale as you open your arms wide to the sides.

**REPS:** After three inhalations forward, switch your breathing pattern to an exhalation on the hug and an inhalation as arms open for three. Notice the difference.

## SHAVING

LUNGE VARIATION

**A**
- Bring your hands together overhead and form a triangle by pressing the thumbs and index fingers together.

**B**
- Bend and straighten the elbows, maintaining tension on the band throughout.

**REPS:** Try three shaves inhaling on the extension and exhaling on the release, then switch the breathing pattern for three and compare.

# BUTTERFLY

**A**

- Start with your arms wide to the sides of the room.

**B**

- Inhale with control as you twist your torso to the left, bringing your right arm

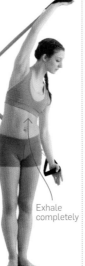

overhead (biceps to your ear) and your left arm just behind you (hand by your bottom).

- Maintain equal tension on both bands as you twist.

- Exhale slowly as you return to the starting position and repeat the twist to the other side.

**REPS:** Complete two sets of Butterfly twists with inhalation on the twist, and then switch the breathing pattern and perform two sets exhaling on the twists.

Exhale completely

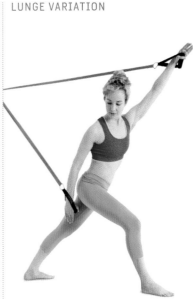

# BOXING

**A**

- Start with your fists up at your shoulders, elbows wide.

- Lean into the spring tension, hingeing from the ankles only.

**B**

- Extend one arm forward at a time, "punching" the air.

- Work on stabilizing the side that is not punching so that there is little to no rotation in the body as you box.

**REPS:** Complete one set of five boxings with slow, methodical control and then one set of five with heat and pace without losing the element of control.

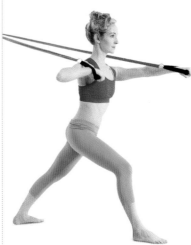
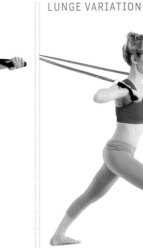

# *Pilates Props: Bands*

## "PUSHUPS"

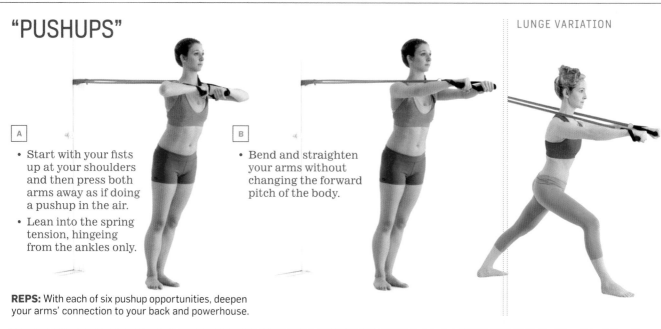

**A**

- Start with your fists up at your shoulders and then press both arms away as if doing a pushup in the air.
- Lean into the spring tension, hingeing from the ankles only.

**B**

- Bend and straighten your arms without changing the forward pitch of the body.

**REPS:** With each of six pushup opportunities, deepen your arms' connection to your back and powerhouse.

## CHEST EXPANSION

LUNGE VARIATION

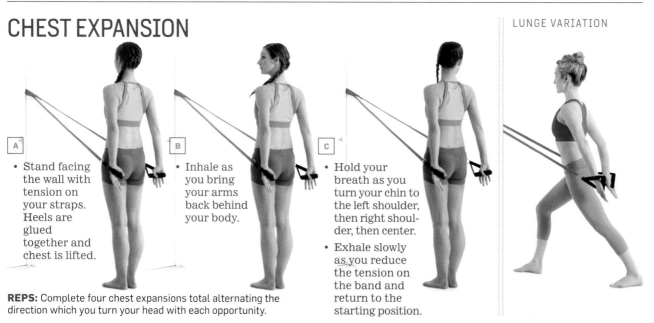

**A**

- Stand facing the wall with tension on your straps. Heels are glued together and chest is lifted.

**B**

- Inhale as you bring your arms back behind your body.

**C**

- Hold your breath as you turn your chin to the left shoulder, then right shoulder, then center.
- Exhale slowly as you reduce the tension on the band and return to the starting position.

**REPS:** Complete four chest expansions total alternating the direction which you turn your head with each opportunity.

# TWISTING CURLS

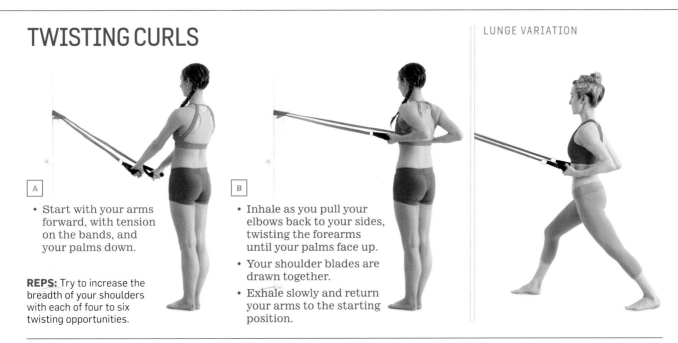

**A**
- Start with your arms forward, with tension on the bands, and your palms down.

**REPS:** Try to increase the breadth of your shoulders with each of four to six twisting opportunities.

**B**
- Inhale as you pull your elbows back to your sides, twisting the forearms until your palms face up.
- Your shoulder blades are drawn together.
- Exhale slowly and return your arms to the starting position.

# COMBO

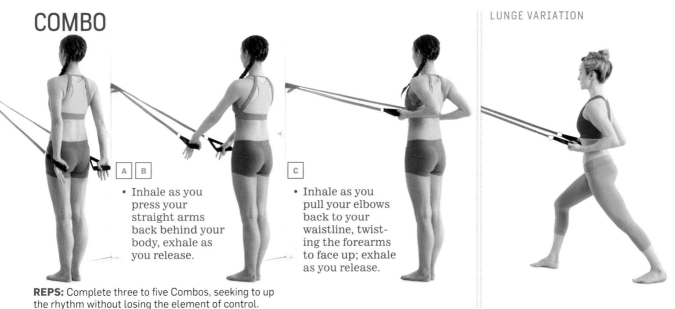

**A** **B**
- Inhale as you press your straight arms back behind your body, exhale as you release.

**C**
- Inhale as you pull your elbows back to your waistline, twisting the forearms to face up; exhale as you release.

**REPS:** Complete three to five Combos, seeking to up the rhythm without losing the element of control.

# *Pilates Props: Bands*

## SQUATS

NOTE: *Squatting with proper technique strengthens your back, core, hips, thighs, and glutes, all of which contribute to the base of support for perfect posture.*

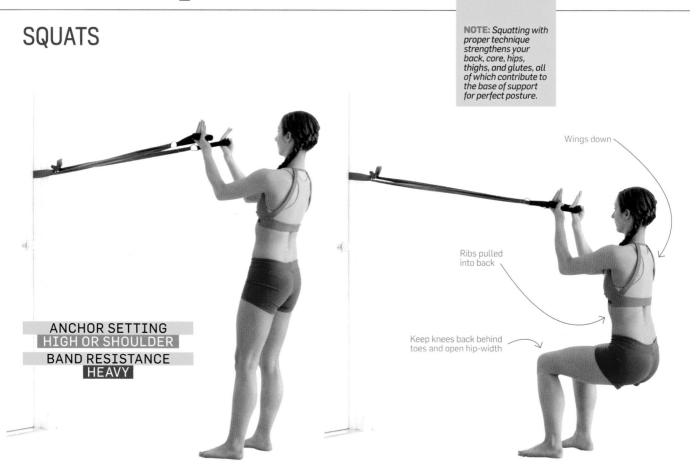

**ANCHOR SETTING**
**HIGH OR SHOULDER**
**BAND RESISTANCE**
**HEAVY**

Wings down

Ribs pulled into back

Keep knees back behind toes and open hip-width

 **A**

- Stand facing the anchor, with parallel feet open to hip-width.
- Walk back to where you can support some of your body weight when leaning backward with your arms bent to 90 degrees.

 **B**

- Inhale as you bend your knees and slide down an invisible wall behind you to as close to right angles in your hips as you can manage with control.
- Your knees remain in line with your hips and directly over your ankles.
- Exhale slowly as you rise up and release some of the tension from the bands.

**REPS:** Reestablish tension and go again. Give yourself three to five chances to master your squat. If you're able to go lower than 90° with proper form you have permission to go as low as you can manage with control and still get back up again. There should NEVER be pain in your knees from a squat!

# STANDING SIDE KICKS: INNER THIGHS

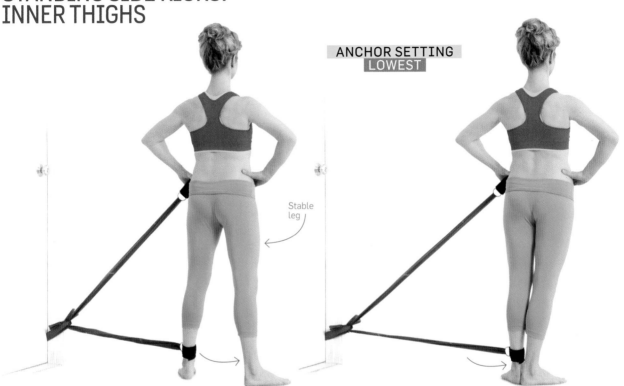

**ANCHOR SETTING**
LOWEST

Stable leg

**ALTERNATE SETUP**

## Hands Behind Head

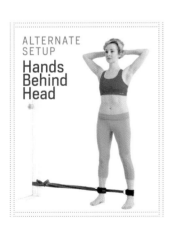

**A**

- Stand sideways on your mat and slip your inside ankle through one band (you can put both bands onto the ankle for more resistance) while holding the other band in your inside hand.

- Sidestep until your outside foot is at the far end of the mat (away from the anchor) and your inside foot is shoulder-width away with sufficient tension on the band.

- Your legs and feet are slightly turned out and your hands are on your hips.

**B**

- Inhale powerfully as you draw your inner heel to your outer, closing the legs tightly.

- Exhale as you slowly resist the release of the tension and return your inside foot to the starting position.

**REPS:** Repeat five times, growing taller and more stable with each opportunity. After five Inner Thigh moves, without removing the band from your ankle, turn your body to face the other side of the room and immediately do five Outer Thigh moves (below), then switch ankles.

211

## STANDING SIDE KICKS: OUTER THIGHS

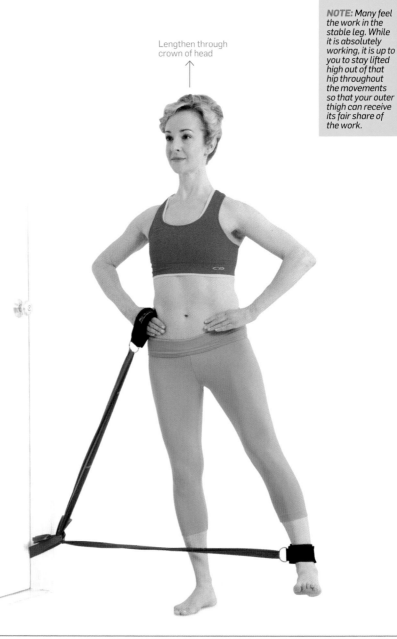

Lengthen through crown of head

A

- After your last Inner Thighs squeeze, pivot toward the band, placing what was your outer foot on the inside of your band foot. (The outer foot has now become the inner foot.)
- Switch the band to your new inside hand and sidestep away from the door to where there is sufficient tension.
- Your legs and feet are parallel and your hands are on your hips, one arm with band tension and the other acting.
- Inhale as you lift your outer foot off the mat and press your thigh out to the side, balancing (not collapsing!) on your inside leg.
- Exhale as you return your feet together with control. Your feet and legs remain parallel throughout. Do not allow the lifted foot to sickle (hang) inward.
- Maintain long lines of tension in the muscles of your body.

**ANCHOR SETTING**
**LOWEST**

**NOTE:** *Many feel the work in the stable leg. While it is absolutely working, it is up to you to stay lifted high out of that hip throughout the movements so that your outer thigh can receive its fair share of the work.*

**REPS:** Press out five times with increasing length and strength in the body. After five outer thigh moves, switch band to opposite ankle and repeat inner and outer thigh sequence on other leg.

# BICEPS CURLS: UNDERHAND

**ANCHOR SETTING**
**LOWEST**

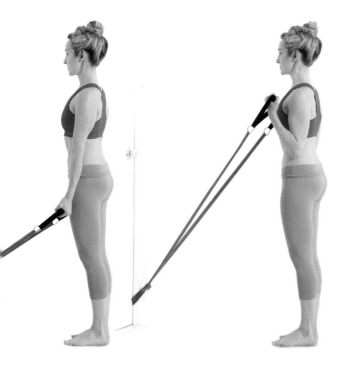

# BICEPS CURLS: OVERHAND

**ANCHOR SETTING**
**LOWEST**

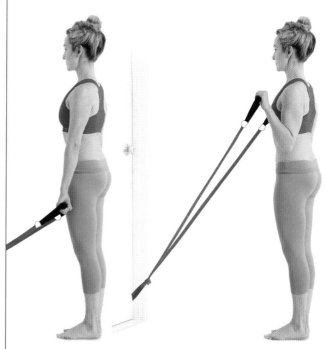

**A**
- Stand facing the anchor with the bands in hand and step back to where there is desired tension from the bands when your arms are bent.

**B**
- Inhale and curl your hands to your shoulders, palms forward, with your arms glued tightly to your ribs; exhale and uncurl your arms until they straighten.

**REPS:** Complete five Biceps Curls, improving one postural aspect with each set. For an additional benefit, add pulling back on the band with straight arms like Chest Expansion (page 208) (your palms remain facing forward) at the end of each curl.

**A** **B**
- Perform this exercise like Biceps Curls: Underhand, only this time keep your palms facing down or back throughout.

**REPS:** Complete five sets of overhand curl. For an additional benefit, add pulling back on the band with straight arms like Chest Expansion (page 208) (palms face back) at the end of each curl.

# Balls as Barrels and Beyond

Let me say loud and clear that there was never such thing as a "Pilates ball." In Joe's day, the only ball he would have had to work with was a medicine ball, and it would not have been used the way we use the balls in fitness today. That said, you'll find many fun and creative ways to incorporate balls into your Pilates workout to challenge stability and increase supported range of motion, particularly in extension.

In the studio, using Pilates barrels feels delicious: There are no springs or resistance to fight with, simply a wonderful shape over which to bend. The function of the barrel is its shape (curved to support spinal flexion and extension), but a Pilates barrel is fixed, whereas a stability ball moves with you. So when working "over" the ball, you must remember to keep your abdominals pulled in and up to ensure you remain glued to the surface.

The arc of the larger stability balls have the nearest measure to the arc of the Pilates barrels. But since the balls aren't fixed like those of the Pilates barrels, I've put together a variety of exercises you would find on many different studio apparatus, and I've listed the piece most associated with the exercise.

Just finding balance on the ball will call all your core muscles into play, so make sure to have some fun and experiment (safely).

# >THE BIG BALL

## ROLL-BACK

From the Cadillac

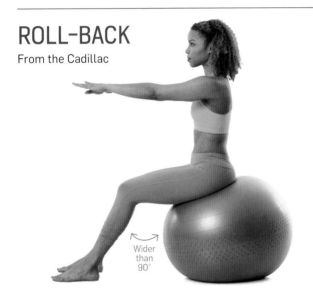

Wider than 90°

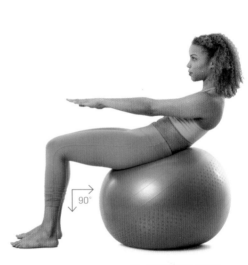

90°

**NOTE:** *The ab work of the Roll-Back and the Hundred can be intensified by squeezing a prop between your knees.*

**A**

- Sit tall in the middle of your ball with your feet flat on the mat, your heels approximately 1½ feet from the ball (the bent leg–thigh angle should be wider than 90 degrees).
- The knees are open hip-width.
- Reach your arms forward, at shoulder-height, and either hold a weighted pole or pretend to hold a weighted pole. (Remember, your body doesn't know the difference.)

**B**

- Inhale slowly as you sit taller and slowly exhale as you curl your bottom under and roll the ball toward your heels from the action of articulating your spine.
- Hold a position around your midback (behind the abs) where you feel work taking place to hold you there.
- (Trembling abs are welcome here! We call this "the Tremor of Truth.")

PROGRESSION
### One-Legged Roll-Back

From the reclined position of Roll-Back, see if you can lift one leg without losing your powerhouse connection.

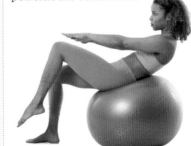

**REPS:** Stay for a count of three. Repeat this sequence five times, deepening your lower-back connection to the ball with each opportunity.

# THE HUNDRED

From the Mat

- Sit tall in the middle of your ball with your feet flat on the mat, your heels approximately 1½ feet from the ball (the bent leg–thigh angle should be wider than 90 degrees).
- The legs can be open hip-width.
- Or, to challenge yourself further, squeeze your knees and feet tightly together.
- As with the Roll-Back, curl under and roll to place your bottom on the ball where the work can be felt in your abs.

B  C

- Stay there and pump your arms up and down over your thighs for a count of 100 (see the Hundred, page 63).
- The ball will bounce under you as you pump, so control the movements as best you can.

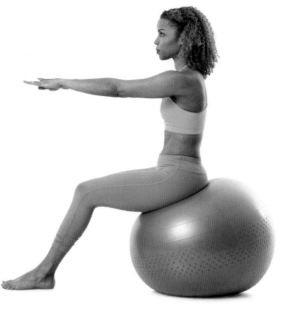

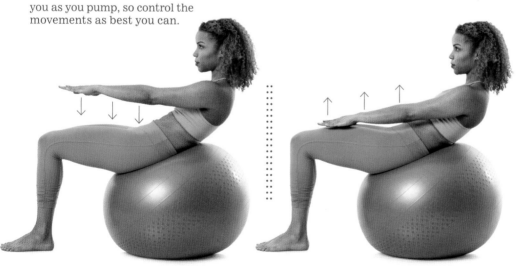

## THE TREMOR OF TRUTH

A distinguished teacher at re:AB Pilates named Cary Regan often calls the trembling of the muscles, "The Tremor of Truth," which I love. I took the saying out West and they returned the favor by giving me a new favorite, "You can't fake the shake." In both cases, what we're experiencing is a muscle working at its max. Take the quake as a sign that you're working deep, but know when to back off before driving your muscles to the point of exhaustion.

# *Pilates Props: Balls as Barrels and Beyond*

## PUSH-THROUGH

From the Cadillac

**A**

- Sit tall in Spine Stretch position (see page 68) with the ball positioned between your legs and your hands on either side of the ball.

**B**

- Inhale to grow taller in your waist, and exhale slowly as you round into yourself while simultaneously rolling the ball forward.

**C**

- Roll back and draw abs away from the ball.

**D**

- Lift the ball overhead, reaching up and slightly forward of center.
- Return to a round back and replace the ball between your legs.

**REPS:** Repeat this sequence five times, creating a more long and stable center with each opportunity.

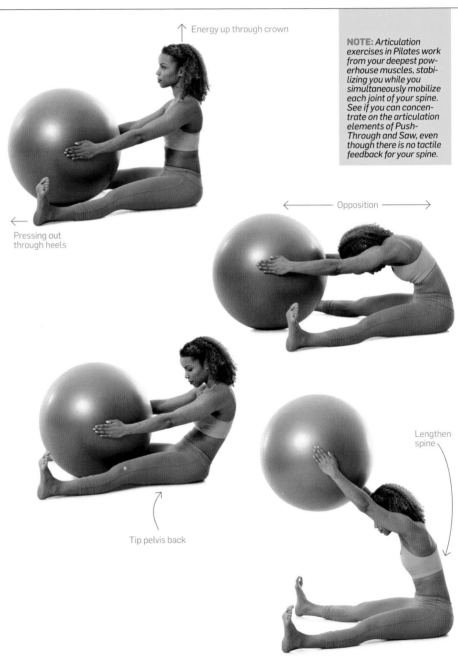

Energy up through crown

Pressing out through heels

**NOTE:** *Articulation exercises in Pilates work from your deepest powerhouse muscles, stabilizing you while you simultaneously mobilize each joint of your spine. See if you can concentrate on the articulation elements of Push-Through and Saw, even though there is no tactile feedback for your spine.*

Opposition

Tip pelvis back

Lengthen spine

# SAW
From the Mat

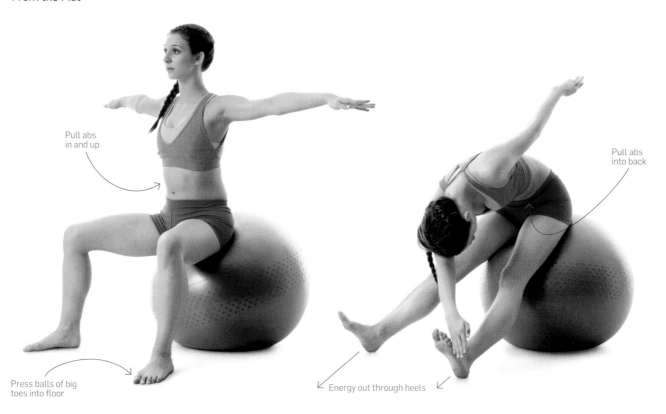

Pull abs
in and up

Pull abs
into back

Press balls of big
toes into floor

Energy out through heels

**A**

- Sit tall on top of the forward portion of your ball (that is, not directly in the center) and, with bent knees, open your legs wider than your mat, turning out in your feet and knees (the bent leg-thigh angle should be wider than 90 degrees).
- Open your arms wide to the sides of the room and draw the shoulder blades together and inhale slowly as you twist left.

**B**

- Exhale slowly as you round forward over your left leg while simultaneously rolling the ball back until your legs are straight.

**REPS:** Inhale slowly to return to the starting position and then repeat the sequence to the right. Complete three sets.

## SWAN

From the Ladder Barrel

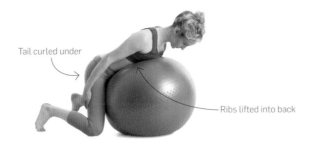

Tail curled under

Ribs lifted into back

### SETUP POSITION

- Lie over the ball with your knees bent on the mat and your legs and feet open mat-width with your toes curled. (Make sure you have enough grip under your feet so you don't slip backward.)
- Place your hands, palms down, on the backs of your thighs.

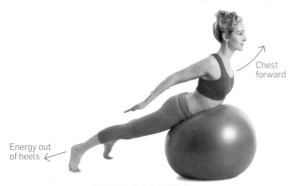

Chest forward

Energy out of heels

## FLIGHTLESS SWAN

- Inhale slowly as you straighten your legs and lift your chest up off the ball, extending your spine.
- To work more upper back and shoulder: Allow your hands to lift off the backs of the thighs and reach farther back for your heels.
- To create more mobility in the chest and shoulders: Slide your hands back to the inner thighs and use the position to broaden your chest.
- Exhale completely as you return to the starting position over the ball.

**REPS:** Repeat three times, lifting more and more from abs with each opportunity.

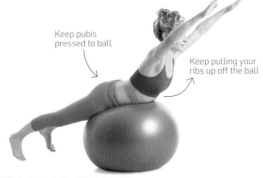

Keep pubis pressed to ball

Keep pulling your ribs up off the ball

## FLYING SWAN

- Inhale, slowly straightening your legs as you lift your chest up and off the ball.
- Bring your arms forward and reach for the front wall.
- Exhale slowly as you return to the bent-knee starting position.

**REPS:** Repeat three times, increasing fluidity and control with each opportunity.

# SINGLE-LEG KICKS

From the Mat

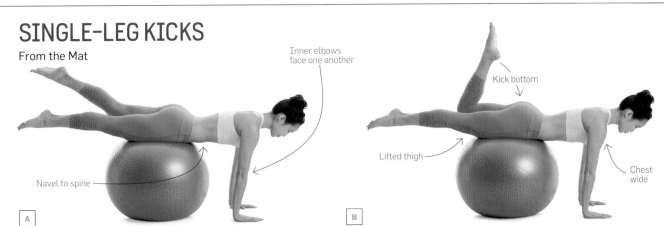

**A**

- Lie over the ball with your palms on the mat and roll forward until your pelvis is almost off the front of the ball and your body is in a plank position, with your legs squeezing together tightly and your chest broad and lifted.

**B**

- Inhale and lift one thigh off the ball, then bend the knee and kick your bottom.
- Exhale with control as you straighten the leg back out and return the thigh to the ball.

**REPS:** Repeat with the other leg. Continue switching sides until you have completed three kicks on each side.

---

# SWIMMING

From the Spine Corrector

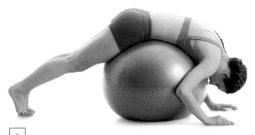

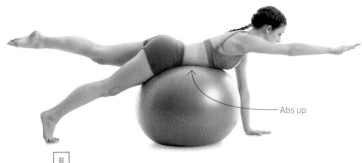

**A**

- Lie over the ball with your navel centered on top.
- Straighten your legs and place the balls of your feet on the mat and your thighs as close together as you can manage while staying balanced.

**B**

- Inhale slowly as you simultaneously lift your right arm and left leg.
- Exhale with control as you replace them. Inhale slowly as you lift your left arm and right leg.
- Exhale with control and replace them.

**REPS:** After five sets, allow your body to hang over the ball in flexion to counter the extension of swimming. Continue switching in alternate pairs, trying to get lighter and lighter on your hands with each iteration.

# *Pilates Props: Balls as Barrels and Beyond*

## KNEELING SIDE KICKS
From the Mat

### STARTING POSITION

- Lie over the ball on your side and bend your bottom knee while keeping your top knee straight.
- "Hug" the ball between your bent bottom arm (palm against the side of the ball) and bent bottom leg.
- Place your top palm behind the base of your head with your elbow wide.
- Lift the top leg to hip-height without allowing your hips to roll back on the ball (the underside of the body is aligned: shoulder to ribs to hip).
- Once the starting position is established, follow the movement instructions for any of the Kneeling Side Kicks (page 129).

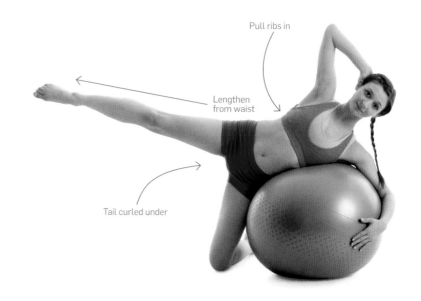

Pull ribs in

Lengthen from waist

Tail curled under

---

## SIDE BENDS
From the Mat

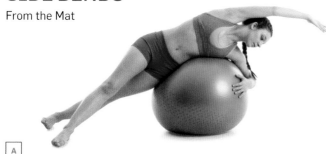

A

B

- From the Kneeling Side Kicks starting position, place your top foot on the front edge of the mat and straighten your bottom leg, placing your bottom foot on the back edge of the mat.
- "Hug" the ball with your bottom arm and reach your top arm alongside your ear as you drape yourself over the top of the ball.
- Turn your head to face the mat.

- Inhale slowly as you bring the top arm to the side body, turn your chin to your top shoulder, and lift the upper body up off the ball, reaching the top hand for the end of the mat between your feet.
- Exhale with control as you return to the starting position.

**REPS:** Complete five Side Bends on each side, using every opportunity available to experience a complete contraction and expansion of the waistline.

# PELVIC LIFT

From the Reformer

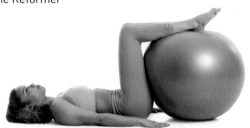

**A**

- Lie on your back on the mat with your arms long by your sides and your legs over the top of the ball.
- Wiggle toward it until the ball is nestled behind your thighs.
- With your knees and feet held together tightly, exhale completely as you squeeze the ball tightly by bringing your heels toward your bottom.

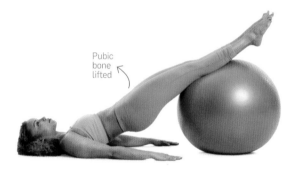

Pubic bone lifted

**B**

- Inhale with control as you release the squeeze and roll the ball away, lifting your hips off the mat.
- Hold your breath and the lifted position and then exhale slowly as you roll back to the mat one vertebra at a time and squeeze the ball to your bottom.

**REPS:** Repeat six times, working the back of the thigh (hamstrings) concentrically and then eccentrically.

# SHOULDER ROLL-DOWN

From the Cadillac

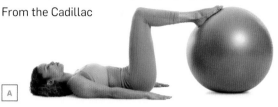

**A**

- Lie on your back on the mat with your arms long by your sides and the soles of your feet pressed against the front "edge" of the ball and your hips at 90°.

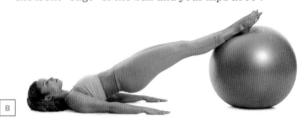

**B**

- Inhale fully as you roll the ball away until your legs are straight and lift your pubic bone into the air.

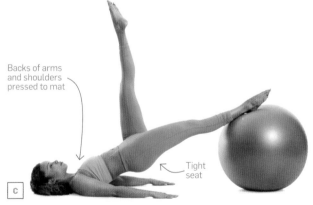

Backs of arms and shoulders pressed to mat

Tight seat

**C**

- Exhale with control and kick one leg straight up without dropping in your hips, inhale and replace the foot to the ball; switch legs.
- Exhale kick, inhale return. Exhale completely as you roll back down to the mat one vertebra at a time and bring the ball back to the starting position.

**REPS:** Repeat the sequence three times.

# *Pilates Props: Balls as Barrels and Beyond*

## BACK STRETCH OVER BALL

From the Ladder Barrel

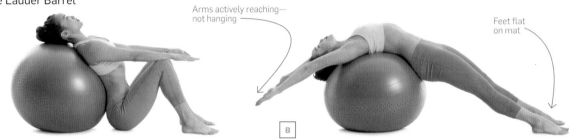

Arms actively reaching—
not hanging

Feet flat
on mat

**A**

- Sit on the mat with your back against the ball and your knees bent deeply.
- Your feet are as close to your bottom as possible and open shoulder-width.
- Place your straight arms on top of your knees with your palms facing down.

**B**

- Inhale with control as you push off your feet and roll the ball backward, lifting your arms overhead and allowing the base of your head to rest on the ball.
- Exhale with control and reverse the roll, bringing your arms back to the tops of your knees but leaving the base of your head on the ball.

**REPS:** Complete five Back Stretches, pulling your navel deeper in and up the spine with each extension.

## PULLUPS

From the Wunda Chair

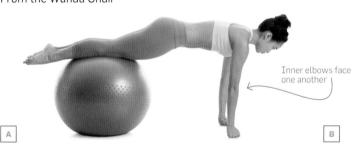

Inner elbows face
one another

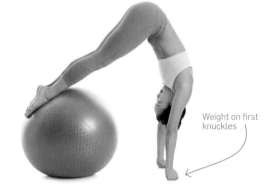

Weight on first
knuckles

**A**

- Lie over the ball with your hands on the mat and roll the ball forward until your knees are almost off the front and your shins are pressing into the top of the ball.
- Make your hands into fists, with the wrists aligned directly beneath the shoulders.

**REPS:** Give yourself three chances to reach the highest point on the handstand position, and use this exercise as a gauge of increasing strength over the time of your Pilates practice.

**B**

- Inhale slowly as you begin pressing down into your first knuckles and pulling up in your abdominal muscles.
- Let this be the impetus to lift your hips and pike your body in the air.
- Work on keeping your shoulders over the wrists and deepening the scoop of the abs.
- Exhale with control as you lower your body to the starting plank position.

# ARM WEIGHTS ON THE BALL

There are many different arm exercise variations you might try over the ball. I have chosen three from the mat, but you can try others.

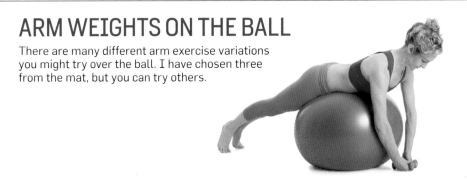

**NOTE:** *Draw parallels between similar exercises from mat, bands, and balls. Once the principles of a movement are understood, the rest is simply a pattern change, or choreography. The work of the powerhouse remains the same.*

## SETUP POSITION

- Lie over the ball with your navel centered on top.
- Straighten your legs and place the balls of your feet on the mat, your heels together and toes apart.
- Your heels and thighs are squeezing together tightly.

## THE BUG

page 108

Crack a walnut

Open and close arms with resistance

## BOXING

page 109

Send one arm forward and one back and alternate

Keep ribs lifted

## TRICEPS EXTENSIONS

page 135

Triceps lifted

Bend and straighten elbows with arms lifted behind you

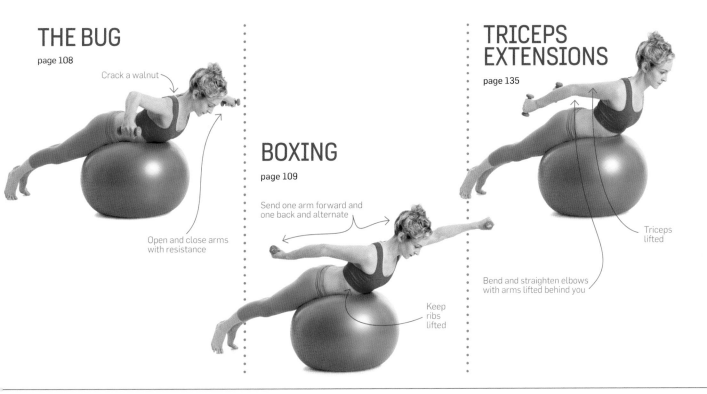

# Balls as Barrels and Beyond

## >THE MEDIUM BALL

Balls that are 8 to 10 inches round can be used as stabilizers when squeezed between your hands, knees, or ankles or used as support behind your head, neck, or lower back. To get as much powerhouse work as possible, use the ball's instability to your advantage. The following exercises challenge your balance and deepen supported extension over its inviting curve.

# Arm Series

This series works on mobilizing your shoulders and working your arms onto the back. Using a medium ball behind the head and neck supports the delicate cervical vertebrae while allowing you to open your chest and work your shoulders in a new plane of movement.

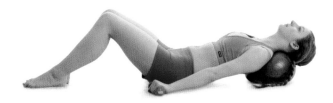

## SETUP POSITION

- Place the ball behind your upper back and roll down on the ball (your bottom toward your heels) until the ball is positioned between your shoulders and neck.
- Your head is resting comfortably; the neck is in supported extension (in other words, allow your head to hang back a bit over the back of the ball).
- This series can be done with or without light weights.
- Your knees and feet can remain open to hip-width or—for an added powerhouse challenge—squeeze tightly together, with or without a prop between knees.

## SCISSORS

**NOTE:** *Think of this move like a backstroke in the pool.*

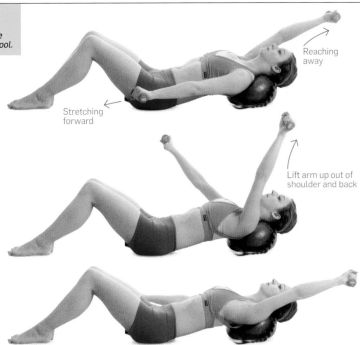

Reaching away

Stretching forward

Lift arm up out of shoulder and back

- Lift your arm straight up and back overhead while other arm reaches forward, long by your side.
- Find the oppositional tension of the arms reaching away from one another.

- Switch arms with control.
- Allow the arm reaching back to bring your blade with it for a delicious shoulder and upper back mobilizer.

**REPS:** Complete five sets, maintaining powerhouse stability as you seek to open the fronts of your shoulders more with each move.

# *Pilates Props: Balls as Barrels and Beyond*

## CIRCLES

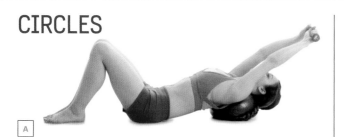

A

- Bring both arms up and back overhead.

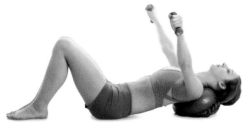

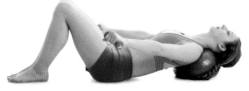

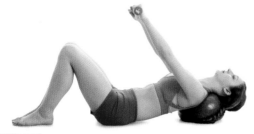

B  C  D

- open to the width that is within your control, and circle your arms around and together.
- Look to deepen the scoop of your abdominals with each lift of your arms.

**REPS:** Complete five circles in one direction and then reverse directions for five circles.

## WINGS

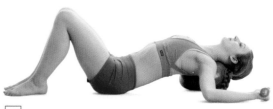

A

- Bring both arms up and back overhead until your hands touch the floor and then bend your elbows to right angles at shoulder-height.
- Take three complete breaths, allowing the backs of your forearms to rest on the mat.

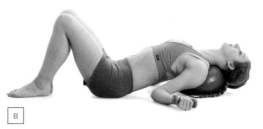

B

- With the back of your hands on the mat and your elbows bent to 90 degrees, bring your elbows toward your side body.

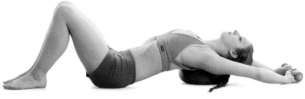

C

- Slide them up and overhead until your hands meet (or as far as possible without discomfort).

**REPS:** Try six slow and controlled movements of your wings, maintaining your powerhouse engagement.

# Leg Series

This series helps to mobilize your hips. Using a medium ball behind your sacrum supports your lower back while providing an opportunity to open the fronts of your hips and thighs. Raising your hips off the mat allows you to work your leg below floor level.

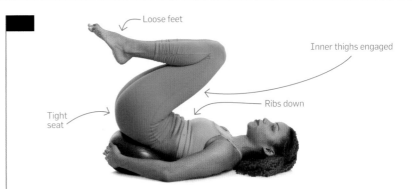

Loose feet

Inner thighs engaged

Tight seat

Ribs down

## SETUP POSITION

- Lying on your back with your knees bent and your feet flat on the mat, lift your pelvis and position the ball between your tail and lower back (against the sacrum).
- Bend your knees into your chest and wrap your hands around the front of the ball with wide elbows flat on the mat.

## SCISSORS

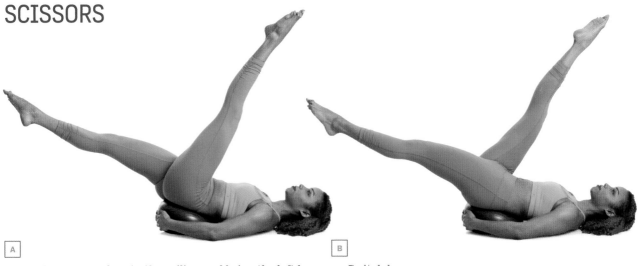

A

- Straighten your legs to the ceiling and bring the left leg forward, reaching it away from your center.

B

- Switch legs.
- The inner thighs remain in close proximity to one another, working inner-thigh strength.

**REPS:** Continue switching legs for five sets of Scissors, working to elongate waist with each reach of the legs.

# Pilates Props: Balls as Barrels and Beyond

## HELICOPTER

The Helicopter is a Scissors/Circles combination.

- Starting with the left leg forward and the right leg back, scissor your legs twice, ending with the left leg forward again.
- Then circle the left leg to the left and the right leg to the right, bringing them back to a Scissor position with the right leg forward.

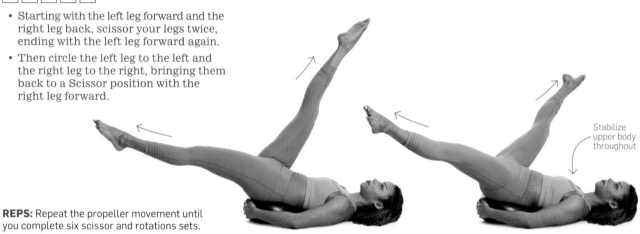

Stabilize upper body throughout

**REPS:** Repeat the propeller movement until you complete six scissor and rotations sets.

## BICYCLE

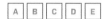

- Straighten your legs to the ceiling and send your left leg forward, reaching it away from your center.
- Bend your left knee and slide your foot on the floor toward your bottom, bringing your knee toward your center as you reach your right leg away and repeat the sequence.

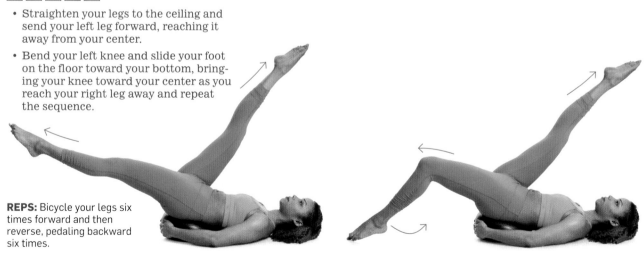

**REPS:** Bicycle your legs six times forward and then reverse, pedaling backward six times.

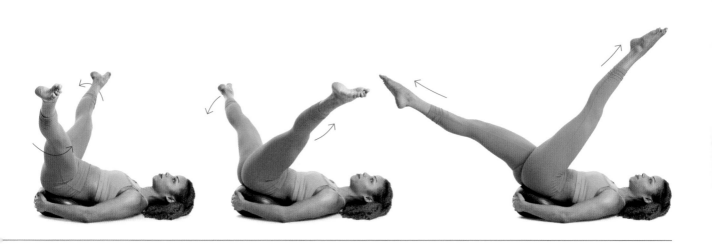

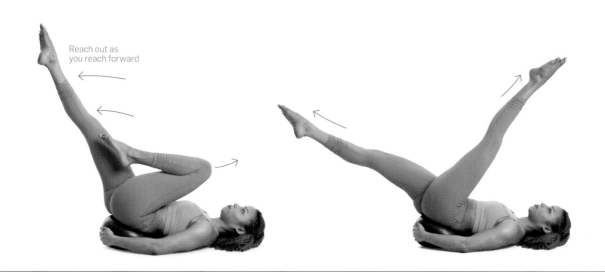

Reach out as
you reach forward

# Steps as Chairs

While the Pilates chairs may be better known for offering spring and pedal work, you can use their flat tops to challenge your center of gravity. When you don't have access to Pilates apparatus, a low, sturdy step or a platform about 12 by 12 by 12 inches would be the best substitute, but you can make do with a sturdy yoga brick or block. With the proper amount of concentration, precision, and centering, you may actually find that less is more.

# GOING UP FRONT

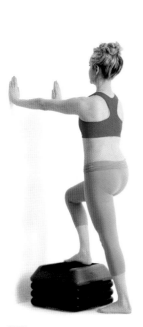

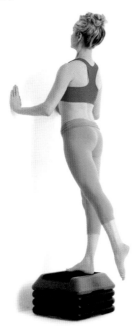

**A**

- Position the step about a foot from the wall (you should be able to palm the wall) in a position that allows your entire foot to fit on its surface.

- Place your right foot squarely on the block and your palms against the wall at shoulder-height.

**B**

- Inhale and step up, making sure the hip-knee-ankle-foot alignment feels ideal.

- Do not allow your knee or ankle to roll in. Maintain square hips.

- At the top, lift your leg out behind you while you lift your chest in opposition (like a standing Swan).

- Exhale and slowly lower your foot to the floor with control.

**REPS:** Step up front five times before switching sides, making sure to improve the stepping leg alignment and maintain a long waist throughout.

# GOING DOWN FRONT

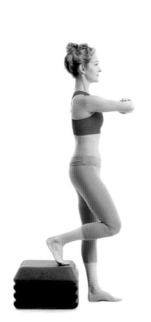

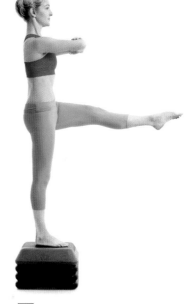

**A**

- Stand on the step with one foot and your back to the wall.

- Fold your arms, genie-style, in front of your chest and inhale slowly as you bend your standing knee and reach your free foot to the floor in front of the block.

**B**

- Exhale with control as you press back up to standing and lift your free leg up in front of you.

- Make sure your knee-over-foot alignment is meticulous (do not roll in or out on the foot, ankle, or knee).

- The abs are pulling in and up throughout so gravity cannot have its way with you.

**REPS:** Step down to the front five times before switching legs. Work on controlling your descent by lifting up in opposition from your abs and chest.

# *Pilates Props: Steps as Chairs*

## GOING UP SIDE

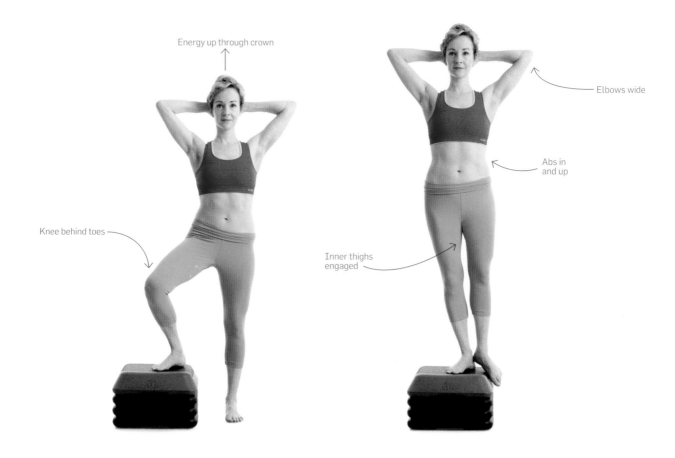

Energy up through crown

Elbows wide

Abs in and up

Knee behind toes

Inner thighs engaged

**A**

- Turn sideways to the wall and place your stepping foot on the diagonal of the step.
- Your hands are behind your head, or on your waist, and your chest is lifted.

**B**

- Inhale and step up, drawing the inner thighs tightly together without turning your hips or shoulders toward the wall.
- Exhale as you slowly lower your foot to the floor with control.

**REPS:** Step up to the side five times before switching sides, making sure that your bottom stays underneath you and your box remains square.

# SHRUNKEN MAT

One of my favorite exercise adaptations is to perform some of the more challenging abdominal strengtheners on top of a yoga block or step to test one's control on a smaller center of gravity.

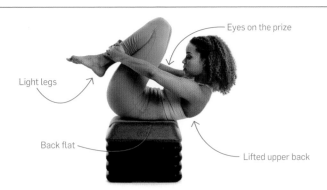

Eyes on the prize

Light legs

Back flat

Lifted upper back

## SETUP POSITION

- Roll back onto the block with your tailbone just off the front edge and your navel directly over the center of the block.
- If needed, you can prep for this series by propping yourself up on your elbows on the mat behind you and going through the leg portions of the exercise patterns.
- However, once those arms are off the ground, may your powerhouse be with you.

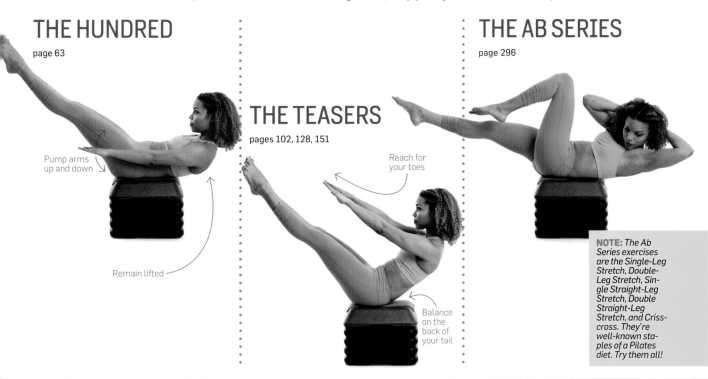

# THE HUNDRED

page 63

Pump arms up and down

Remain lifted

# THE TEASERS

pages 102, 128, 151

Reach for your toes

Balance on the back of your tail

# THE AB SERIES

page 296

**NOTE:** *The Ab Series exercises are the Single-Leg Stretch, Double-Leg Stretch, Single Straight-Leg Stretch, Double Straight-Leg Stretch, and Criss-cross. They're well-known staples of a Pilates diet. Try them all!*

# Pilates Props: Steps as Chairs

## FOOTWORK IV

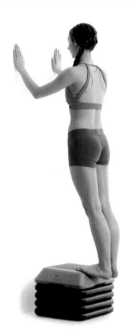 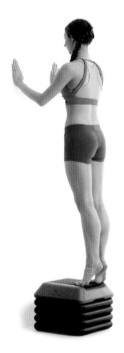 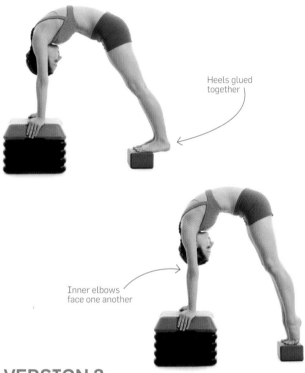

Heels glued together

Inner elbows face one another

### VERSION 1

**A**

- Place the step or yoga block about 6 inches away from the wall.
- Step up with the balls of your feet on the block and your heels squeezing together and off the back edge (without tipping the block).
- Your hands can be against the wall for support.

**B**

- Inhale and lift your heels up, squeezing them together and creating one leg from two.
- Exhale, slowly lowering your heels below block-height to stretch the backs of your legs without tipping the block over.
- Inhale as you lift your heels again.

**REPS:** Continue ten times, with the intention of getting lighter and lighter on your feet and deeper and deeper into your inner thighs and lifted abs.

### VERSION 2

**A**

- Round forward and place your hands on a step and then step your feet up on a block with your heels together and off the back edge (without tipping the block).
- With your hands turned out and holding the outer edges of the step, round forward until your shoulders are over your wrists.

**B**

- With your heels lifted high and your abs pulled up far into your spine as if you were doing a handstand, exhale slowly as you lower your heels without moving your shoulders or upper back from over your wrists.
- Inhale and lift your heels up again.

**REPS:** Continue lowering and lifting your heels ten times, with the intention of getting lighter and lighter on your feet and deeper and deeper into your scoped abs.

# RUNNING

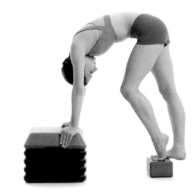

## VERSION 1

- As in Footwork IV version 1, only this time, open your heels to parallel and lower one heel at a time for ten reps.

## VERSION 2

- As in Footwork IV version 2, only this time, open your heels to parallel and lower one heel at a time, for ten reps.

## ASYMMETRICAL PUSHUPS

(page 174)

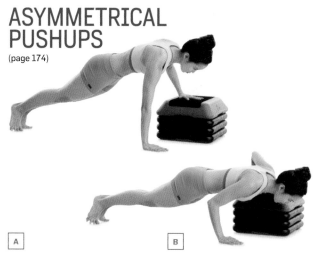

A

B

- One hand is on the step or yoga block, one hand is on the floor.

- Complete two rounds of three pushups on your right side, then move the block to the other side and complete two more rounds.

## INCLINE PUSHUPS AND PLANKS

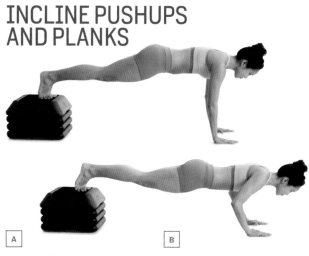

A

B

- Your body is in plank with the balls of your feet on the front edge of the step or yoga block (toes off).

- Keeping elbows tight to sides and heels over toes, perform as many reps as you are able while maintaining proper form and control.

# Tension Rings and Things

Besides being a genius with springs, Joe was a master at creating new ways to use tension to change a body or enhance a workout. One particular piece was called the "Pilates magic circle." As lore tells, it was fashioned from the metal bands (or hoops) that wrapped around wooden kegs. These circular metal structures, layered within one another and with wooden blocks screwed into their sides, were the very first "thigh master," only with many more uses.

# >MAGIC CIRCLE

## SITTING: MAGIC CIRCLE BETWEEN THE KNEES

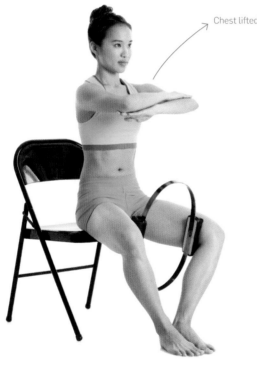

Chest lifted

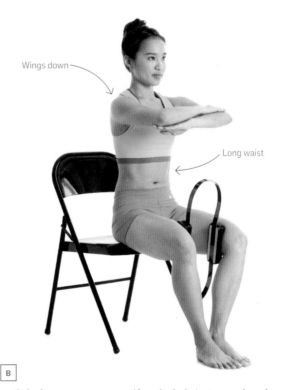

Wings down

Long waist

**A**

- Sit on the front edge of a bed or chair (where your legs can be at right angles to your hips) and place the ring between your inner thighs just above your knees.
- Sit tall with your arms folded, genie-style, in front of your chest and walk the feet together.

**B**

- Inhale as you squeeze the circle into an oval and hold for a count of three.
- Exhale with control as you release the tension of the ring.

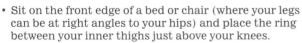

**REPS:** Repeat the squeeze-and-release sequence three to five times, lengthening your waist with each opportunity.

# *Pilates Props: Tension Rings and Things*

## SITTING: MAGIC CIRCLE BETWEEN THE FEET

**NOTE:** *For anyone with weak feet or collapsed arches this inverted position will open a world of new sensation in the ankles and calves. Try to connect the feeling of lifting your arches to engaging through your inner thighs.*

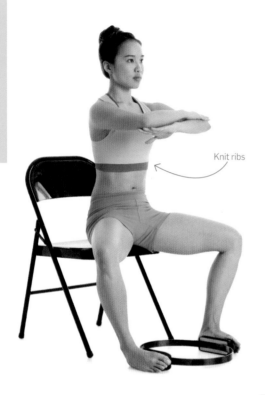

Knit ribs

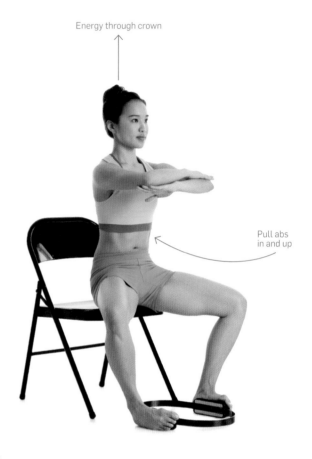

Energy through crown

Pull abs in and up

**A**

- Place the ring flat on the floor and turn your feet so that the soles are pressed against the pads of the circle.
- Allow your knees to open past hip-width but do not allow them to fall completely open.
- Sit tall with your arms folded, genie-style, in front of your chest.

**B**

- Inhale as you squeeze the circle, holding for a count of three.
- Exhale with control as you release the tension of the ring.

**REPS:** Repeat the squeeze-and-release sequence three to five times.

**NOTE:** *The deep neck flexors often get ignored and can contribute to neck and shoulder problems. Try this: Hold the circle pad under your chin, with both hands layered underneath the other pad, elbows wide and head level. Press the back of your tongue to the roof of your mouth and the circle up into your chin, hold for a count of three, and release. Repeat three times.*

# SITTING: MAGIC CIRCLE AGAINST THE HEAD (ISOMETRIC SERIES)

For this series involving the delicate vertebrae of the cervical spine (your neck), the movements are very small but potent. As the circle is pressed toward your head, you are stabilizing the movement of the head with your neck muscles and so you should not see your head move off its centerline of balance. Start slowly and see how it feels later, because the effects of improperly executed isometrics can creep up on you throughout the day.

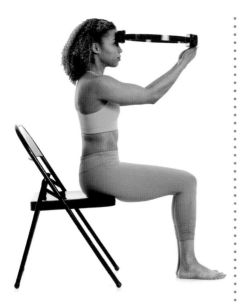

## FRONT

- Sit tall with your inner thighs squeezed together and hold the near circle pad against your forehead with both hands layered around the far pad.

**REPS:** Press and hold for a count of three, then release. Repeat three times.

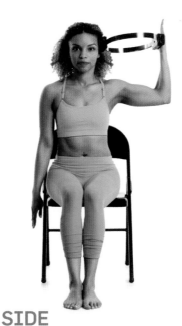

## SIDE

- Sit tall with your inner thighs squeezed together and hold the circle with your left hand so that one pad sits against the left side of your head.
- If needed, reach your right hand overhead and secure the circle.

**REPS:** Press and hold for a count of three and release. Repeat three times and then switch sides.

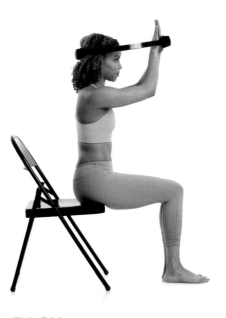

## BACK

- Sit tall with your inner thighs squeezed together and place your head inside the circle, with the back of your head against the back pad of the circle and both hands layered on the inside pad of the front of the circle.

**REPS:** Press and hold for a count of three and release. Repeat three times.

241

# *Pilates Props: Tension Rings and Things*

## STANDING: MAGIC CIRCLE BETWEEN THE HEELS OF THE HANDS

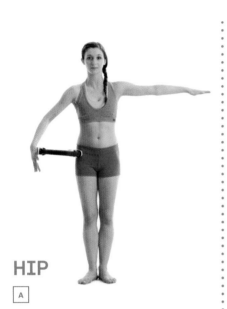

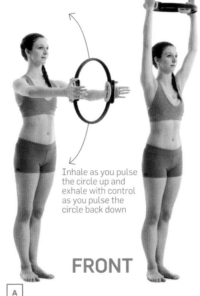

Inhale as you pulse the circle up and exhale with control as you pulse the circle back down

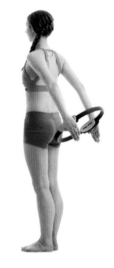

### HIP

**A**

- Stand tall with your heels together and toes apart and hold the circle against the side of one hip with the heel of your hand, the elbow bent and wide.
- With a lifted chest and low shoulders, inhale and press the circle toward your hip.
- Hold for a count of three and then exhale slowly as you release the tension of the ring.

**REPS:** Complete four circle presses and then switch sides.

### FRONT

**A**

- Stand tall with your heels together and toes apart and hold the circle out in front of you at shoulder-height with elbows slightly bent and lifted.
- Inhale and squeeze the circle.
- Exhale slowly as you release.

**B**

- After three to five squeezes, lift your arms overhead and repeat.
- Then lower your arms in front of your hips and repeat.
- Squeeze the circle in eight to ten sharp pulselike movements as you lift it up through all three positions (low, middle, high) and back down again.

**REPS:** Repeat the pulsing three times.

### BACK

**A**

- Stand tall with your heels together and toes apart and hold the circle between the heels of your hands behind your back with your shoulders wide and chest lifted.
- Pitch slightly forward from the ankle so the whole body leans into the wind.
- Inhale and squeeze the ring behind you.
- Any movement? Hold it for a count of three and then exhale slowly as you "release" the ring.

**REPS:** Do your best to repeat this three to five times or until sufficiently humbled.

# STANDING: MAGIC CIRCLE BETWEEN THE ANKLES

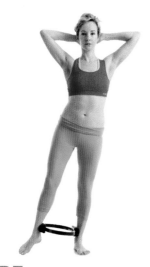

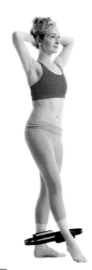

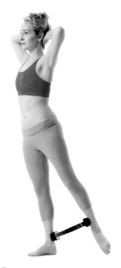

## SIDE

 **A**

- Stand tall and place the circle pads between your upper ankles.
- Open your arms wide to the sides of the room or behind your head, with your chest lifted and shoulder blades drawn together.
- Shift your weight slightly to a standing leg (your choice) and lift the other foot off the mat.

 **B**

- Inhale and squeeze the circle by bringing the lifted heel toward the stable one and holding for a count of three.
- Exhale with control as you release the ring.

**REPS:** Repeat three to five times, and do not switch until after Front and Back have been completed on one leg.

## FRONT

 **A**

- Roll the circle forward until the pad is pressed between the front of one ankle and the heel of the other.
- The front foot is lifted off the mat and the body is tall and stable.

 **B**

- Inhale and draw your front heel backward, squeezing the circle and holding for a count of three.
- Exhale with control as you release the ring.

**REPS:** Repeat three to five times.

## BACK

**A**

- After the last Front squeeze, rock forward until the front foot is flat on the mat and the back foot is lifted off the ground.

**B**

- Inhale and squeeze the back foot toward the stable leg, holding for a count of three.
- Exhale slowly as you release the tension of the ring.

**REPS:** Repeat three to five times. Now switch legs and repeat the entire Side, Front, Back series.

# Magic Circle Mat

The magic circle can add a wonderful challenge to a mat workout by incorporating it into the existing exercises. It serves to help stabilize the body parts that are holding it, forcing the work of the moving body parts to be more exact. I have also added the Tensatoner, where possible, as another alternative.

**4**
Single-Leg
Circles
(page 122)

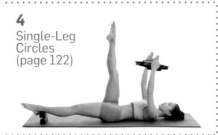

**5**
Rolling Like a Ball
(page 91)

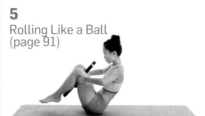

**6**
Single-Leg Stretch (page 66)

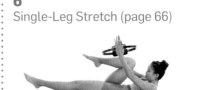

**10**
Crisscross (page 123)

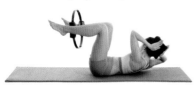

**11**
Spine Stretch (page 68)

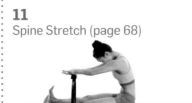

**12**
Open-Leg
Rocker
(page 123)

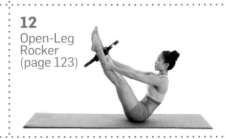

**16**
Single-Leg Kicks (page 70)

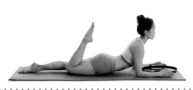

**17**
Double-Leg Kicks (page 97)

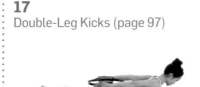

**18**
Neckpull (page 125)

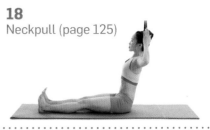

**22**
Double-Leg Lifts and Beats
(page 101)

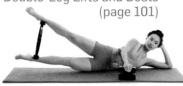

**23**
Teaser I, II, III
(pages 102, 128)

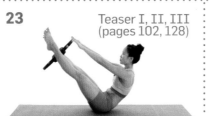

**24**
Hip Twist
(or Hip
Circles)
(page 128)

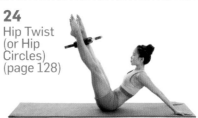

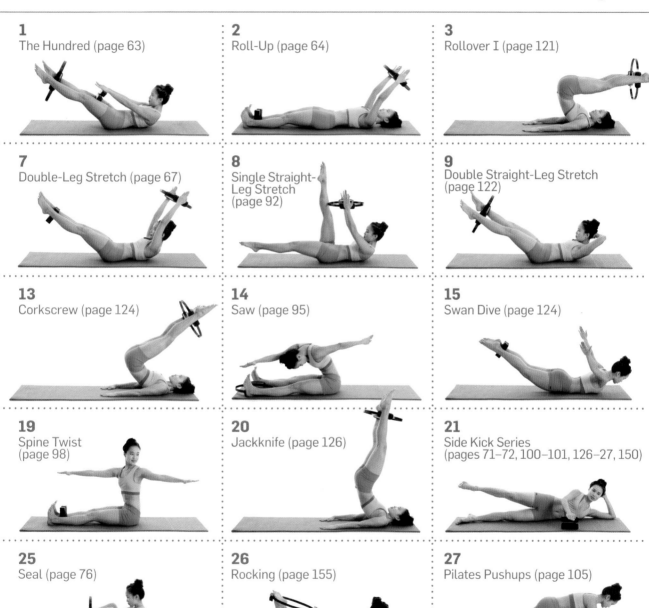

**1**
The Hundred (page 63)

**2**
Roll-Up (page 64)

**3**
Rollover I (page 121)

**7**
Double-Leg Stretch (page 67)

**8**
Single Straight-Leg Stretch (page 92)

**9**
Double Straight-Leg Stretch (page 122)

**13**
Corkscrew (page 124)

**14**
Saw (page 95)

**15**
Swan Dive (page 124)

**19**
Spine Twist (page 98)

**20**
Jackknife (page 126)

**21**
Side Kick Series (pages 71–72, 100–101, 126–27, 150)

**25**
Seal (page 76)

**26**
Rocking (page 155)

**27**
Pilates Pushups (page 105)

# Tension Rings and Things

## > TENSATONER

The size and shape of the magic circle are perfect for shoulder-wide exercises, but it is not always the ideal prop to get into smaller places needing tone and stability. We often use balls or pillows to try to compensate, but they are missing the all-important resistance component.

Enter the Tensatoner, an adaptable prop suitable for situations where the pro-portion and instability of the magic circle won't do. The Tensatoner not only provides resistance and stability for matwork exer-cises but also doubles as a foot corrector and even as a pushup aid. It's also another portable prop small enough for travel, and taking some-thing with you promotes oppor-tunities for work-outs anywhere.

## ASYMMETRICAL PUSHUP PRESS

- Place the Tensatoner on your step or yoga block and stand alongside it.
- Round forward and place one hand on the top pad of the toner and one on the floor.

**NOTE:** *If you have a weaker side, begin there and then come back to it again after working the stronger side.*

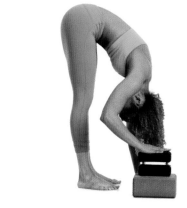

- Keeping your shoulder weight over your hands, walk your feet back until you are in a plank position with the Tensatoner spring closed.

Abs up

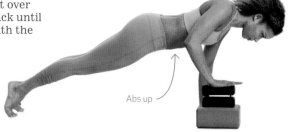

- Hold your plank as you release the press of the spring without shifting your weight.
- Press and release the spring three more times and then, holding the spring closed, walk your feet back into your hands and roll up to standing.

Square off as much as possible

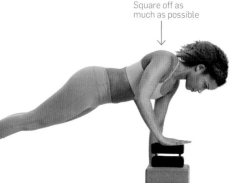

**REPS:** Repeat the sequence on the other side.

# *Pilates Props: Tension Rings and Things*

## FOOT PRESS

**NOTE:** *The Tensatoner can be used in nearly every way the magic circle can, including the isometrics on page 241.*

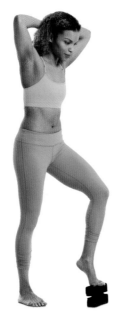

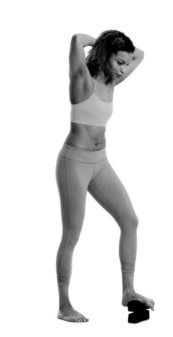

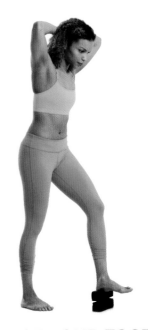

### BALL OF YOUR FOOT

 **A**

- Stand with the ball of your foot on the top pad of the Tensatoner (your heel can be planted or lifted) and your other foot flat on the floor.

- Your hands can be on your hips, open wide to your sides, or layered behind the base of your head.

- Inhale as you press down and close the toner spring, using the press of the spring to lift your abdominals in and up in order to take all pressure off the hip, knee, and ankle joints of the standing leg.

### ARCH OF YOUR FOOT

 **A**

- Next, place the arch of the foot on the top pad and repeat the sequence, allowing your toes to curl forward over the front edge of the toner and your heel to curl back over the back edge like the foot of a bird on a perch.

### HEEL OF YOUR FOOT

 **A**

- Last, place the heel of your foot on the pad (your toes can be planted on the floor or lifted) and repeat the press sequence.

**REPS:** Hold for a count of three and then release. Repeat this five times. When one side is complete, switch feet.

# TABLETOP PRESS

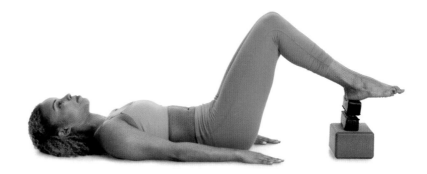

### A

- Place the Tensatoner on your step or yoga block and lie on your back with your feet together and arches rounded over the top pad.
- Your arms are long by your sides and pressed firmly to the mat.

### B

- Inhale and press the toner spring closed.
- With the spring held closed, roll your pelvis up off the mat and hold at the top, pubic bone pressing toward the ceiling.
- Exhale with control as you slowly roll back down to the mat one vertebra at a time, keeping the spring closed.
- When your sacrum reaches the mat, release the tension on the spring.

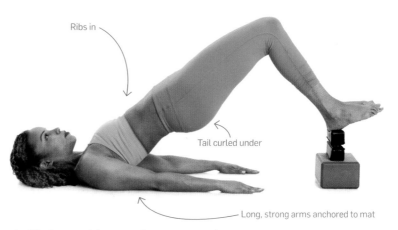

Ribs in

Tail curled under

Long, strong arms anchored to mat

**REPS:** Complete five Tabletop Presses, making sure the lift of your pelvis comes from your powerhouse and not your back (there should not be an arch in your lower back when you are at the top of the press.

PROGRESSION
## Tabletop One-Leg Press
Repeat the entire sequence of Tabletop Press with one leg reaching up and the other pressing the Tensatoner closed.

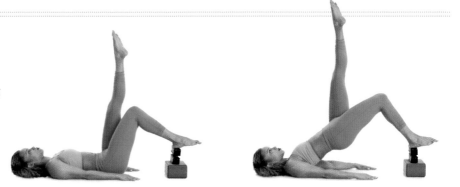

249

# *Pilates Props: Tension Rings and Things*

## STANDING PRESS

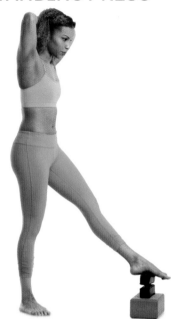
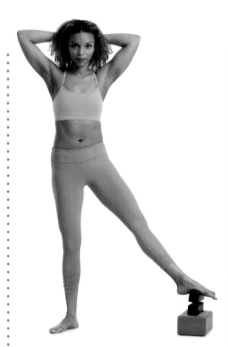
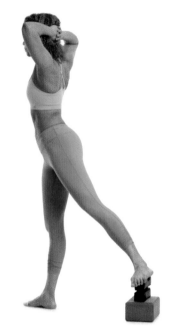

### FRONT

- Place the Tensatoner on your step or yoga block and reach the arch of one foot over the top pad.
- Hands are layered behind your head, on your hips, or open wide to the sides.
- Inhale as you press the spring of the toner closed and hold for a count of three. Exhale and release.
- Legs are straight but knees remain unlocked.

### SIDE

- Turn sideways to the Tensatoner with the arch of one foot over the top pad and inner thigh turned out at your hip.
- Layer your hands behind your head and inhale as you press the spring of the toner closed, targeting your inner thighs, and hold for a count of three.
- Exhale and release.
- Grow longer in the waistline with each press.

### BACK

- Turn to face away from the Tensatoner and turn your foot so that your heel and arch are on top of the top pad. Unless you are extremely limber, this will undoubtedly rotate your pelvis.
- Stay as squared off as possible with your heel connected to toner.
- Hands are layered behind your head, on your hips, or open wide to the sides.
- Inhale as you press the spring of the toner closed and hold for a count of three. Exhale and release.
- Legs are straight but knees remain unlocked.

**REPS:** Perform three presses to the front, pivot 90° and perform three side presses, then turn to the back to perform three presses there. You can switch legs while facing back and repeat the sequence from the back.

# SITTING LEG-PRESS FRONT

A

- Place the Tensatoner on your step or yoga block and sit with your legs straight and the back of one ankle on the top pad.
- Sit tall with your fingertips pressing into the floor behind you.
- Inhale and press on the pad, closing the spring of the toner, and hold for a count of three.
- Exhale and release.

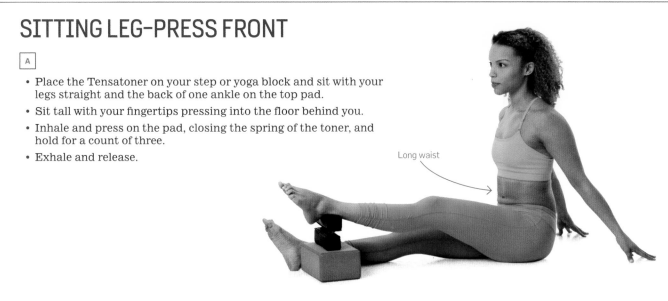

Long waist

**REPS:** Repeat this three times, working to lift your waist up in opposition to the press of your leg. Repeat on the other side.

# SIDE-LYING LEG PRESS

A

- Place the Tensatoner on your step or yoga block and lie on your side with your legs straight and the inside of your top ankle on the toner pad.
- Your bottom leg is lengthened on the floor in front of the block.
- Layer your hands behind the base of your head as you would for the Side Kicks Series (page 71).
- Inhale and press on the pad, closing the spring of the toner and hold for a count of three.
- Exhale and release.

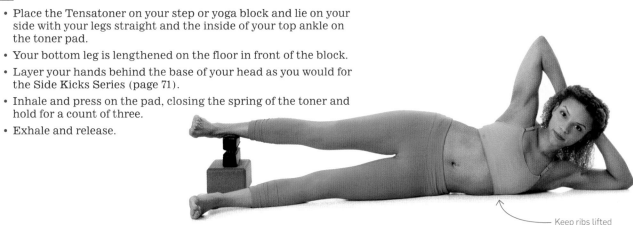

Keep ribs lifted

**REPS:** Repeat this three times, working to elongate your waist in opposition to the press of your leg. Repeat on the other side.

# FOOTWORK

Romana used to say: "You can't build a sturdy structure on a shoddy foundation." When working out in a properly equipped Pilates studio with a teacher trained in the entire system of Pilates, you would find yourself with much more access to weighted strength-building exercises for the feet and ankles. To compensate for some of that missing resistance, we need to add a tour of duty for your tootsies.

## HOW CAN WE BEST SUPPORT OURSELVES ON OUR FEET?

The first step (no pun intended!) is to balance between the three points of contact with the ground:

- Heel
- Ball of the baby toe
- Ball of the big toe

The next step is to balance the three arches of support:

- Transverse arch: runs across the ball of the foot
- Medial arch: runs the inner length of the underside of the foot
- Lateral arch: runs the outer length of the underside of the foot

According to a *New York Times* article, about 75 percent of people in the United States have foot pain at some time in their lives—and most of this pain is caused by shoes that don't fit properly or that squeeze our feet into unnatural shapes. Yes, I'm talking about your favorite stilettos! Here are just some of the problems that weak feet and ankles can cause:

- Excessive pronation (feet rolling in, collapsed arches)
- Excessive supination (feet rolling out)
- Hip, knee, lower-back, and shoulder and neck pain
- ACL tears
- Plantar fasciitis
- Achilles tendonitis
- Shin splints
- Ankle sprains or stress fractures
- Bunions, corns, callouses; toes that stick up or out to the side

**ASSESS:** NOT SURPRISINGLY, HIGH HEELS ARE THE WORST FOR MAINTAINING THE INTEGRITY OF YOUR FEET. BAREFOOT IS THE BEST. BAREFOOT IN THE SAND IS THE ULTIMATE. WHAT A GREAT REASON TO HIT THE BEACH! EVEN IF YOU DON'T HAVE SAND NEARBY, TRY WALKING AROUND BAREFOOT AND ON YOUR TOES FOR 5 MINUTES A DAY.

# MEET YOUR FEET >>>

The foot is a complex structure of 26 bones (plus 2 sesamoid bones) and 33 joints, layered with an intertwining web of more than 120 muscles, ligaments, and nerves. Because your feet are very small in comparison with the rest of your body (even if you wear size 10s), the impact of each step exerts tremendous force upon them. The force imposed on your feet daily is about 50 percent greater than your body weight. During a typical day, we spend about 4 hours on our feet and, ideally, take 8,000 to 10,000 steps. That's several hundred tons of force every day! If your feet aren't strong and flexible enough, you may experience problems throughout your entire body.

**OUCH!** *Many in the barefoot running community aptly refer to shoes as "little foot coffins" because of the damage the wrong footwear can do to our bodies. You can begin to make changes by simply changing your shoes often (remember Mr. Rogers?). And socks count, too—make sure they fit properly and that you take them off often.*

## DORSAL VIEW

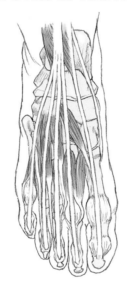

## ANTERIOR VIEW

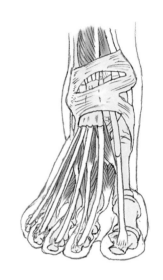

## POSTERIOR VIEW

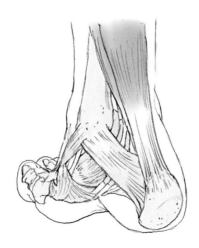

## PLANTAR VIEW

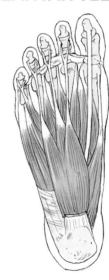

# Tension Rings and Things

## > FOOT CORRECTORS

Joe Pilates designed a few unique devices meant to bring strength and awareness to our feet. Besides the Foot Corrector and Toe Exerciser, seen in the chart on page 9, he also fashioned steel insoles to be strapped to the soles of your feet so you could remain connected during your Reformer and spring work.

Many of these strengtheners can be done while brushing your teeth, at your desk, waiting for traffic lights to change, or in front of the TV. Sometimes, I begin a client session using Joe's Foot Corrector before starting work on the big apparatus. Why? Because once we can connect your foundation to your powerhouse, you can work from a place of coordination.

As you go through all of the exercises in this book, determine how well your feet are connected to your center. Simulate Joe's Toe Corrector at home by tying two broccoli bands together. Broccoli bands are thicker and stronger than your average rubber bands, so they make for good resistors.

# TEA TOWEL EXERCISE

**A**

- Sit at the front edge of a chair with your legs at a right angle from your body and a small towel spread out on the floor beneath you.
- Place the balls of your feet on the front edge of the towel and spread your toes as wide as possible.
- Next, place your outer toes on the towel, then follow suit from outer to inner toes.

**B**

- Pull the towel toward you by lifting the arch of your foot as you curl your toes.
- Use the ball of your feet to hold the towel under your arch as you lift and spread your toes again and repeat.

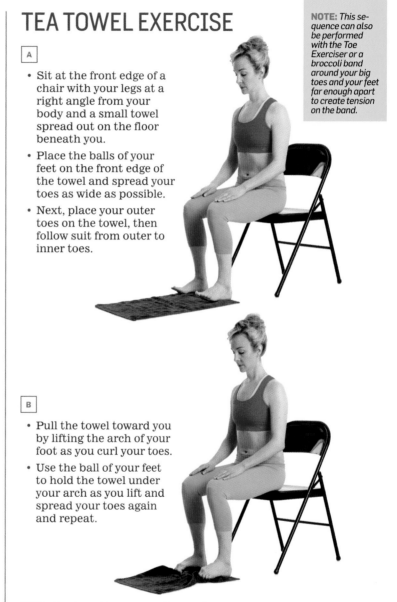

**NOTE:** *This sequence can also be performed with the Toe Exerciser or a broccoli band around your big toes and your feet far enough apart to create tension on the band.*

**REPS:** Continue this pattern until the entire tea towel is bunched under your arch and then reverse the motion, this time lifting the foot at the ankle and curling toes under before pushing the towel away one fold at a time until it is flat again.

# *Pilates Props: Tension Rings and Things*

## 2X4 EXERCISE

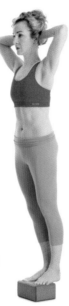

**A**

- Stand with the balls of your feet on a raised surface (like a 2x4 or a stair step or yoga block).

**REPS:** Repeat this sequence three times and then reverse the sequence three times, tracking the movement of your feet and ankles as high up the body as you're able.

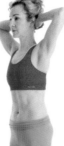

**B**

- Lift your heels and squeeze them together, tightly zipping up your entire midline.
- Hold a wall for balance or layer your hands behind your head.

**NOTE:** *This exercise can also be done without a board or step.*

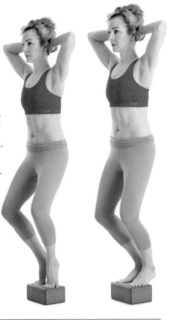

**C** **D**

- Keeping your heels together, bend your knees deeply, opening them to the sides about shoulder-width.
- Stop before your pelvis or torso moves forward or back.
- Hold the balanced position and lower your heels toward the ground.
- Pressing away from the heels, straighten your legs to standing.

## BIG TOE PRESS

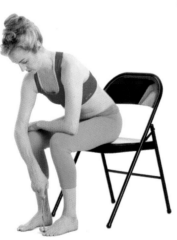

**A**

- Place your big toe through one loop of the band and your finger through the other.

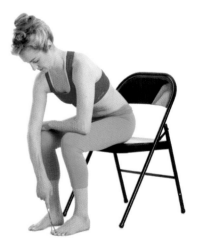

**B**

- With your foot flat on the floor, lift your big toe and then press it back down to the floor against the resistance of the band.
- Notice whether your ankle tries to roll in or out as you do this and whether you can minimize any movement other than that of your big toe.

**REPS:** Press ten times on each foot. For additional benefit, try other toes!

# 10-TOE SPREAD

- Sitting or (preferably) standing with your feet flat on the floor and your big toes through each loop of the band, spread all your toes as wide as possible on the floor against the resistance of the band.

**B**

- Lift your heels.

**REPS:** Do this ten times, maintaining the distance of your toes.

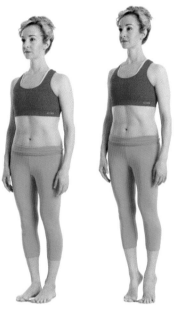

# BIG TOE LIFT

**A**

- Sitting or (preferably) standing with your feet flat on the floor and your big toes through each loop of the band, spread all your toes as wide as possible on the floor against the resistance of the band.

- Press all your toes into the floor, then isolate and lift only your big toes off the floor.

**REPS:** Do this ten times.

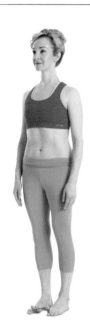

# EIGHT-TOE LIFT

**A**

- Sitting or (preferably) standing with your feet flat on the floor and your big toes through each loop of the band, spread all your toes as wide as possible on the floor against the resistance of the band.

- Press your big toes into the floor and lift the rest of your toes off the floor.

**REPS:** Do this ten times.

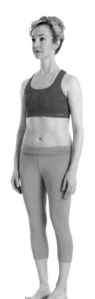

# LONG ARCH STRETCH

**A**

- Stand with your feet shoulder-width apart and your big toes through each loop of the band.

- Bend your knees open slightly to shift your weight to the outer edges of your feet.

**B**

- Keeping weight on the outer foot, lift all your toes and hold for 5 seconds.

**REPS:** Do this five times daily— or as often as you are able.

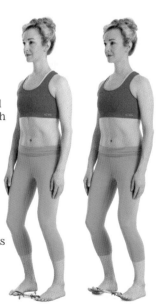

# The Wall: Your Vertical Mat

Finally, the best "prop" you can use without issue or cost is a wall. So long as it's sturdy and straight and can support your body weight, a wall makes a great companion to your workout, especially if you are restricted to being upright for any reason.

Since our perception of our bodies can often be skewed, a wall can be a wonderful way to gauge your posture from a tactile point of view as opposed to trying to "sense" your curves. While some might argue (rightfully) that walls are manmade structures and therefore not the best reflection of our organic selves, they can still be helpful when trying to figure out where you are in space.

## ROLL-DOWN

See page 81.

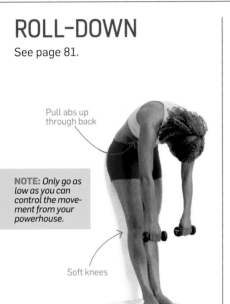

Pull abs up through back

**NOTE:** *Only go as low as you can control the movement from your powerhouse.*

Soft knees

## PUSHOFFS

See page 112.

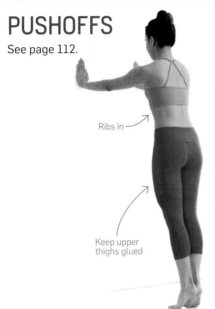

Ribs in

Keep upper thighs glued

## CORNER PUSHOFFS

See page 113.

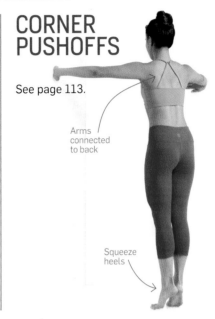

Arms connected to back

Squeeze heels

## ARM CIRCLES

See page 79.

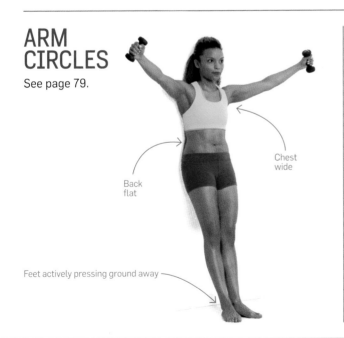

Chest wide

Back flat

Feet actively pressing ground away

## FLUSH WITH CIRCLES

See page 110.

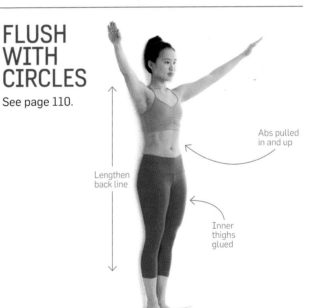

Abs pulled in and up

Lengthen back line

Inner thighs glued

# *Pilates Props: The Wall*

## SQUATS

See page 80.

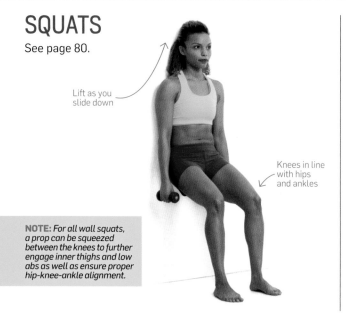

Lift as you slide down

Knees in line with hips and ankles

**NOTE:** *For all wall squats, a prop can be squeezed between the knees to further engage inner thighs and low abs as well as ensure proper hip-knee-ankle alignment.*

## SINGLE-LEG SQUATS

See page 139.

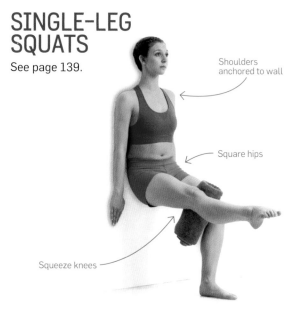

Shoulders anchored to wall

Square hips

Squeeze knees

## SQUATS WITH CIRCLES

See page 111.

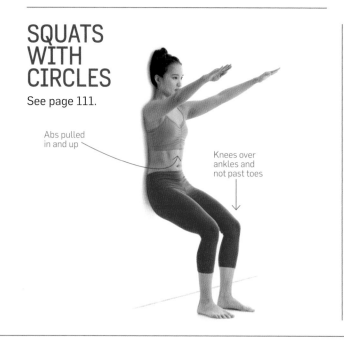

Abs pulled in and up

Knees over ankles and not past toes

## SQUATS WITH WINGS

See page 138.

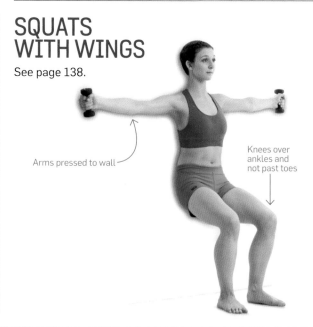

Arms pressed to wall

Knees over ankles and not past toes

## SPINE STRETCH:
## BACK TO THE WALL

See page 67.

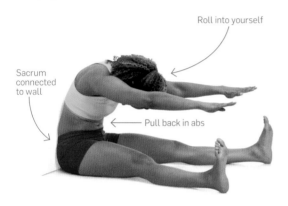

Roll into yourself

Sacrum
connected
to wall

Pull back in abs

## SPINE TWIST:
## FEET TO THE WALL

• Perform the Spine Twist with your heels butted up against a wall for stability and tactile feedback. As you twist, press your heels deeper into the wall, activating the movement from your hips.

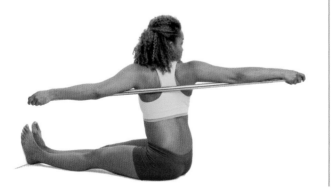

## PELVIC LIFTS:
## DRIVE YOU UP A WALL

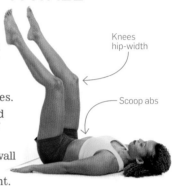

A

• Lie on your back with the bare soles of your feet flat on the wall, knees hip-width, and long arms by your sides.
• Your fingertips should just touch the base of the wall.
• Walk your feet up the wall until your knees are three-quarters straight.

Knees
hip-width

Scoop abs

B

• Opening your chest wide and pressing the backs of your arms firmly into the mat, curl your bottom and roll up until your shins are perpendicular to the wall and you are propped on your upper back.

Backs of arms pressing
actively into mat/floor.

No weight
on neck!

C

• Exhale with control as you roll back down to the starting position, articulating your spine one vertebra at a time.

**REPS:** Drive up the wall five times, holding at the top for three counts each time.

Tight
seat

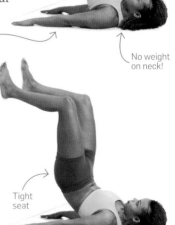

# *Pilates by Posture*

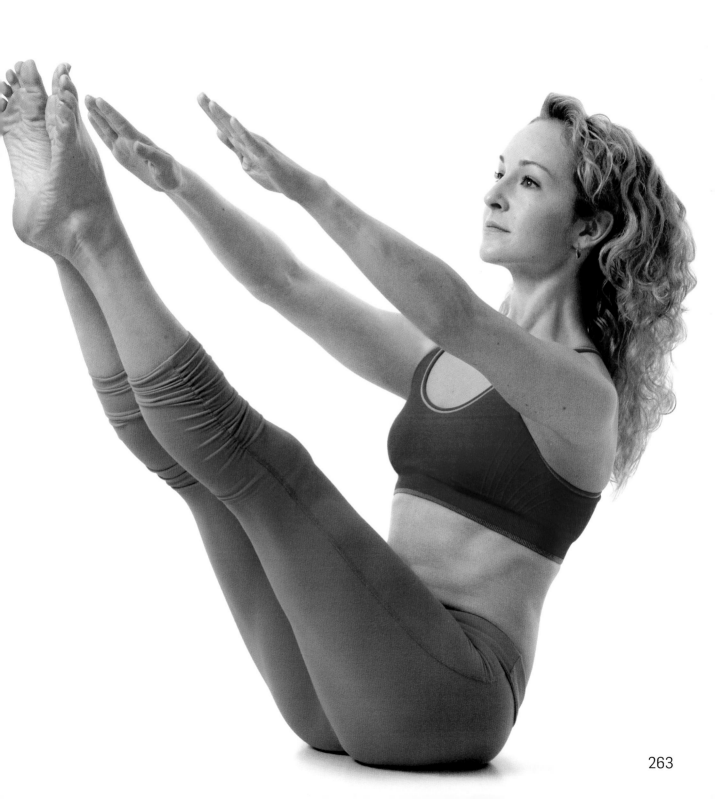

263

# Balance Your Body

If you've made it to this chapter by way of mastering one or two levels of the mat series, you're probably looking for a little more personal attention and insight. Or maybe you're just curious. Either way, welcome! Once we enter the domain of personalizing Pilates for specific body imbalances, goals, and issues, we need to sharpen our lens and really hone in on the specifics. To do that, I'm going to ask you to be open to new language about your body that may sound funny, foreign, or downright forensic! But I assure you that the more knowledge you have when it comes to your body, the better you can take care of it, and the better you'll look and feel.

Creating a workout that works for you means figuring out what you actually need! You've hopefully completed the awareness assessment about your mental and spiritual commitment (see "Before You Begin?" on page 15 in Chapter 1). Now let's look at your physical attributes and what you'd like to focus on or improve.

## Take Inventory of Yourself

First things first: It's very difficult to change things if you're not willing to take an objective look at what you're working with physically. I'm going to ask you to stand in front of a mirror and answer the following questions. One of my college majors was figure drawing, and I was trained to see lines and spaces, mass and volume, through artistic rather than judgmental eyes. On first glance, what usually strikes me are three factors: poise, proportion, and posture.

Stand facing a full-length mirror and look for signs of the habits that are currently shaping your physical self:

1. Are your shoulders level? Why might one be higher than the other?

2. Does your head sit upright or tilt to one side? Does your nose face more to one direction than the other? Why would those positions be that way and not the other?

3. Do the spaces between your arms and torso seem equal? If not, what

directions do you need to shift to make them look equal?

**4.** When you look at your hands at rest alongside your torso, do you see only your thumb and index finger or all five knuckles? If more than thumb and index finger show, follow that line up your arm—is there something happening at the elbows and shoulders that is causing that twist at the wrists?

**5.** Are the tops of your hips level? If not, why might one be higher than the other? Do you stand on one leg often? Do you carry things on one hip more than the other?

**6.** Are your kneecaps facing straight ahead, turned out, or turned in? If not straight ahead, can you turn them to face forward and see what else has to adjust to make that happen? Do different muscles begin working?

**7.** Are your ankles straight or do they lean in or out? What happens if you find a way to straighten them: Can you feel more points of your feet on the floor? Do you feel more stable?

**8.** Are your shoulders wide compared to your hips, or vice versa? Do you feel stronger in your upper body or lower body, and could it be related to this proportion?

**9.** Does your torso seem long in proportion to your legs, vice versa, or neither? Do you find that your two halves support one another equally, or does one half bear more of the burden of being upright?

**10.** Overall, what message does your posture reflect? Uplifted and open? Rounded and retracted? Rigid and resolute? Soft and yielding?

Did you discover anything new about your body? Are you able to trace some of your findings back to habits in the way you sit? Stand? Sleep? Carry things? Did you know that standing and sitting tall positively affect the way people feel about themselves and operate in the world? Studies show that assuming an "open and expansive" posture decreases the stress hormone cortisol, increases testosterone, and boosts feelings of power and tolerance for risk—whereas a closed posture has the opposite effect. Food for thought.

Next, read through the sequences in this chapter and try to find ones that work best for you! You can mix and match so long as you are always keeping Pilates's tenets in mind, especially concentration, control, center, breath, and balance. If you need to, refer to Chapter 5: Pilates Primer for a refresher. Remember that all the exercises shown here, whether unique to Pilates or not, can become Pilates-esque when performed with proper intention.

Also, bear in mind that the matwork sequences (the Mains) should follow the order shown due to Joe's intention to balance the body as you go (for instance, after rolling forward, roll backward; after being on your back, you're on your stomach; and so on).

*"More spine, less mind. I find that all exercises improve when the spine is given the lead. The organs and the bones know where they belong in relation to the spine. Everything falls into place in relationship to the spine when it can lead. With this orientation, the exercises and the whole body are longer, lighter, and we can have more fun."*

—Pilates elder Mary Bowen

# YOUR DIVINE SPINE

One of the quintessential qualities of Pilates is its focus on spinal mobility and freedom. Joe is often quoted as saying that a man is as young as his spine is flexible: "If your spine is inflexibly stiff at 30, you are old. If it is completely flexible at 60, you are young."

Gravity is always working to pull us toward the earth, whether we like it or not, but the way we limit the spinal slump is by relying on our muscles—not our joints—to hold us up. Obviously, since the spine is made up of lots of small, individual bones, it needs a little help from its muscle buddies. When we narrow our focus from the hundreds of muscles acting upon one another down to the relative simplicity of 26 spinal segments and then even further down to the curves at work in the spinal column, we find a wonderful way to look at Pilates (and the business of movement in general) that is accessible and digestible.

Since all things are relative, it's hard to know how much movement you're looking for without some guide for what "normal" ranges are. Here are some normal ranges of motion (ROM) for the segments of your spine, as well as four common postural imbalances.

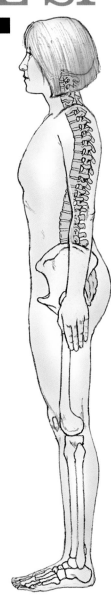

## Ideal Posture

### NORMAL RANGES OF MOTION

- **NECK:** Cervical spine (40° of flexion, 75° of extension, 35° of side bending, and 50° of rotation

- **MIDBACK:** Thoracic spine (45° of flexion, 25° of extension, 20° of side bending, and 35° of rotation)

- **LOWER BACK:** Lumbar spine (60° of flexion, 35° of extension, 20° of side bending, and 5° of rotation)

- **SACRUM AND TAILBONE** (five vertebrae fused into one bone)

*"Good posture can be successfully acquired only when the entire mechanism of the body is under perfect control."*
—Joe Pilates

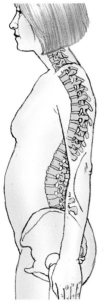

## KYPHOTIC-LORDOTIC POSTURE
**(see page 268)**

- Hip issues due to tight hip flexors (iliopsoas)
- Neck tension (cyclists and spinners: beware)
- Tight chest and upper back
- Weak neck flexors
- Weak/overly long hamstrings and gluteus maximus
- Weak abs

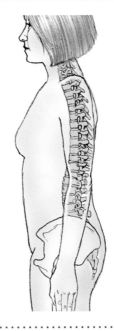

## FLAT-BACK POSTURE
**(see page 274)**

- Tight musculature between the ribs that makes breathing shallow
- Upper abs and accessory muscles of respiration are shortened and tight
- Hamstrings tight
- Hip flexors long and weak
- Increased strain in the forefoot from forward lean
- Knees slightly hyperextended, with plantar-flexed ankles (or slightly flexed with dorsiflexed ankles)

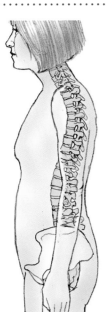

## SWAYBACK POSTURE
**(see page 280)**

- Long, weak upper-back extensors
- Weak neck flexors (limits ROM)
- Shoulders round forward
- Weak serratus anterior (the shoulder-blade anchor)
- Weak lower abs, while upper abs are short and strong
- Long and weak external obliques, short and tight upper fibers of internal obliques
- Tight and/or painful lower back
- Tight and weak glutes
- Tight hamstrings with recurrent strains
- Hyperextended knees
- Plantar fasciitis

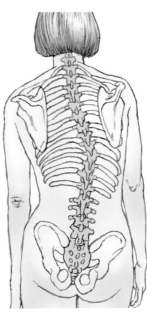

## POSTURAL SCOLIOSIS
**(see page 286)**

- Spinal rotation
- Spinal bend
- Ribs and shoulder blade bulge on one side of the back
- One shoulder hangs lower than the other
- One shoulder blade sits higher than the other
- The pelvis thrusts forward on one side
- One leg may appear shorter than the other
- Hip is "hiked" on one side

# Kyphotic-Lordotic Posture

## IS THIS YOU?

- My head sits forward of my body, and there is an increased inward curve of my neck, making my chin poke forward.
- I have an outward curve in my upper back.
- My shoulders are rounded forward, creating a "sunken chest," with my shoulder blades positioned wide apart (protracted away from the spine).
- I have a large gap between my lower back and the floor when lying on my back, or standing up against a wall, that does not change when I bend forward.
- My pelvis tips forward. (*Note:* Lordotic posture is common in gymnasts and pregnant women.)

## SYMPTOMS

- Hip issues due to tight hip flexors (iliopsoas)
- Neck tension (cyclists and spinners: beware)
- Tight chest and upper back
- Weak neck flexors
- Weak/overly long hamstrings and gluteus maximus
- Weak abs

## TRAINING TIPS

- Work from the bottom up, making sure to properly align the lower body.
- Stretch the hip flexors, neck, chest, and upper back.
- Strengthen the hamstrings, glutes, and abs.
- Use pads or pillows under the head, if needed when prone, to maintain spinal alignment.

# Starters

| 1 | 2 | 3 |

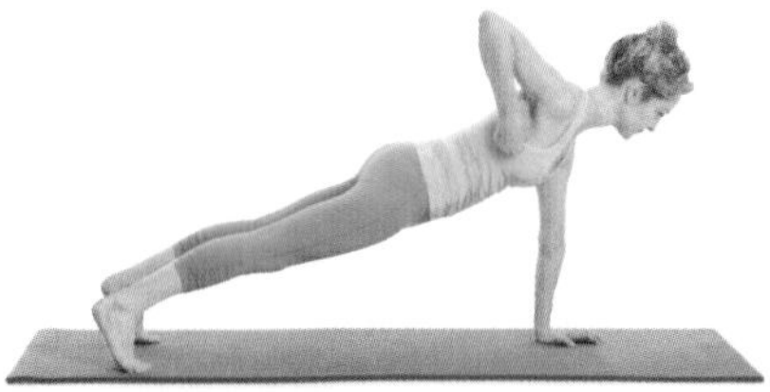

**Pushup
with a Dumbbell Row**
(page 172)

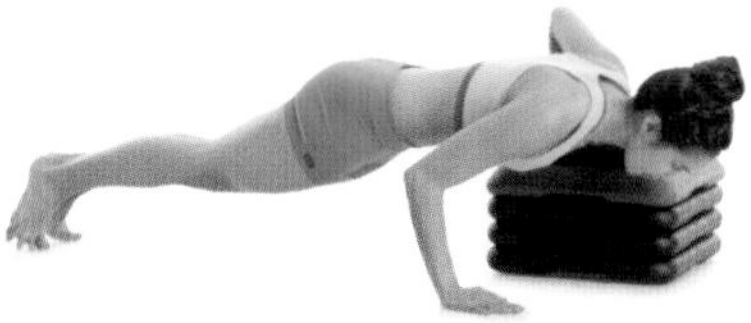

**Asymmetrical
Pushup/Plank**
(page 174)

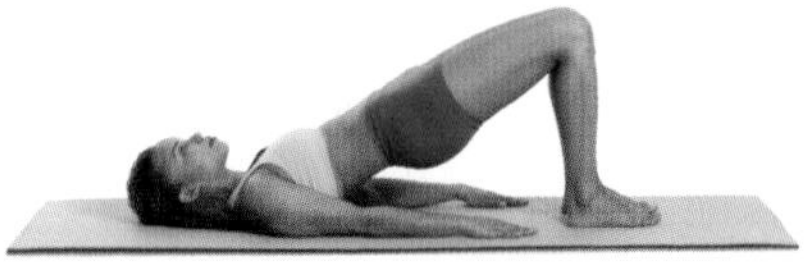

**Pelvic Lift**
(page 60)

# Mains

| 1 | 2 | 3 |

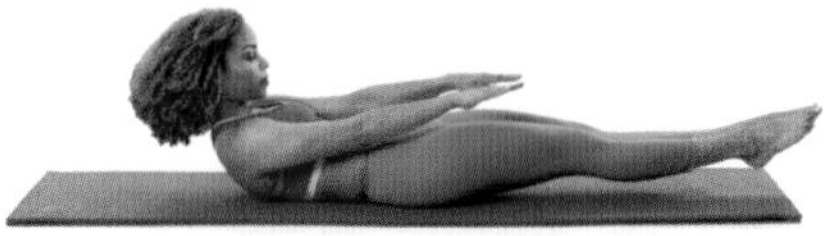

**The Hundred**
(page 63)

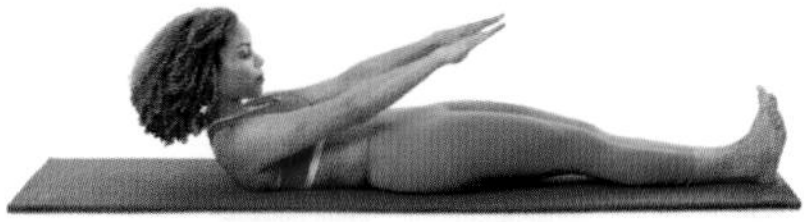

**Roll-Up**
(page 64)

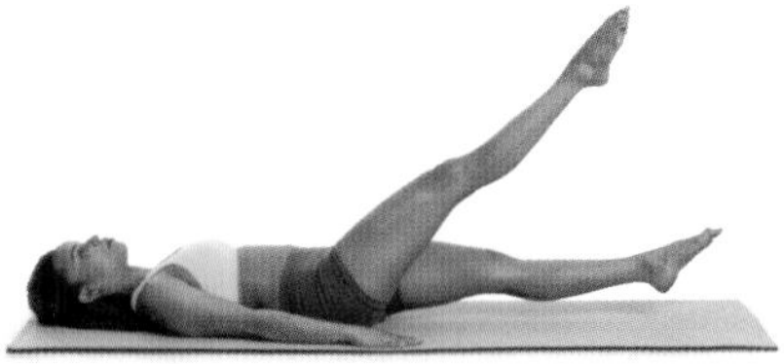

**Single-Leg Circles**
Lower leg lifted
(page 65)

## Mains *cont'd*

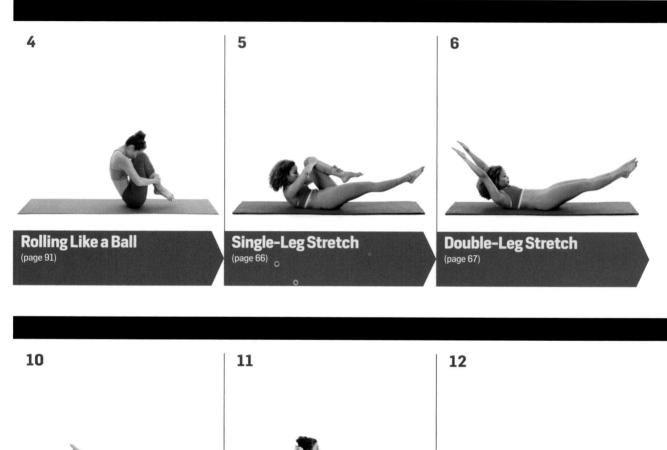

**4**

**Rolling Like a Ball**
(page 91)

**5**

**Single-Leg Stretch**
(page 66)

**6**

**Double-Leg Stretch**
(page 67)

**10**

**Saw**
(page 95)

**11**

**Neckpull**
(page 125)

**12**

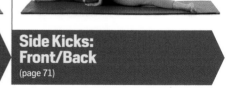

**Side Kicks:
Front/Back**
(page 71)

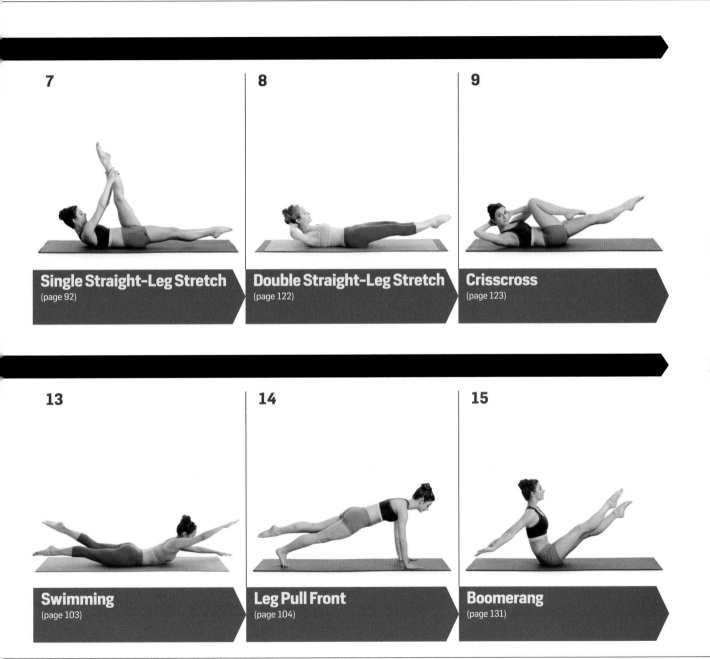

**7**

**Single Straight-Leg Stretch**
(page 92)

**8**

**Double Straight-Leg Stretch**
(page 122)

**9**

**Crisscross**
(page 123)

**13**

**Swimming**
(page 103)

**14**

**Leg Pull Front**
(page 104)

**15**

**Boomerang**
(page 131)

## Mains *cont'd*

## Enders

**16**

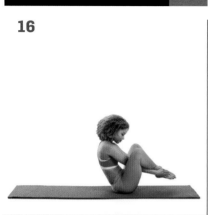

**Seal**
(page 76)

**1**

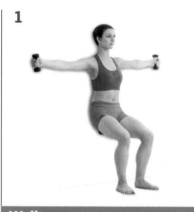

**Wall:
Squats with Wings**
(page 138)

**2**

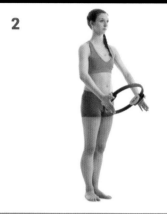

**Standing: Magic Circle
between the Heels of Hands**
(page 242)

**6**

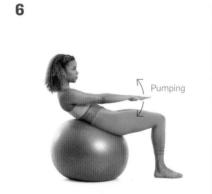

Pumping

**Big Ball:
The Hundred**
(page 217)

**7**

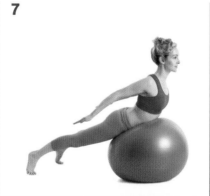

**Big Ball:
Swan**
(page 220)

**8**

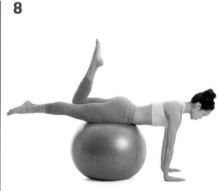

**Big Ball:
Single-Leg Kicks**
(page 221)

**3**

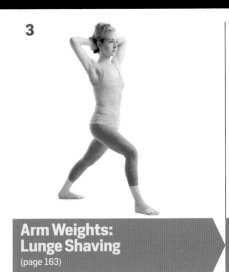

**Arm Weights:
Lunge Shaving**
(page 163)

**4**

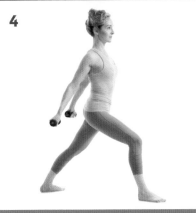

**Arm Weights:
Chest Expansion**
(page 139)

**5**

**Big Ball:
Roll-Back**
(page 216)

**9**

**Big Ball:
Swimming**
(page 221)

**10**

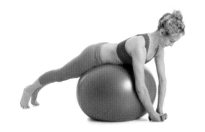

**Big Ball:
Arm Weights on the Ball**
(page 225)

# Flat-Back Posture

## IS THIS YOU?

- I tend to breathe shallowly.
- My pants and jeans may sag a bit in the rear due to my lack of booty.
- I have calluses under the balls of my feet/big toes.
- My shoulders are rounded forward, creating a "sunken chest," with my shoulder blades positioned wide apart (protracted away from the spine).
- My pelvis is tucked under, causing my lower back to be flat, and I hyperextend my knees.
  (*Note:* Notice if your entire body leans forward a bit; this is easier to observe when you try to stand with your back flush against a wall.)

## SYMPTOMS:

- Tight musculature between the ribs that makes breathing shallow
- Upper abs and accessory muscles of respiration are shortened and tight
- Hamstrings tight
- Hip flexors long and weak
- Increased strain in the forefoot from forward lean
- Knees slightly hyper-extended, with plantar-flexed ankles (or slightly flexed with dorsiflexed ankles)

## TRAINING TIPS

- Open the sides of the body around the ribs.
- Loosen the hamstrings.
- Strengthen the hip flexors (iliopsoas).
- Balance the ankles/feet.
- Use pads or pillows under the head, if needed when prone, to maintain spinal alignment.

# Starters

**1**

**Up-Stretch Combo**
(page 119)

**2**

**Pelvic Lift**
(page 60)

# Mains

**1**

**Roll-Up**
(page 64)

**2**

**Rollover I**
(page 121)

**3**

**Single-Leg Circles**
With lower leg lifted
(page 122)

**4**

**Rolling Like a Ball**
(page 91)

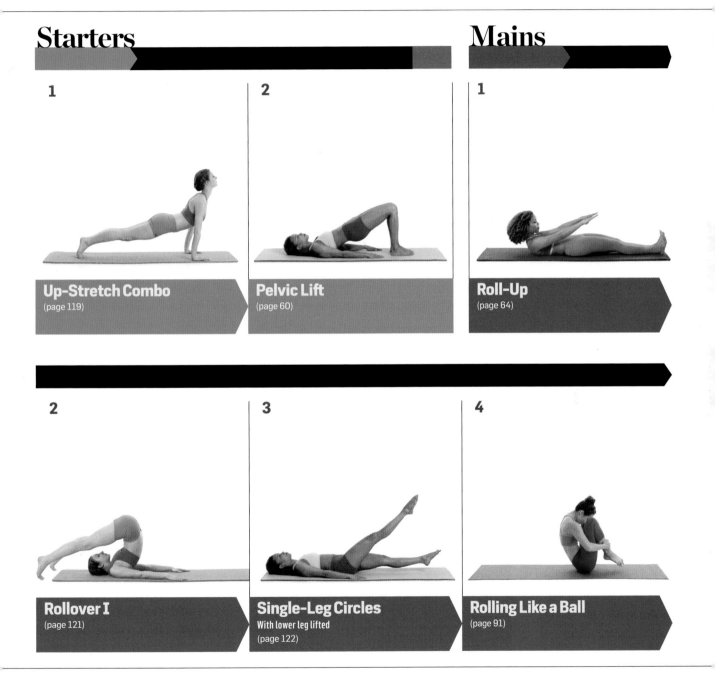

# Pilates by Posture: Flat-Back Posture

## Mains *cont'd*

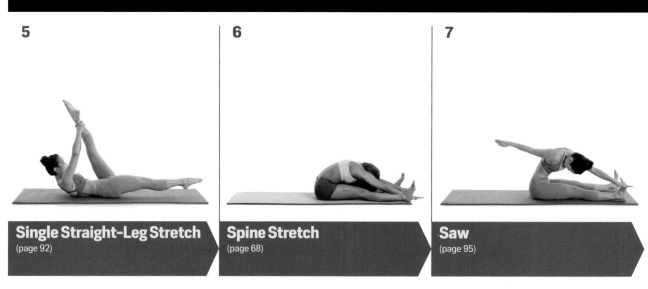

**5**

### Single Straight-Leg Stretch
(page 92)

**6**

### Spine Stretch
(page 68)

**7**

### Saw
(page 95)

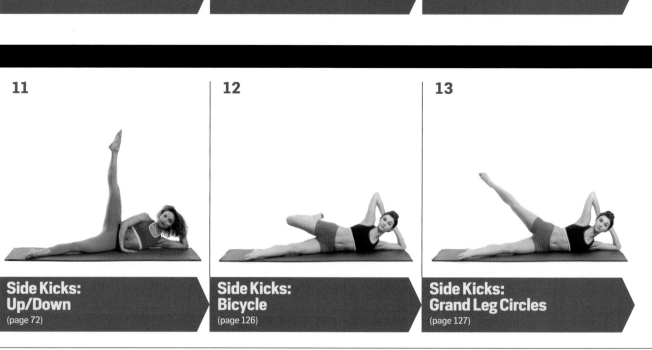

**11**

### Side Kicks: Up/Down
(page 72)

**12**

### Side Kicks: Bicycle
(page 126)

**13**

### Side Kicks: Grand Leg Circles
(page 127)

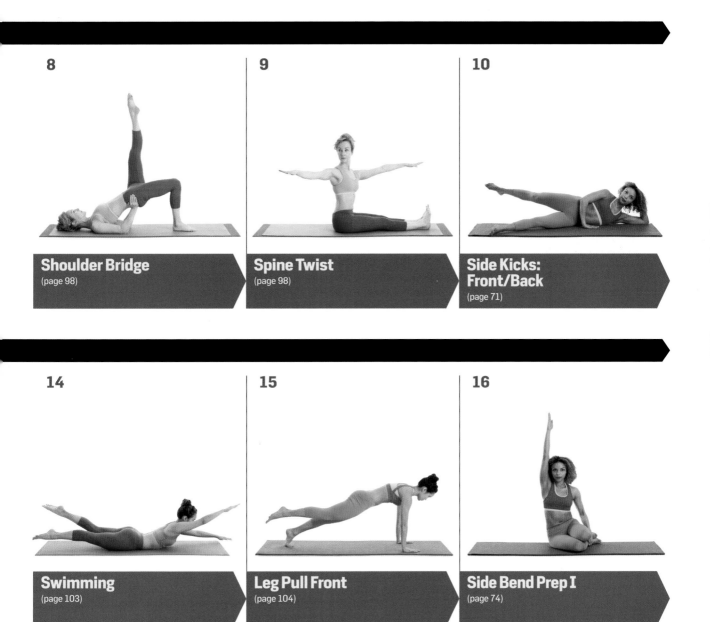

**8**

**Shoulder Bridge**
(page 98)

**9**

**Spine Twist**
(page 98)

**10**

**Side Kicks: Front/Back**
(page 71)

**14**

**Swimming**
(page 103)

**15**

**Leg Pull Front**
(page 104)

**16**

**Side Bend Prep I**
(page 74)

# *Pilates by Posture: Flat-Back Posture*

## Mains *cont'd*

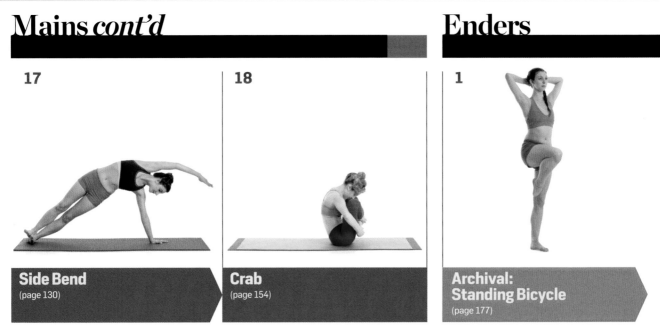

**17**

**Side Bend**
(page 130)

**18**

**Crab**
(page 154)

## Enders

**1**

**Archival:
Standing Bicycle**
(page 177)

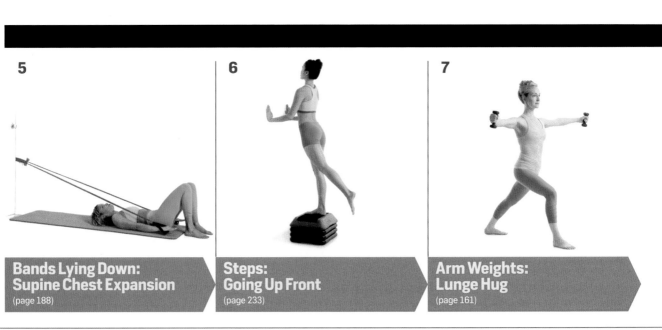

**5**

**Bands Lying Down:
Supine Chest Expansion**
(page 188)

**6**

**Steps:
Going Up Front**
(page 233)

**7**

**Arm Weights:
Lunge Hug**
(page 161)

**2**

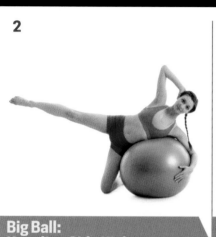

**Big Ball:
Kneeling Side Kicks**
(page 222)

**3**

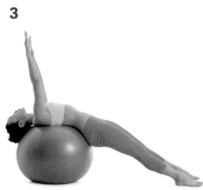

**Big Ball:
Back Stretch over Ball**
(page 224)

**4**

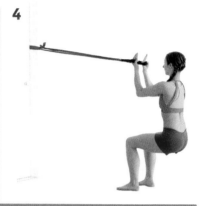

**Bands Standing Up:
Squats**
(page 210)

**8**

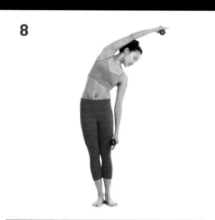

**Arm Weights:
Side Bends**
(page 107)

**9**

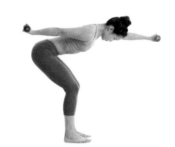

**Arm Weights:
Boxing**
(page 109)

# Swayback Posture

## IS THIS YOU?

- My head sits forward of my body, and there is an increased inward curve of my neck making my chin poke forward.
- My lower back is flat and my hips are swayed forward of my ankle bones, while my ribcage is swayed backward.
- The inward curve of my spine is midspine rather than lower back, and I hyperextend my knees.
(*Note:* Swayback posture is common in runners, teens, ballerinas, and sedentary individuals or people who stand for long periods of time, especially on one leg. It's also common in older adults because of weakened glutes.)

## SYMPTOMS:

- Long and weak upper-back extensors
- Weak neck flexors (limits ROM)
- Shoulders round forward
- Weak serratus anterior (the shoulder-blade anchor)
- Weak lower abs, while upper abs are short and strong
- Tight and/or painful lower back
- Tight and weak glutes
- Tight hamstrings with recurrent strains
- Hyperextended knees
- Plantar fasciitis

## TRAINING TIPS

- Strengthen the psoas, glutes, and external obliques.
- Increase hip flexion.
- Use pads or pillows under the head, if needed when prone, to maintain spinal alignment.

# Starters

**1**

**Wave**
(page 118)

**2**

**Spider Planks**
(page 171)

**3**

**Pelvic Lift**
(page 60)

# Mains

**1**

**The Hundred**
(page 63)

**2**

**Roll-Up**
(page 64)

**3**

**Single-Leg Circles**
With lower leg lifted
(page 65)

## Mains *cont'd*

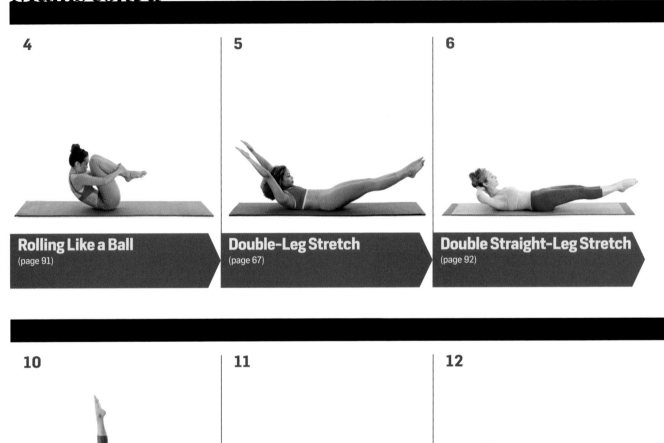

**4**

**Rolling Like a Ball**
(page 91)

**5**

**Double-Leg Stretch**
(page 67)

**6**

**Double Straight-Leg Stretch**
(page 92)

**10**

**Shoulder Bridge**
(page 98)

**11**

**Side Kicks:
Front/Back**
(page 71)

**12**

**Side Kicks:
Grand Leg Circles**
(page 127)

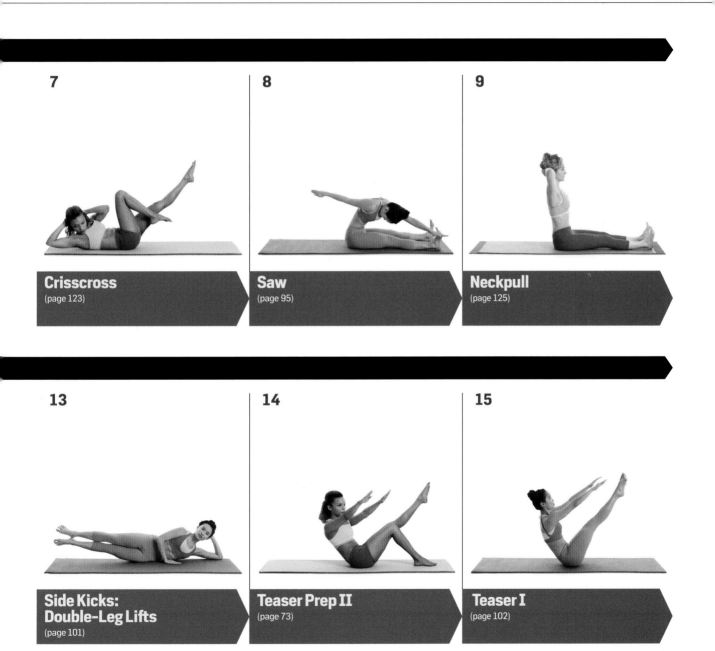

**7**

**Crisscross**
(page 123)

**8**

**Saw**
(page 95)

**9**

**Neckpull**
(page 125)

**13**

**Side Kicks:
Double-Leg Lifts**
(page 101)

**14**

**Teaser Prep II**
(page 73)

**15**

**Teaser I**
(page 102)

# Pilates by Posture: Swayback Posture

## Mains *cont'd*

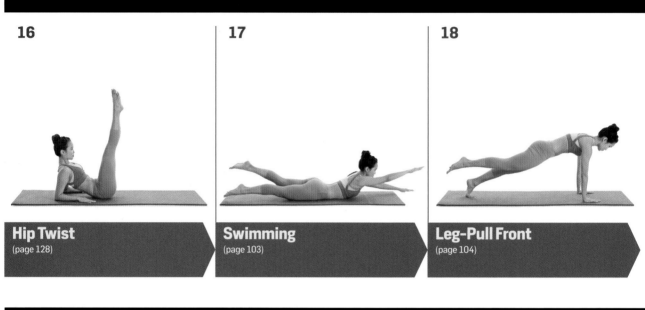

**16**

**Hip Twist**
(page 128)

**17**

**Swimming**
(page 103)

**18**

**Leg-Pull Front**
(page 104)

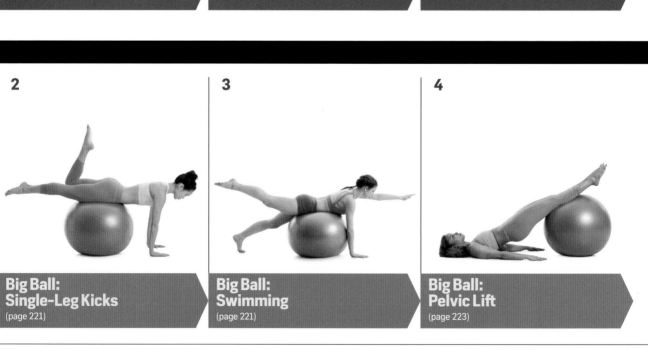

**2**

**Big Ball:
Single-Leg Kicks**
(page 221)

**3**

**Big Ball:
Swimming**
(page 221)

**4**

**Big Ball:
Pelvic Lift**
(page 223)

# Enders

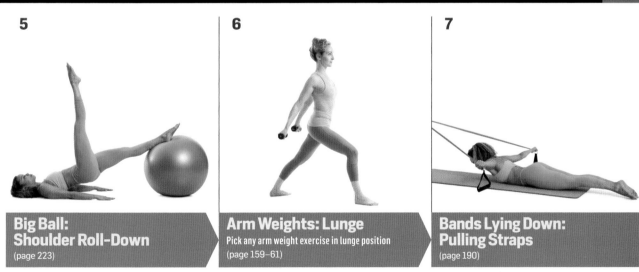

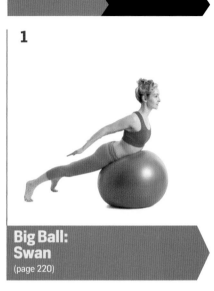

**19**

**Side Bend**
(page 130)

**20**

**Seal**
(page 76)

**1**

**Big Ball:
Swan**
(page 220)

**5**

**Big Ball:
Shoulder Roll-Down**
(page 223)

**6**

**Arm Weights: Lunge**
Pick any arm weight exercise in lunge position
(page 159–61)

**7**

**Bands Lying Down:
Pulling Straps**
(page 190)

# Postural Scoliosis

## IS THIS YOU?

- One of my shoulders or hips may be higher than the other, my head is off center, the gap between my elbows and waist is not even.
- One of my arms hangs longer than the other because of a tilt in my upper body that may make clothes hang unevenly.
- Bending forward, I notice that one side of my ribcage is higher than the other.
- One shoulder blade may be higher due to a "rib hump" that sticks out farther than the other.
  (*Note:* If you have postural scoliosis, the curvature disappears when you sit down as your pelvis automatically becomes level. If it is structural scoliosis, sitting will not make any difference to the visible curvature.)

## SYMPTOMS:

- Spinal rotation
- Spinal bend
- Ribs and shoulder blade bulge on one side of the back
- One shoulder hangs lower than the other
- The pelvis thrusts forward on one side
- One leg may appear shorter than the other
- Hip is "hiked" on one side

## TRAINING TIPS

- Muscle length and strength should be balanced on both the right and left sides of the body.
- Pay extra attention to "squaring the box," forcing the weaker side to catch up.
- If there is a "hollow" place along your back, place a folded hand towel under the hollow side and work your abs into the towel.
- Be conscious of balancing unilateral (same side) repetitive motions in sports as well as repeated bad postural habits.

# Starters

# Mains

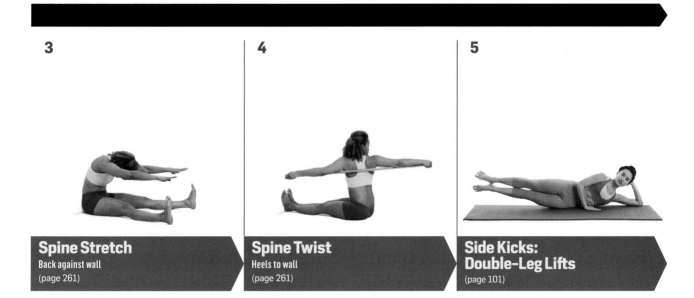

**1**

### Asymmetrical Pushup/Plank
(page 174)

**1**

### The Hundred
(page 63)

**2**

### Single-Leg Circles I
(page 65)

**3**

### Spine Stretch
Back against wall
(page 261)

**4**

### Spine Twist
Heels to wall
(page 261)

**5**

### Side Kicks: Double-Leg Lifts
(page 101)

# Pilates by Posture: Postural Scoliosis

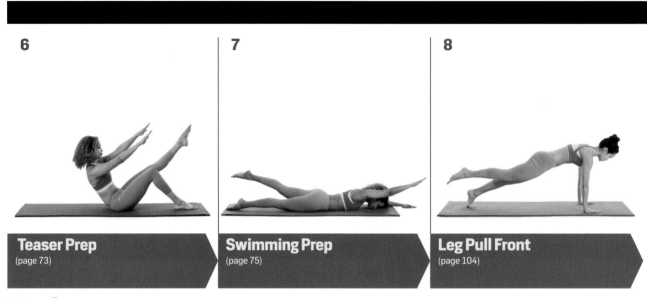

**6**
**Teaser Prep**
(page 73)

**7**
**Swimming Prep**
(page 75)

**8**
**Leg Pull Front**
(page 104)

## Enders

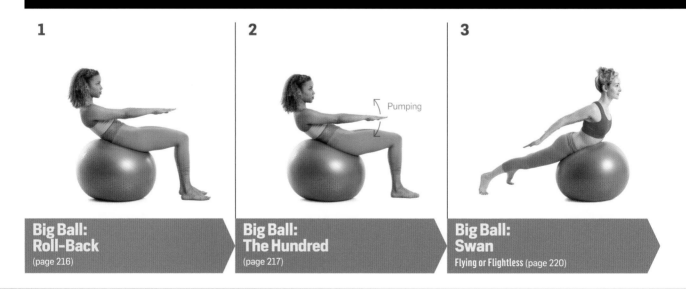

**1**
**Big Ball: Roll-Back**
(page 216)

**2**
Pumping
**Big Ball: The Hundred**
(page 217)

**3**
**Big Ball: Swan**
Flying or Flightless (page 220)

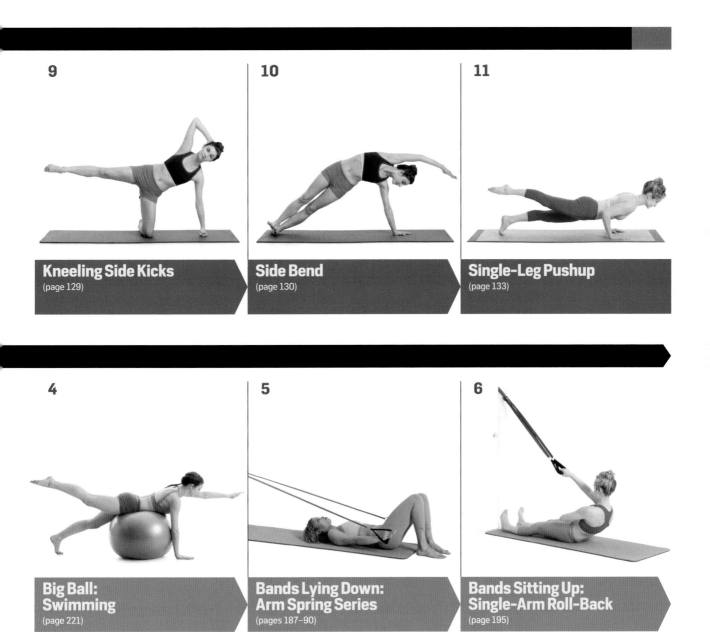

**9**

**Kneeling Side Kicks**
(page 129)

**10**

**Side Bend**
(page 130)

**11**

**Single-Leg Pushup**
(page 133)

**4**

**Big Ball:
Swimming**
(page 221)

**5**

**Bands Lying Down:
Arm Spring Series**
(pages 187–90)

**6**

**Bands Sitting Up:
Single-Arm Roll-Back**
(page 195)

# *Postural Scoliosis*

**7**

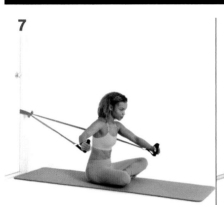

**Bands Sitting Up:
Single-Arm Rowing Hug**
(page 196)

**8**

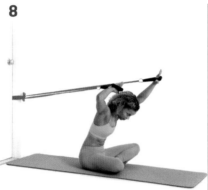

**Bands Sitting Up:
Single-Arm Rowing Shave**
(page 195)

**9**

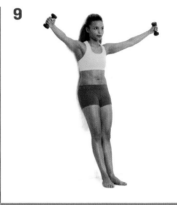

**Wall:
Arm Weight Circles**
Or any Arm Weights (page 79)

**10**

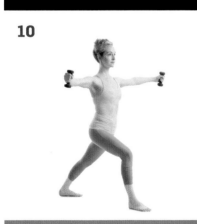

**Arm Weights:
Lunge Hug**
(page 161)

**11**

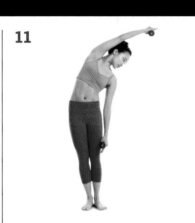

**Arm Weights:
Side Bends**
(page 107)

**12**

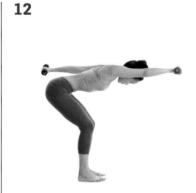

**Arm Weights:
Boxing**
(page 109)

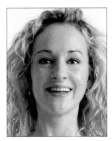

Amber is a recent graduate of Brooke Siler's re:AB Pilates Teacher Training Program.

# Amber Stone

"After dancing my way through college, I spent years 'pushing through the pain' as a professional performing artist. After suffering multiple injuries following a serious car accident, I could no longer deny the wear and tear on my body. I threw myself into an intensive summer Pilates course and fell in love with the system— it steadily began to correct years of misuse.

*My understanding of healthy exercise has deepened through the everyday discipline of Pilates, with its masterful progression, poetic athleticism, and explosive grace.*

Pilates has helped me to restore my body's strength and constantly emboldens me to strive fearlessly for truly balanced health!"

# CHAPTER 9

# *Pinpoint Pilates*

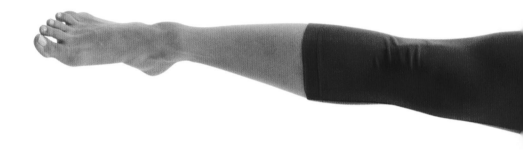

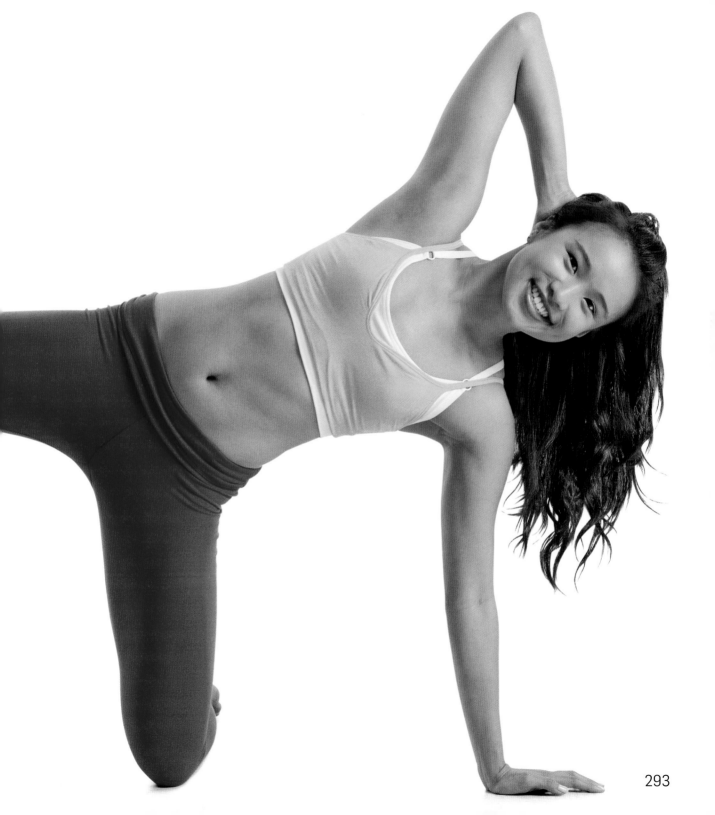

# Target and Tune-up

What makes Pilates so uniquely effective is getting our whole body under our full control without compartmentalization. However, when creating a session for a client, we, the teachers, will steer the direction of the session toward those exercises that are best suited to each student's particular needs. Oftentimes, that means finding those areas people need to work to bring their body into more balance and honing in on exercises that more greatly emphasize those particular areas. We never stop asking for the entire body to be working as a united whole; we simply pick a point or two to drive home. The following are "areas of the body" most targeted for tune-ups. Even if you don't see your particular favorite listed, do not for one second believe that it is not also receiving its quota of strength-building work. Pilates is an equal-opportunity investor in your musculature, and these series are simply pointing your mental and physical attention in a particular direction to encourage those muscles to catch up to their teammates.

Pinpoint workouts are simply a matter of knowing the muscles you want to work and then following their actions. When people tell me they "don't know how to work their abs," I know it's mostly a matter of not knowing what muscles are in there and what their jobs are. Once you know that muscle ends are pulled toward one another for strengthening, pulled away from one another for lengthening, and held in between for stabilization, then you are well on your way to eradicating "I don't know how" from your vocabulary.

I've sorted through the Pilates matwork to find the exercises and their variations that best fulfill the requirements above to create a Mains series for you. I've also added targeted Starters and Enders that you can choose to add to your workout depending on how you're feeling that day and your time constraints. For best results, do what feels right for your body and keep your mind focused on the muscle task at hand. If the work of an exercise seems to be escaping from the pinpointed area you're looking for, simply use your mind to coax it back into the fold.

# Abs

As you're aware by now, all Pilates moves are fueled by the abdominal muscles of the powerhouse. However, sometimes we still manage to use less desirable and less efficient muscles to achieve the exercise "picture." Here you'll get a better understanding of where your abdominal muscles are and what they do. And I have created a workout for you with selected exercises that make escaping abdominal use impossible.

## KEY MUSCLES OF YOUR ABS

* Rectus abdominis (your six-pack) pulls chest and pubic bone toward one another (as in a Roll-Up).

* Internal and external obliques draw together opposing ribs and hips (as in the Saw).

* Transversus abdominis cinches your midsection like a corset. (It owns the majority share in "Pull abs in and up.")

* Psoas flexes torso to thigh and thigh to torso (as in the Teasers).

*"The Pilates system is based on the idea that you consider the whole body, which means that the routine is not just to focus on an injury or a problem; the routine uses the whole body in every exercise."*
—Pilates elder Bruce King

# *Pinpoint Pilates: Abs*

## Starters

**1**

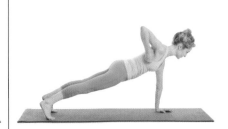

**Knee-Ins**
(page 169)

**2**

**Mountain Climbers**
(page 169)

**3**

**Pushup
with a Dumbbell Row**
(page 172)

**4**

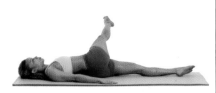

**Single-Leg Circles I:
Hip Off**
(page 65)

**5**

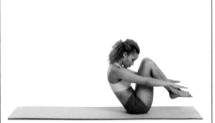

**Rolling Like a Ball**
Hands free
(page 91)

**6**

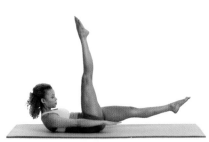

**Single-Leg Stretch**
Hands free
(page 66)

# Mains

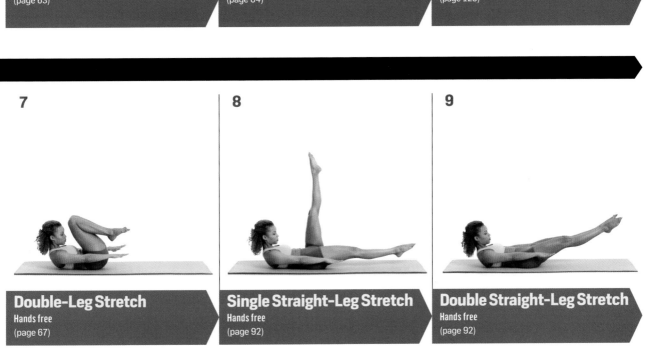

**1**

**The Hundred**
(page 63)

**2**

**Roll-Up**
(page 64)

**3**

**Rollover I**
(page 123)

**7**

**Double-Leg Stretch**
Hands free
(page 67)

**8**

**Single Straight-Leg Stretch**
Hands free
(page 92)

**9**

**Double Straight-Leg Stretch**
Hands free
(page 92)

## Mains *cont'd*

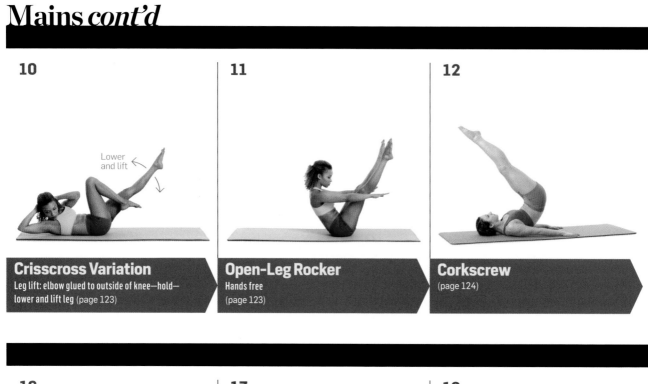

**10**

Lower and lift

**Crisscross Variation**
Leg lift: elbow glued to outside of knee—hold—lower and lift leg (page 123)

**11**

**Open-Leg Rocker**
Hands free
(page 123)

**12**

**Corkscrew**
(page 124)

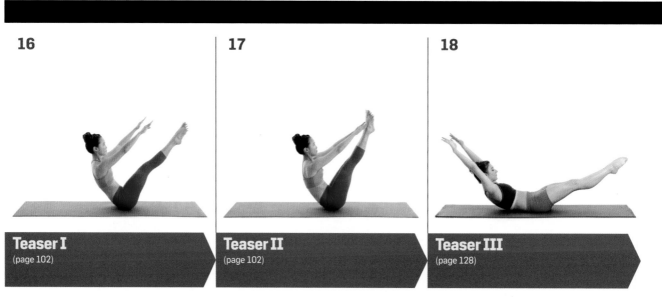

**16**

**Teaser I**
(page 102)

**17**

**Teaser II**
(page 102)

**18**

**Teaser III**
(page 128)

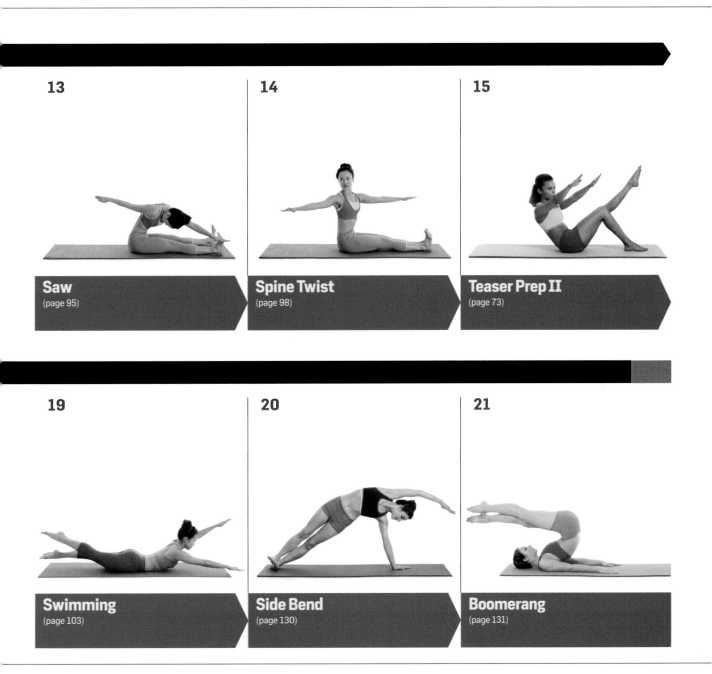

**13**

**Saw**
(page 95)

**14**

**Spine Twist**
(page 98)

**15**

**Teaser Prep II**
(page 73)

**19**

**Swimming**
(page 103)

**20**

**Side Bend**
(page 130)

**21**

**Boomerang**
(page 131)

# *Pinpoint Pilates: Abs*

## Enders

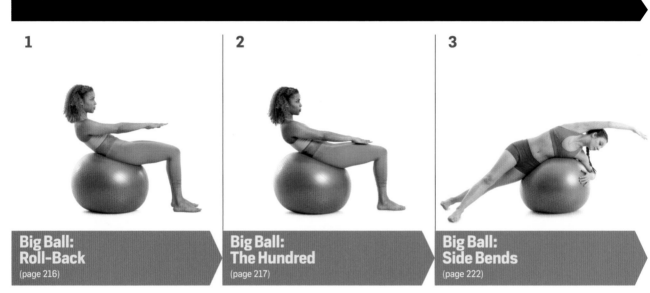

**1**

**Big Ball:**
**Roll-Back**
(page 216)

**2**

**Big Ball:**
**The Hundred**
(page 217)

**3**

**Big Ball:**
**Side Bends**
(page 222)

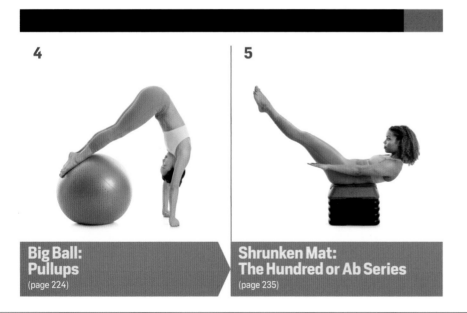

**4**

**Big Ball:**
**Pullups**
(page 224)

**5**

**Shrunken Mat:**
**The Hundred or Ab Series**
(page 235)

# Back

Since your back is, obviously, directly behind your front, these two areas directly affect one another, and so many of the exercises from the abs section are repeated here. Your back muscles and abdominal muscles work best with the cooperation of the other. Think of these two muscular sides of the body as a set of suspenders: If the front suspender is pulled short, then the back suspender will correspondingly be stretched long and lock out into its held position, and vice versa. To stay upright and comfortable with as little effort as possible, it's critical that we balance the two sides.

## KEY MUSCLES OF YOUR BACK

- Erector spinae group extends and side bends the spine, tips the pelvis forward (as in Rocking, Side Bends).

- Upper trapezius extends, rotates, and side bends the head; lifts your scapular "wings."

- Middle trapezius brings the shoulder blades together ("Cracks the walnut").

- Lower trapezius brings the scapular "wings" down.

- Latissimus dorsi brings the arm into the body, brings the arm back, and rotates the arm toward the midline of the body (as when lifting the arms behind you in the Boomerang).

- Quadratus lumborum "hip-hikes" (lifts the side of the hip to the rib), extends, and side bends the spine (as in the Side Bends).

# Pinpoint Pilates: Back

## Starters

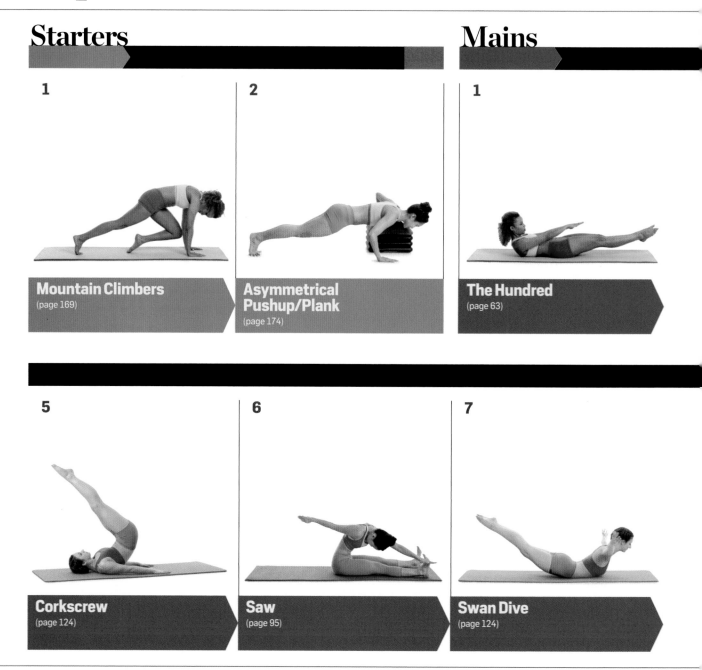

**1**

**Mountain Climbers**
(page 169)

**2**

**Asymmetrical Pushup/Plank**
(page 174)

## Mains

**1**

**The Hundred**
(page 63)

**5**

**Corkscrew**
(page 124)

**6**

**Saw**
(page 95)

**7**

**Swan Dive**
(page 124)

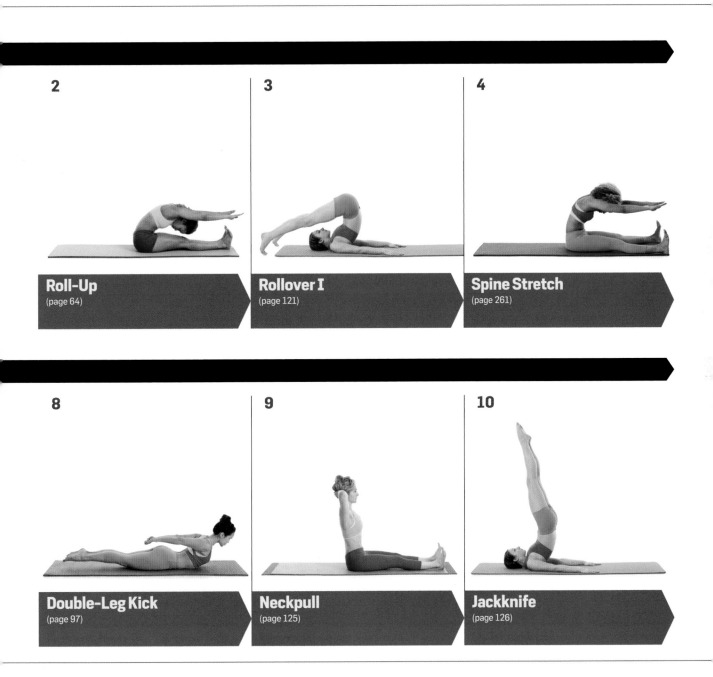

**2**

**Roll-Up**
(page 64)

**3**

**Rollover I**
(page 121)

**4**

**Spine Stretch**
(page 261)

**8**

**Double-Leg Kick**
(page 97)

**9**

**Neckpull**
(page 125)

**10**

**Jackknife**
(page 126)

## Mains *cont'd*

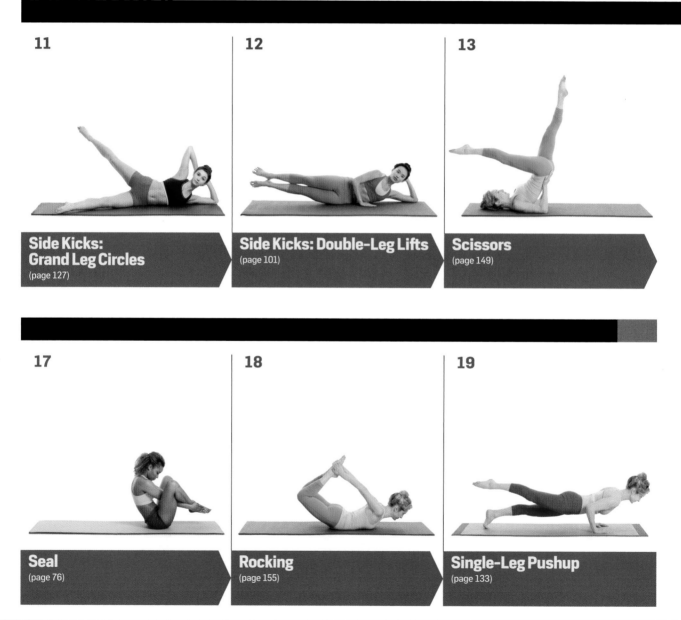

**11**

Side Kicks:
Grand Leg Circles
(page 127)

**12**

Side Kicks: Double-Leg Lifts
(page 101)

**13**

Scissors
(page 149)

**17**

Seal
(page 76)

**18**

Rocking
(page 155)

**19**

Single-Leg Pushup
(page 133)

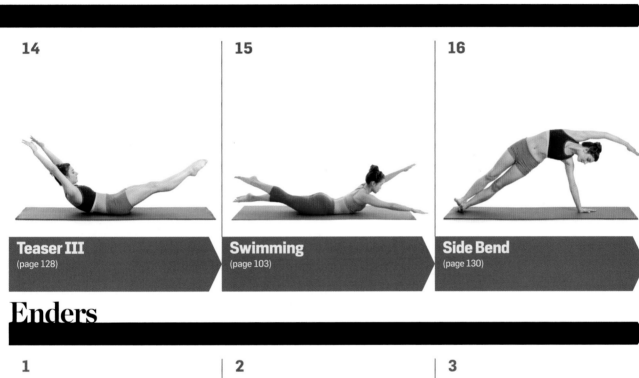

**14**

**Teaser III**
(page 128)

**15**

**Swimming**
(page 103)

**16**

**Side Bend**
(page 130)

# Enders

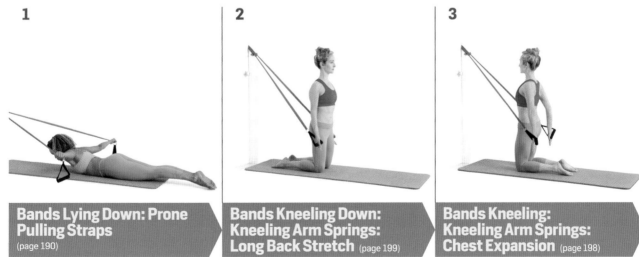

**1**

**Bands Lying Down: Prone Pulling Straps**
(page 190)

**2**

**Bands Kneeling Down: Kneeling Arm Springs: Long Back Stretch** (page 199)

**3**

**Bands Kneeling: Kneeling Arm Springs: Chest Expansion** (page 198)

# *Pinpoint Pilates: Back*

## Enders *cont'd*

**4**

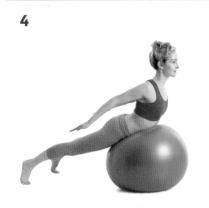

**Big Ball:
Flightless Swan**
(page 220)

**5**

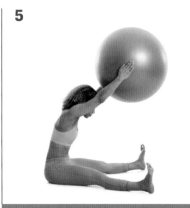

**Big Ball:
Push-Through**
(page 218)

**6**

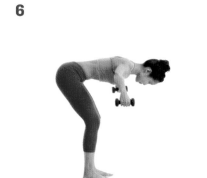

**Arm Weights**
Any "tabletop" variation, such as the Bug
(page 108)

**7**

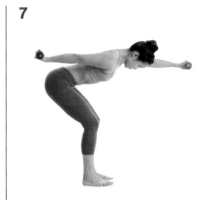

**Arm Weights: Boxing**
(page 109)

# Glutes

Everyone either has, or wishes they had, a naturally great backside. But you may not realize that if you weren't gifted one from the start, you can certainly create one now. To sculpt the perfect posterior, you'll want to strengthen from the top and the bottom without gripping. Tightening your tush on some exercises may be easier said than done; however, if you want that shapely derriere, you'll need to remember where to squeeze. For best results, work from the backs of the upper inner thighs (you could squeeze a tennis ball back there until you get the hang of it) and then follow the sequence with your attention tuned to your tush at all times.

## KEY MUSCLES OF YOUR GLUTES

- Gluteus maximus, medius, and minimus turn your thighs out in the sockets, extend your thighs behind you, and pull your thighs away from the midline of the body (as in the back swing phase of Side Kicks: Bicycle).

- Glutes also tip your pelvis under you (as in a Roll-Back).

# *Pinpoint Pilates: Glutes*

## Starters

**1**

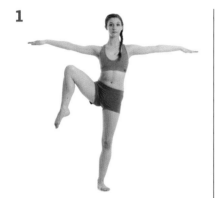

**Archival:
Knees to Elbows Side**
(page 177)

**2**

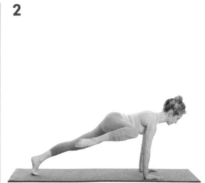

**Spider Planks**
(page 171)

**3**

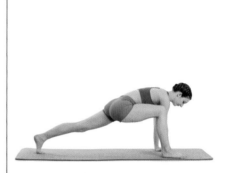

**Side-Sweeper**
(page 169)

**3**

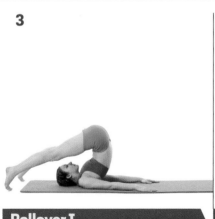

**Rollover I**
Legs wide
(page 121)

**4**

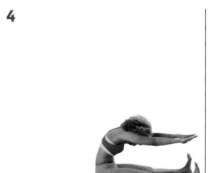

**Spine Stretch**
(page 68)

**5**

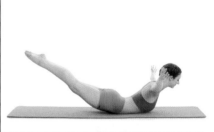

**Swan Dive**
(page 124)

# Mains

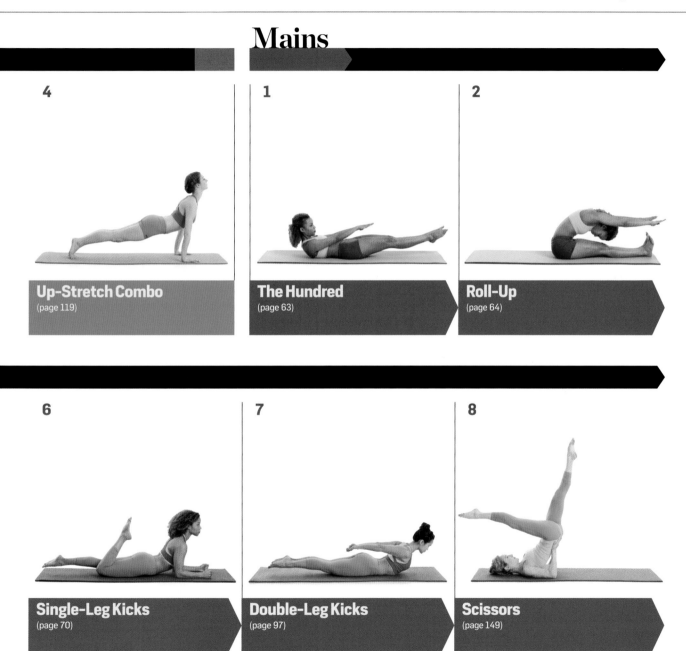

**4**

**Up-Stretch Combo**
(page 119)

**1**

**The Hundred**
(page 63)

**2**

**Roll-Up**
(page 64)

**6**

**Single-Leg Kicks**
(page 70)

**7**

**Double-Leg Kicks**
(page 97)

**8**

**Scissors**
(page 149)

# *Pinpoint Pilates: Glutes*

## Mains *cont'd*

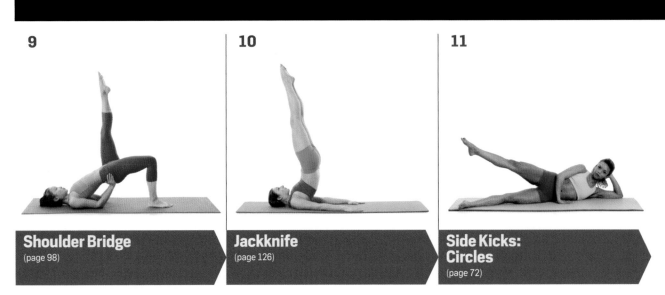

**9**
**Shoulder Bridge**
(page 98)

**10**
**Jackknife**
(page 126)

**11**
**Side Kicks: Circles**
(page 72)

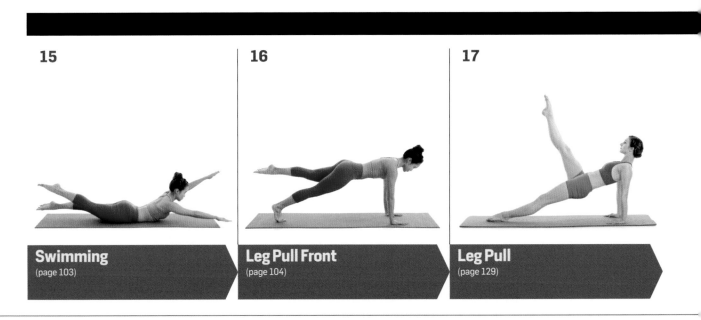

**15**
**Swimming**
(page 103)

**16**
**Leg Pull Front**
(page 104)

**17**
**Leg Pull**
(page 129)

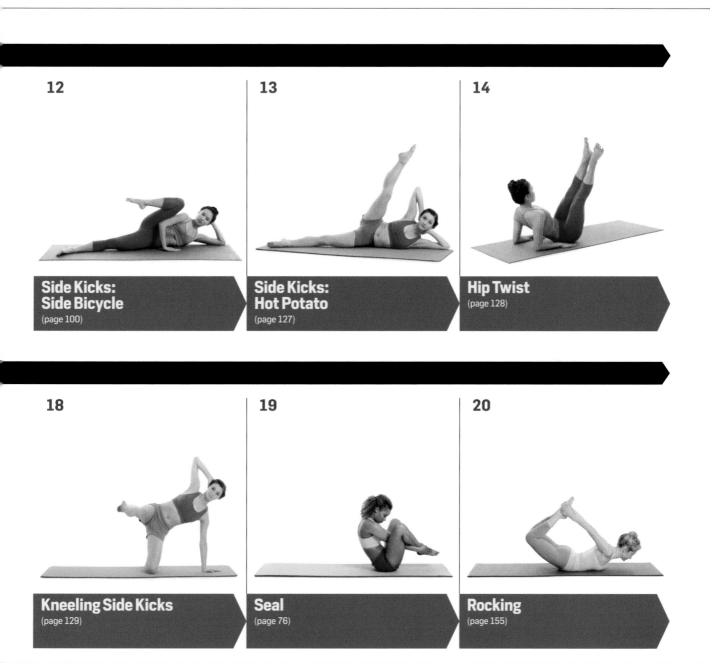

**12**

**Side Kicks:
Side Bicycle**
(page 100)

**13**

**Side Kicks:
Hot Potato**
(page 127)

**14**

**Hip Twist**
(page 128)

**18**

**Kneeling Side Kicks**
(page 129)

**19**

**Seal**
(page 76)

**20**

**Rocking**
(page 155)

# Pinpoint Pilates: Glutes

## Mains *cont'd*

**21**

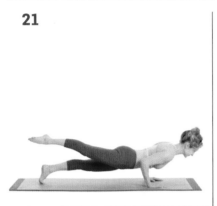

**Single-Leg Pushups**
(page 133)

## Enders

**1**

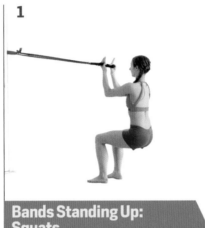

**Bands Standing Up: Squats**
(page 210)

**2**

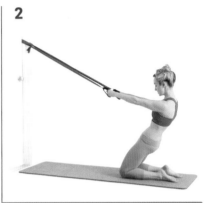

**Bands Kneeling: Kneeling Arm Springs: Thigh Stretch**
(page 200)

**6**

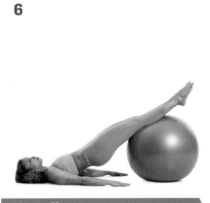

**Big Ball: Pelvic Lift**
(page 223)

**7**

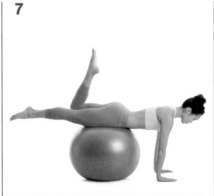

**Big Ball: Single-Leg Kicks**
(page 221)

**8**

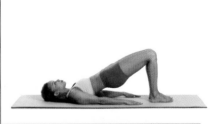

**Pelvic Lift**
(page 60)

**3**

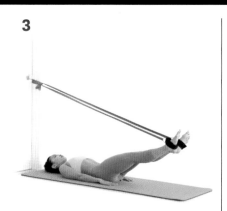

**Bands Lying Down:
Leg Spring Series**
(any or all on pages 192–93)

**4**

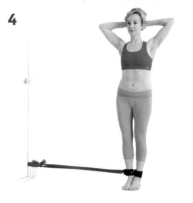

**Bands Standing Up: Standing
Side Kicks: Inner Thighs
and Outer Thighs** (page 211)

**5**

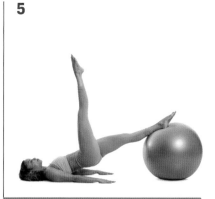

**Big Ball:
Shoulder Roll-Down**
(page 223)

**9**

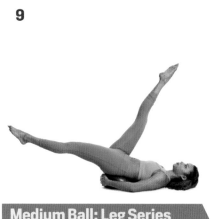

**Medium Ball: Leg Series**
Circles, Helicopter
(pages 229–31)

**10**

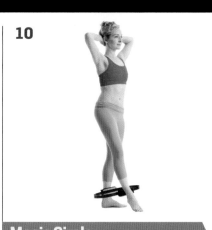

**Magic Circle
Between Ankles**
(front, side, and back on page 243)

**11**

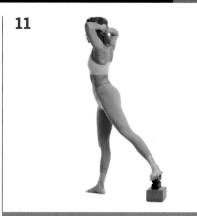

**Tensatoner Press Down Back**
(page 250)

# Arms

Between Madonna and Michelle Obama, beautiful, buff arms have caused quite a stir recently. Whether you're into tightly toned triceps or bulging biceps, or you just want to be able to arm wrestle with ease, you'll want to know the best way to go when it comes to flexing your guns. In Pilates, we see arms as extensions of your back, so when you're performing the recommended exercises, make sure you can find the deeper connection from your arms all the way down to the back of your powerhouse.

## KEY MUSCLES OF YOUR ARMS

- Biceps bend the elbow and flex the upper arm at the shoulder (as in Biceps Curl).

- Triceps straighten the elbow and extend the upper arm at the shoulder (bring it behind you, as in Triceps Extension).

- Deltoids are arm lifters in all directions, especially out to the sides (as in Wall: Squats with Wings).

# Starters

**1**

**Wave**
(page 118)

**2**

**Asymmetrical Pushup/Plank**
(page 174)

**3**

**Pushup with a Dumbbell Row**
(page 172)

# Mains

**4**

**Superman Plank**
(page 171)

**5**

**Side Planks**
(page 171)

**1**

**The Hundred: With Weighted Pole**
(page 63)

## Mains *cont'd*

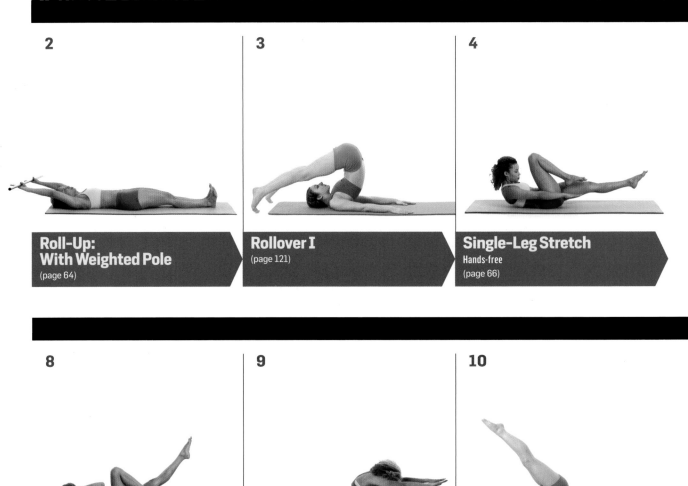

**2**

**Roll-Up:
With Weighted Pole**
(page 64)

**3**

**Rollover I**
(page 121)

**4**

**Single-Leg Stretch**
Hands-free
(page 66)

**8**

**Crisscross**
(page 123)

**9**

**Spine Stretch**
(page 68)

**10**

**Corkscrew**
(page 124)

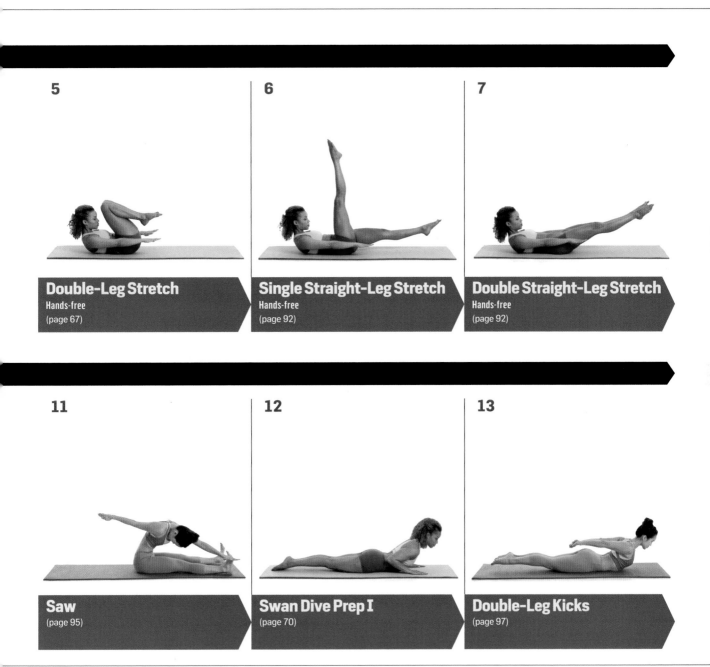

**5**

**Double-Leg Stretch**
Hands-free
(page 67)

**6**

**Single Straight-Leg Stretch**
Hands-free
(page 92)

**7**

**Double Straight-Leg Stretch**
Hands-free
(page 92)

**11**

**Saw**
(page 95)

**12**

**Swan Dive Prep I**
(page 70)

**13**

**Double-Leg Kicks**
(page 97)

# Pinpoint Pilates: Arms

## Mains *cont'd*

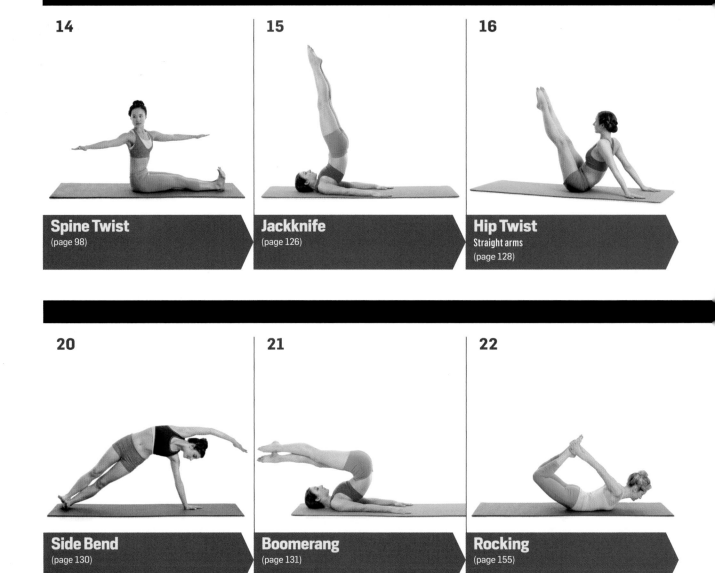

**14**

**Spine Twist**
(page 98)

**15**

**Jackknife**
(page 126)

**16**

**Hip Twist**
Straight arms
(page 128)

**20**

**Side Bend**
(page 130)

**21**

**Boomerang**
(page 131)

**22**

**Rocking**
(page 155)

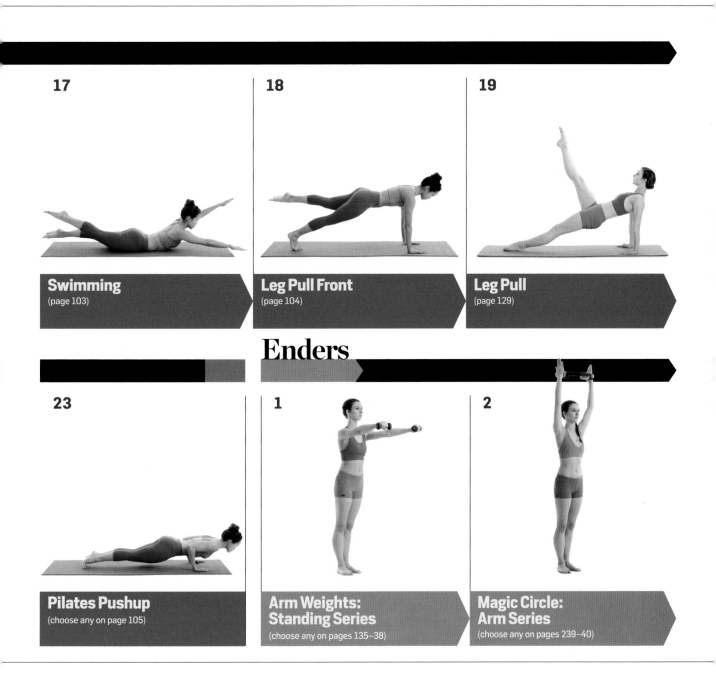

**17**

**Swimming**
(page 103)

**18**

**Leg Pull Front**
(page 104)

**19**

**Leg Pull**
(page 129)

# Enders

**23**

**Pilates Pushup**
(choose any on page 105)

**1**

**Arm Weights:
Standing Series**
(choose any on pages 135–38)

**2**

**Magic Circle:
Arm Series**
(choose any on pages 239–40)

## Enders *cont'd*

**3**

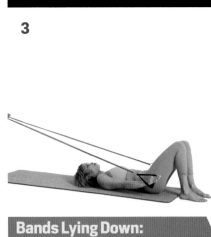

**Bands Lying Down:
Arm Spring Series**
(pages 187–90)

**4**

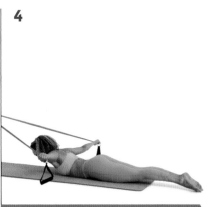

**Bands Lying Down:
Prone: Pulling Straps**
(page 190)

**5**

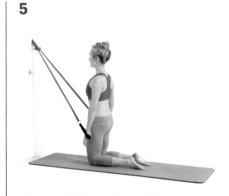

**Bands Kneeling Down:
Kneeling Arm Springs:
Chest Expansion** (page 198)

**9**

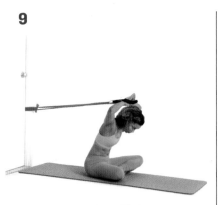

**Bands Sitting Up:
Rowing Shave**
(page 195)

**10**

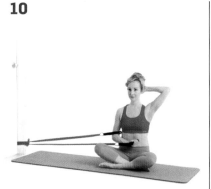

**Bands Sitting Up:
Door Closers:
Internal Rotators** (page 197)

**11**

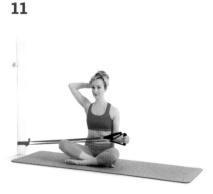

**Bands Sitting Up:
Door Openers:
External Rotators** (page 197)

**6**

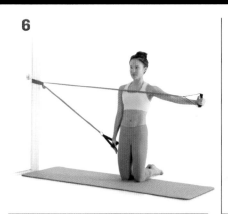

**Bands Kneeling Down:
Swakate Series**
(any or all on pages 202–3)

**7**

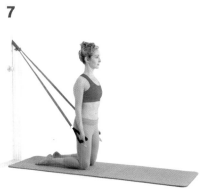

**Bands Kneeling Down:
Kneeling Arms Springs:
Long Back Stretch** (page 199)

**8**

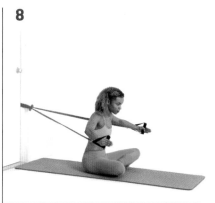

**Bands Sitting Up:
Rowing Hug**
(page 196)

**12**

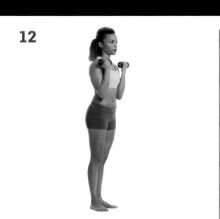

**Biceps Curls**
(pages 82–83)

**13**

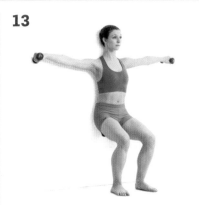

**Wall:
Squats with Wings**
(page 138)

**14**

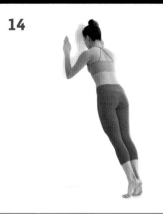

**Wall:
Pushoffs**
(page 112)

# Thighs

Because of the way we move on a daily basis, there are thigh muscles that get more action than others. For example, walking, running, and going up and down stairs can all draw from many more muscles than they do. However, most people predominantly use their quadriceps muscles because that's where it's easiest to default in your thinking. Of course, Pilates asks you to widen the scope of your thinking. Thus, when trying the following sequence, make sure to include all the muscles of the thigh—front, back, and sides— so you can work from a place of balance and efficiency.

## KEY MUSCLES OF YOUR THIGHS

- Hamstrings bend your knee, bring your thigh backward, tip your pelvis under you (posterior) (as in Single-Leg Kicks done properly).

- Quadriceps femoris ("quads") straighten your knees, flex your thigh at the hip, tip your pelvis forward (anterior). ("Soften your knees" translates to lessening the work coming from your quads and spreading the wealth.)

- Adductors bring your thighs toward your midline ("squeeze your inner thighs together tightly").

- Abductor group (TFL/ sartorious) moves your thighs away from your midline (as in Side Kicks: Up/Down).

# Starters

**1**

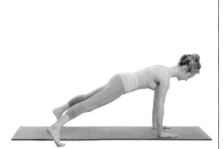

**Plank Jacks**
(page 170)

**2**

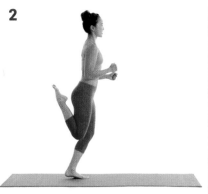

**Jogging Knees Up/Heels Up**
(page 89)

**3**

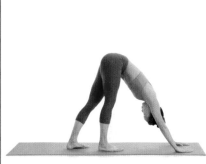

**Elephant Planks**
(page 87)

**4**

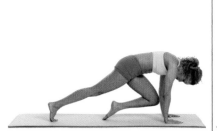

**Mountain Climbers**
(page 169)

**5**

**Squat-Thrusts**
(page 172)

# Mains

**1**

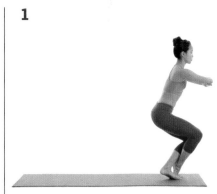

**Lowering Down to the Mat**
(page 91)

# *Pinpoint Pilates: Thighs*

## Mains *cont'd*

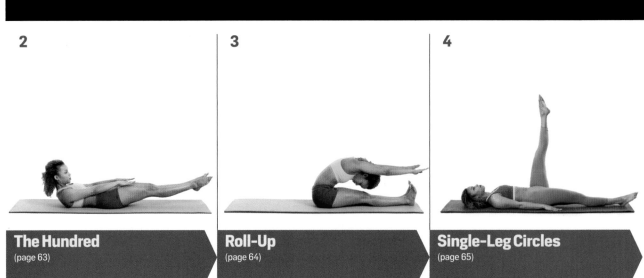

**2**
**The Hundred**
(page 63)

**3**
**Roll-Up**
(page 64)

**4**
**Single-Leg Circles**
(page 65)

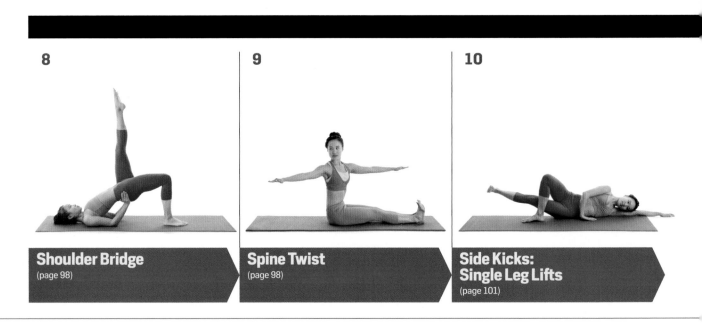

**8**
**Shoulder Bridge**
(page 98)

**9**
**Spine Twist**
(page 98)

**10**
**Side Kicks:
Single Leg Lifts**
(page 101)

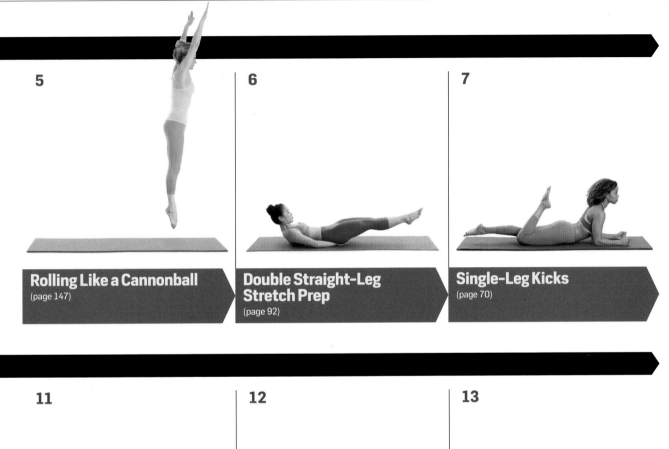

**5**

**Rolling Like a Cannonball**
(page 147)

**6**

**Double Straight-Leg
Stretch Prep**
(page 92)

**7**

**Single-Leg Kicks**
(page 70)

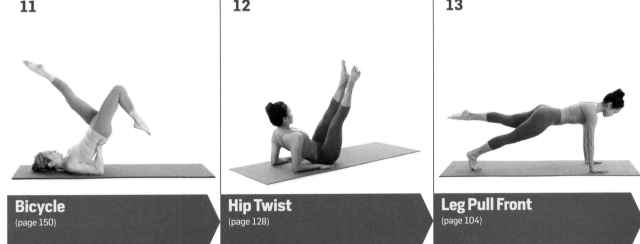

**11**

**Bicycle**
(page 150)

**12**

**Hip Twist**
(page 128)

**13**

**Leg Pull Front**
(page 104)

# *Pinpoint Pilates: Thighs*

## Mains *cont'd*

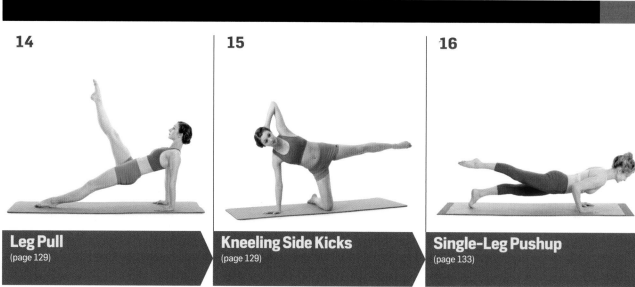

**14**

**Leg Pull**
(page 129)

**15**

**Kneeling Side Kicks**
(page 129)

**16**

**Single-Leg Pushup**
(page 133)

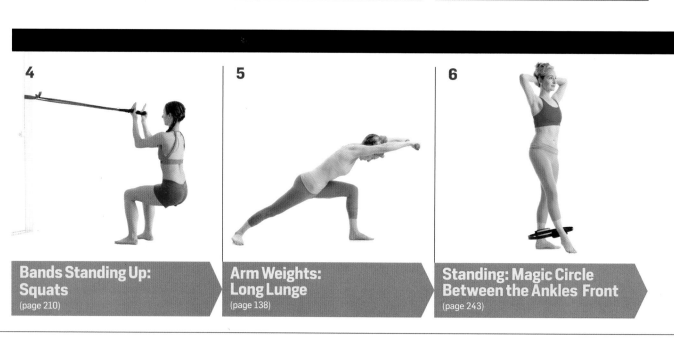

**4**

**Bands Standing Up: Squats**
(page 210)

**5**

**Arm Weights: Long Lunge**
(page 138)

**6**

**Standing: Magic Circle Between the Ankles Front**
(page 243)

# Enders

**1**

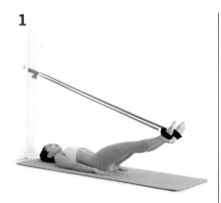

**Bands Lying Down:
Leg Springs**
(any or all on pages 192–93)

**2**

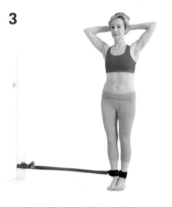

**Bands Kneeling Down:
Thigh Stretch**
(page 200)

**3**

**Bands Standing Up:
Inner Thighs**
(page 211)

**7**

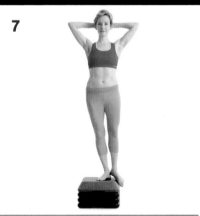

**Steps: Going Up Side**
(page 234)

**8**

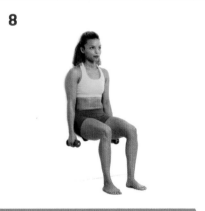

**Wall:
Squats**
(page 80)

**9**

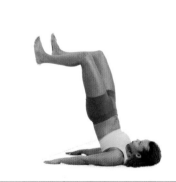

**Pelvic Lifts:
Drive You Up a Wall**
(page 261)

# Legs/Feet

The connection of your legs to your feet is a critical one, because any and all compensatory patterns happening down below eventually creep their way steadily upward into knees, hips, and onward. By maintaining a strong and supple lower leg, your connection to the earth is rooted and you are better able to manage the building blocks of your body stacked above. During this series, stay very aware of your feet: Point and flex from the ankle on as many occasions as you can, and, when flat on the mat, make sure all points of the foot are pressing evenly. Refer to "Meet Your Feet" on page 253 for more on how to press into all points of the foot.

## KEY MUSCLES OF YOUR LEGS/FEET

- Gastrocnemius and soleus (calf muscles): Both point the foot at the ankle, and the gastroc also bends the knee.

- Fibularis group (outside of lower leg): Two of these muscles point the foot and one of them flexes it. All three evert (roll the ankles in) and stabilize the ankle when strong.

- Tibialis and extensors (shin muscles): All flex the foot at the ankle.

# Starters

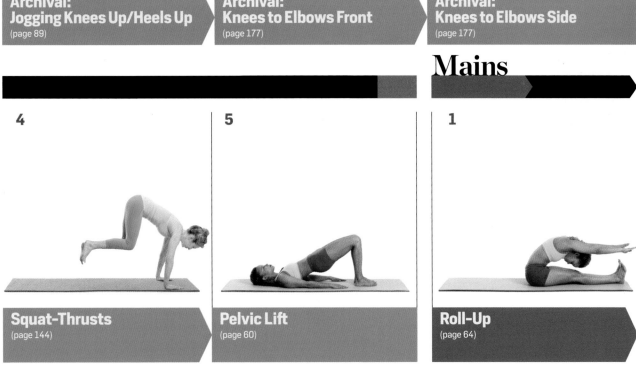

**1**

**Archival:
Jogging Knees Up/Heels Up**
(page 89)

**2**

**Archival:
Knees to Elbows Front**
(page 177)

**3**

**Archival:
Knees to Elbows Side**
(page 177)

# Mains

**4**

**Squat-Thrusts**
(page 144)

**5**

**Pelvic Lift**
(page 60)

**1**

**Roll-Up**
(page 64)

# Pinpoint Pilates: Legs and Feet

## Mains *cont'd*

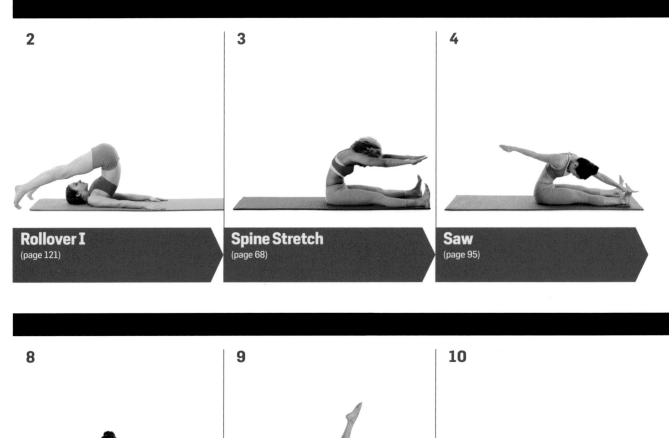

**2**

**Rollover I**
(page 121)

**3**

**Spine Stretch**
(page 68)

**4**

**Saw**
(page 95)

**8**

**Spine Twist**
(page 98)

**9**

**Side Kicks: Up/Down**
(page 72)

**10**

**Side Kicks: Bicycle**
(page 126)

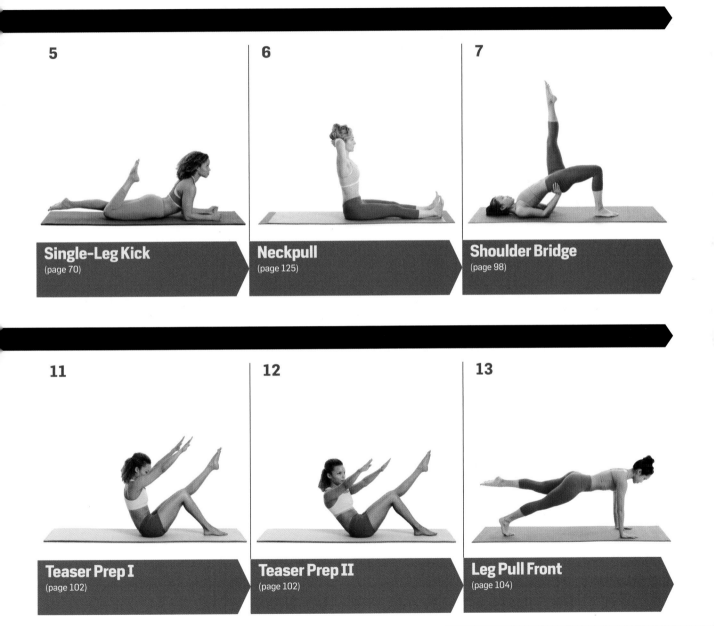

**5**

**Single-Leg Kick**
(page 70)

**6**

**Neckpull**
(page 125)

**7**

**Shoulder Bridge**
(page 98)

**11**

**Teaser Prep I**
(page 102)

**12**

**Teaser Prep II**
(page 102)

**13**

**Leg Pull Front**
(page 104)

# *Pinpoint Pilates: Legs and Feet*

## Mains *cont'd*

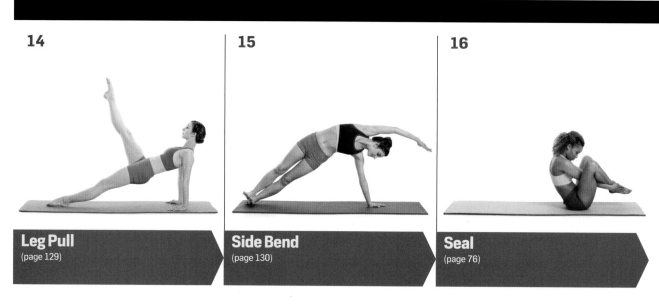

**14**

**Leg Pull**
(page 129)

**15**

**Side Bend**
(page 130)

**16**

**Seal**
(page 76)

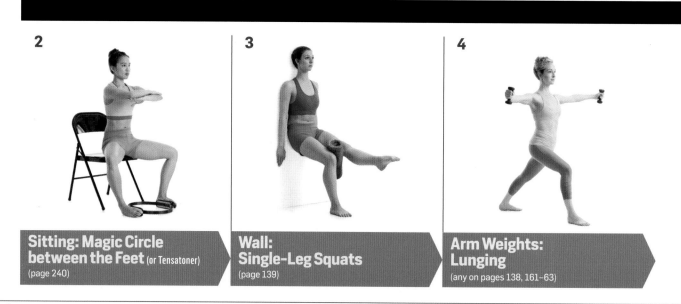

**2**

**Sitting: Magic Circle between the Feet** (or Tensatoner)
(page 240)

**3**

**Wall: Single-Leg Squats**
(page 139)

**4**

**Arm Weights: Lunging**
(any on pages 138, 161–63)

# Enders

**17**

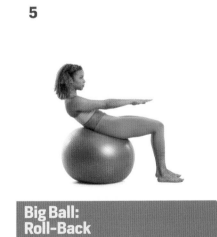

**Pilates Pushup**
(page 105)

**18**

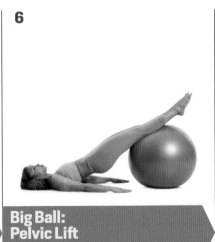

**Single-Leg Pushup**
(page 133)

**1**

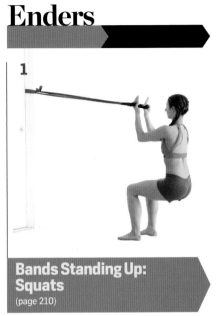

**Bands Standing Up:
Squats**
(page 210)

**5**

**Big Ball:
Roll-Back**
(page 216)

**6**

**Big Ball:
Pelvic Lift**
(page 223)

**7**

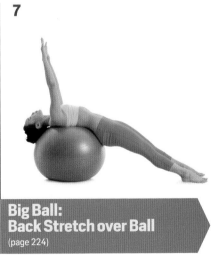

**Big Ball:
Back Stretch over Ball**
(page 224)

# Pinpoint Pilates: Legs and Feet

## Enders cont'd

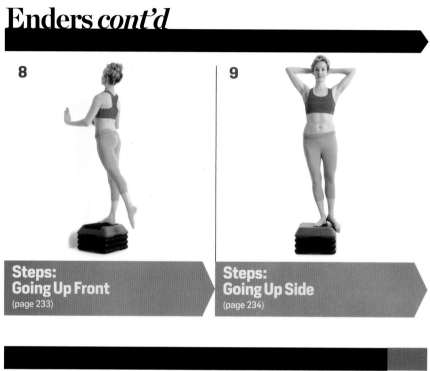

**8**

**Steps:
Going Up Front**
(page 233)

**9**

**Steps:
Going Up Side**
(page 234)

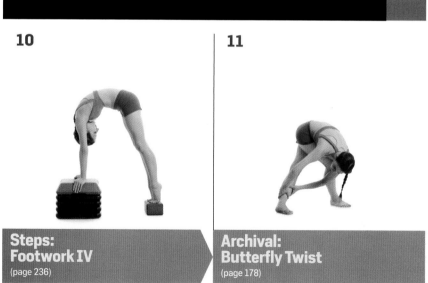

**10**

**Steps:
Footwork IV**
(page 236)

**11**

**Archival:
Butterfly Twist**
(page 178)

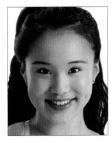

Katie is a current trainee of Brooke Siler's re:AB Pilates Teacher Training Program.

# Katie Yip

"Coming from a background in competitive soccer, I was surprised at how much Pilates challenged me physically, mentally, and emotionally. My weaknesses became apparent, and I realized how little control I actually had over my body.

*Through my studies and practice, I have learned that Pilates is more than just a form of exercise; it has taught me to take responsibility for myself and to exercise discipline and control in all facets of my life.*

It has given me the confidence to achieve whatever I set out to accomplish because I am no longer confined by my body's limitations. With Pilates under your belt, who's to say what you can't do?"

CHAPTER 10
# *Pilates by Purpose*

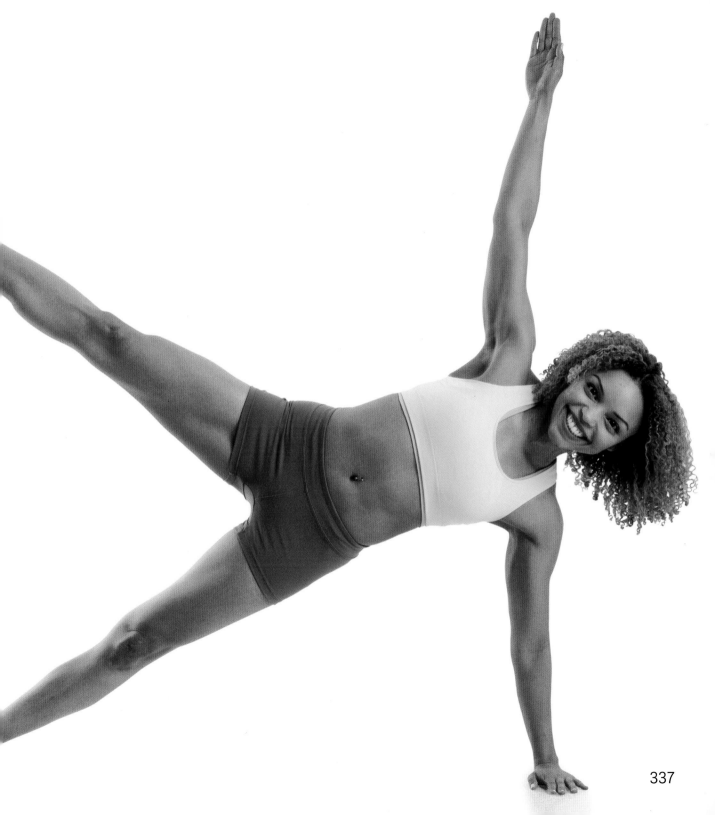

337

# Fitness Goals

This chapter is goal oriented. You should be able to track your progress as you practice. In fact, you may want to come up with some small ability tests for yourself (such as how long you can hold your breath, how long you can hold a plank position, etc.). Write the answers down. After trying your selected series three or four times a week (more if you're game!), check again and see if you are making strides toward your goal.

To help you choose a series to start, I've created a quick awareness test. If you answer yes to a statement, try the corresponding workouts to help improve you in that area. If you have many categories to work on, simply choose one to focus on today and see if it's a good fit.

## Fitness Awareness Test

1. I tend to be cold all the time. A

2. I get winded walking up a flight of stairs. A B

3. I have a job that has me sitting most of the day. A C

4. I tend to hold my breath throughout the day or breathe in a very shallow manner. B

5. My shoulders tend to round forward, and my chest is slightly concave. B

6. I get stitches (side pains) if/when I run. B

7. I can't reach the middle of my back between my shoulder blades. C

8. I feel stiff most of the time. C

9. I can't touch my toes. C

10. I can touch my toes easily. D

11. I am called Gumby by friends. D

12. I can't do a pushup. D

13. I frequently trip over things. D

A = **Better Calorie Burn**

B = **Better Endurance Series**

C = **Better Flexibility Series**

D = **Better Strength Series**

# Better Cardio and Calorie Burn

Quite simply, the more you work and build your muscles, the more calories you burn. Add weighted moves (like pushups and planks) as transitions for an even bigger fat-blasting effect!

* Do not stop the rhythm of your workout.

* Add lots of up-and-down movements (i.e., go from mat to standing whenever the opportunity arises).

* Lifting your arms up above your heart forces your heart to pump harder.

* Add resistance to build muscle.

* Work on making transitions seamless and efficient. (For example, have your weights ready to go so there is no stopping.)

* This series will eventually take under 20 minutes to complete.

*"A few well-designed movements, properly performed in a balanced sequence, are worth hours of doing sloppy calisthentics or forced contortion."* —Joe Pilates

# *Pilates by Purpose: Better Cardio and Calorie Burn*

## Starters

**1**

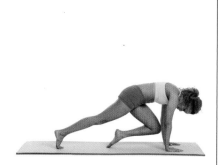

**Mountain Climbers**
(page 169)

**2**

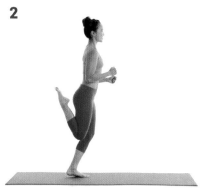

**Jogging Knees Up/Heels Up**
(page 89)

**3**

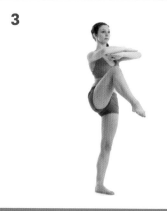

**Archival:
Knees to Elbows Front**
(page 177)

## Mains

**1**

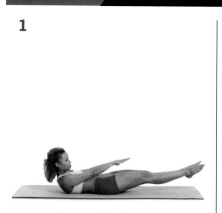

**The Hundred**
(page 63)

**2**

**Roll-Up**
(page 64)

**3**

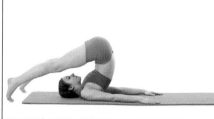

**Rollover I**
(page 123)

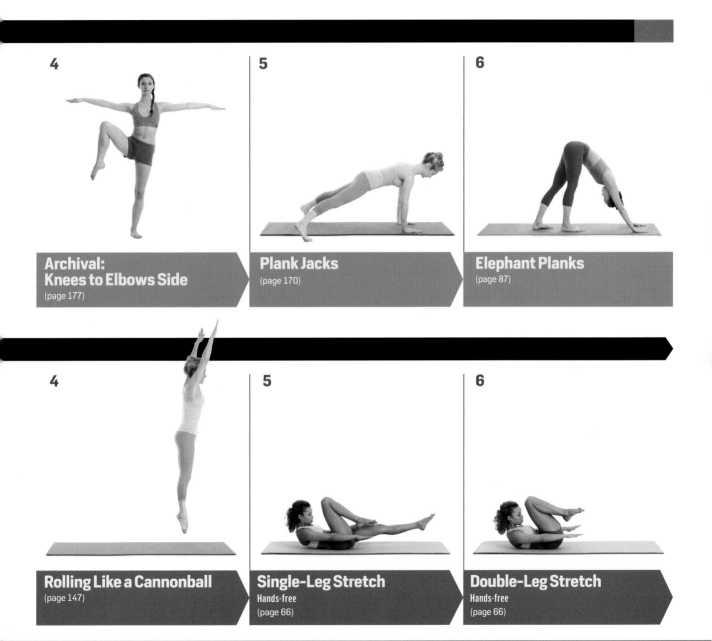

**4**

**Archival:
Knees to Elbows Side**
(page 177)

**5**

**Plank Jacks**
(page 170)

**6**

**Elephant Planks**
(page 87)

**4**

**Rolling Like a Cannonball**
(page 147)

**5**

**Single-Leg Stretch**
Hands-free
(page 66)

**6**

**Double-Leg Stretch**
Hands-free
(page 66)

## Mains *cont'd*

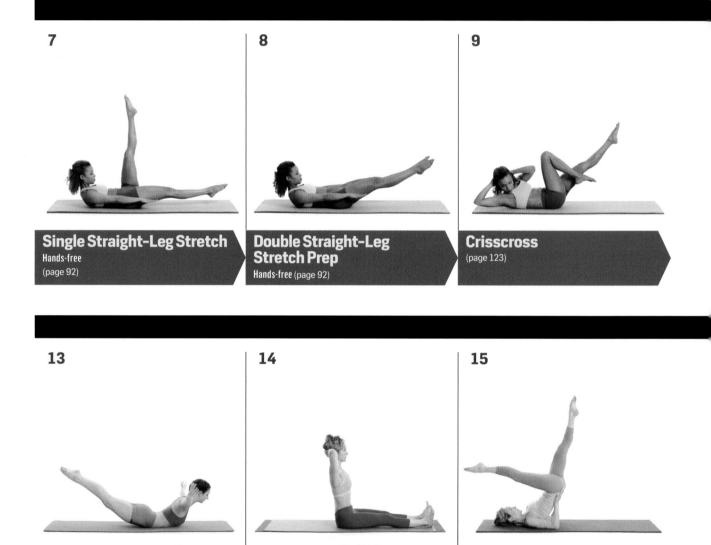

**7**

**Single Straight-Leg Stretch**
Hands-free
(page 92)

**8**

**Double Straight-Leg Stretch Prep**
Hands-free (page 92)

**9**

**Crisscross**
(page 123)

**13**

**Swan Dive**
(page 124)

**14**

**Neckpull**
(page 125)

**15**

**Scissors**
(page 149)

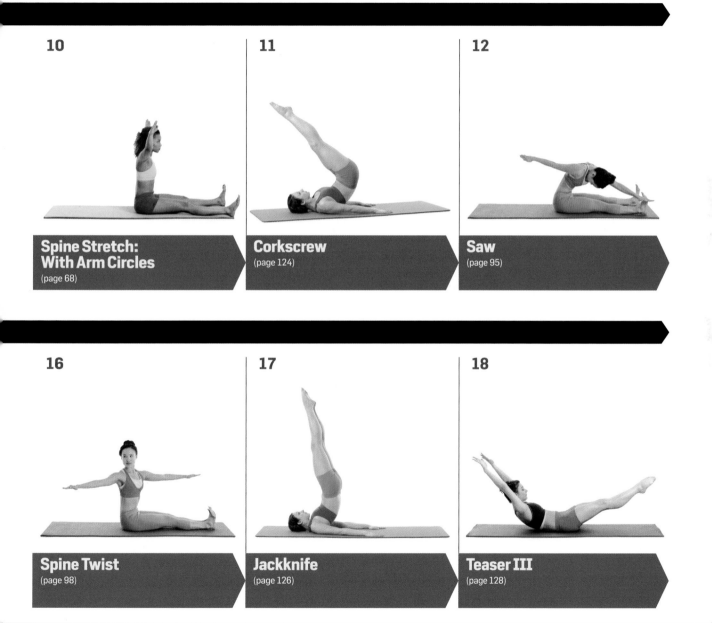

**10**
**Spine Stretch: With Arm Circles**
(page 68)

**11**
**Corkscrew**
(page 124)

**12**
**Saw**
(page 95)

**16**
**Spine Twist**
(page 98)

**17**
**Jackknife**
(page 126)

**18**
**Teaser III**
(page 128)

# Pilates by Purpose: Better Cardio and Calorie Burn

## Mains *cont'd*

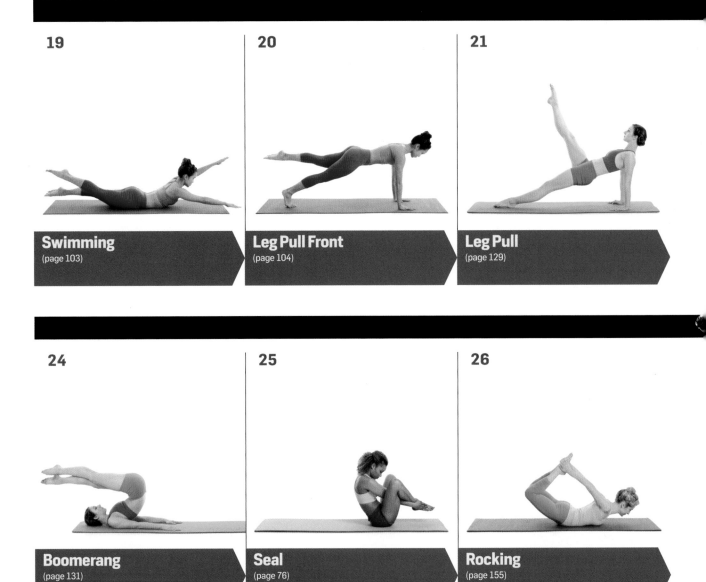

**19**

**Swimming**
(page 103)

**20**

**Leg Pull Front**
(page 104)

**21**

**Leg Pull**
(page 129)

**24**

**Boomerang**
(page 131)

**25**

**Seal**
(page 76)

**26**

**Rocking**
(page 155)

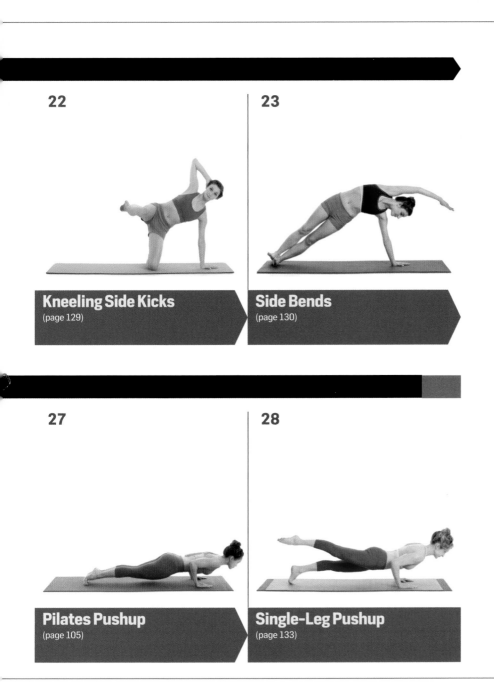

**22**

**Kneeling Side Kicks**
(page 129)

**23**

**Side Bends**
(page 130)

**27**

**Pilates Pushup**
(page 105)

**28**

**Single-Leg Pushup**
(page 133)

## TRAINER'S TIP

Another factor in increasing your oxygen capacity (maximum $VO_2$) is increasing the mitochondrial density within your muscle cells. "Mitochondria are the little powerhouses of the cell that allow for the conversion of oxygen into energy. The more mitochondria you have, the more oxygen you can utilize. Most research shows that it's the short, highly intense efforts that improve mitochondrial density, and you really don't get much benefit once you've trained for more than 1 hour at a low intensity," says Ben Greenfield, MS, a triathlete expert trainer.

# *Pilates by Purpose: Better Cardio and Calorie Burn*

## Enders

**1**

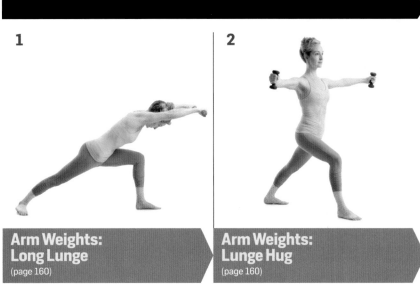

**Arm Weights:
Long Lunge**
(page 160)

**2**

**Arm Weights:
Lunge Hug**
(page 160)

**3**

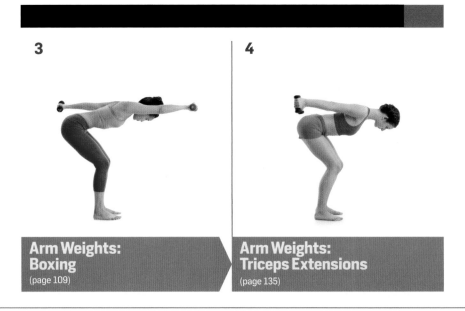

**Arm Weights:
Boxing**
(page 109)

**4**

**Arm Weights:
Triceps Extensions**
(page 135)

# Better Breathing and Endurance

Most breathing and endurance issues come from poor postural habits that compress and stiffen the musculature around your chest, neck, and ribcage, making it hard to breathe. When your respiratory muscles are weak, it is difficult to create enough volume, within the chest cavity.

## TRAINING TIPS

- Create space around your upper back, chest, and side body.

- Create space around your ribs, neck, and shoulders.

- Try different breathing patterns (holding the inspiration or holding the expiration).

- Use the rhythm of your breath to guide the movements.

- Change the rhythm from steady to fast every other exercise.

- Use your muscles to induce full exhalations and allow inhalations to "happen."

## EXPERT VOICE

The simplest way to understand the mechanics of breathing is to recognize that it is the shape-change of the belly and chest cavities. Because the spine is the back of both cavities, spinal and breath movement are inextricably linked.

Another way I like to say it is: "Breath is how we mobilize the space in our bodies, and posture is how we stabilize our bodies in space."

Therefore, well-coordinated breath is synonymous with well-coordinated postural support because you cannot have one without the other. That is why a natural system of exercise, whether it's Pilates, yoga, or any another breath-centered method, is the best way to have efficient posture, freer breath, and more graceful movement.

—LESLIE KAMINOFF,
yoga educator

# *Pilates by Purpose: Better Breathing and Endurance*

## Starters

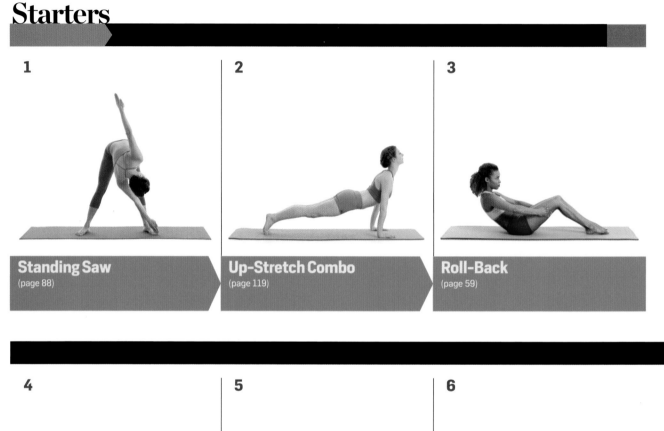

**1**

**Standing Saw**
(page 88)

**2**

**Up-Stretch Combo**
(page 119)

**3**

**Roll-Back**
(page 59)

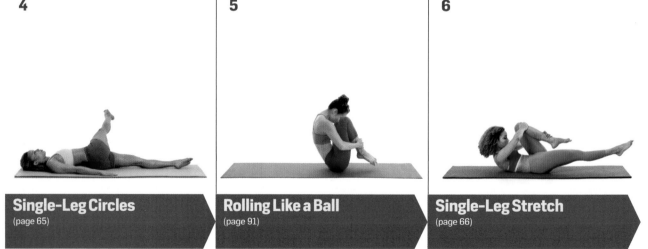

**4**

**Single-Leg Circles**
(page 65)

**5**

**Rolling Like a Ball**
(page 91)

**6**

**Single-Leg Stretch**
(page 66)

# Mains

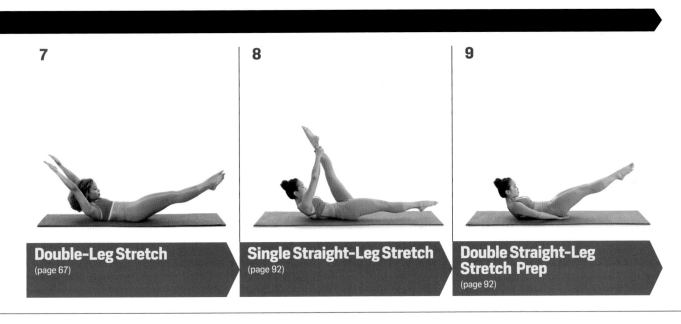

**1**

**The Hundred**
(page 63)

**2**

**Roll-Up**
(page 64)

**3**

**Rollover I**
(page 121)

**7**

**Double-Leg Stretch**
(page 67)

**8**

**Single Straight-Leg Stretch**
(page 92)

**9**

**Double Straight-Leg Stretch Prep**
(page 92)

## Mains *cont'd*

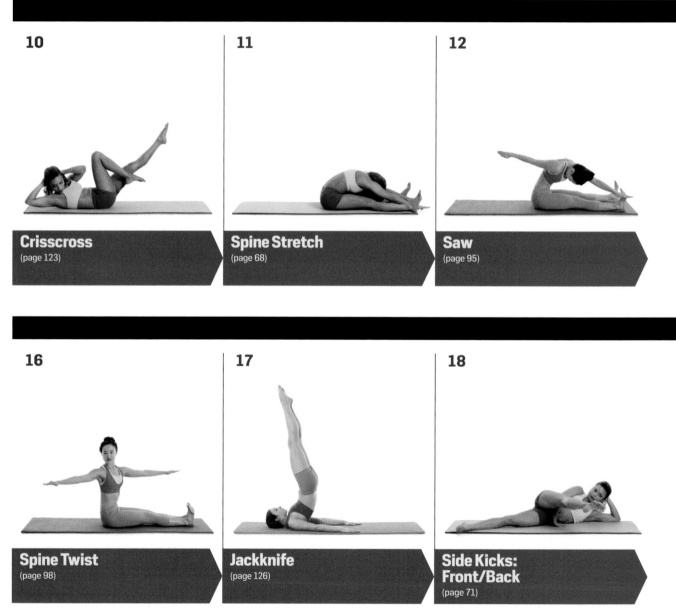

**10**

**Crisscross**
(page 123)

**11**

**Spine Stretch**
(page 68)

**12**

**Saw**
(page 95)

**16**

**Spine Twist**
(page 98)

**17**

**Jackknife**
(page 126)

**18**

**Side Kicks: Front/Back**
(page 71)

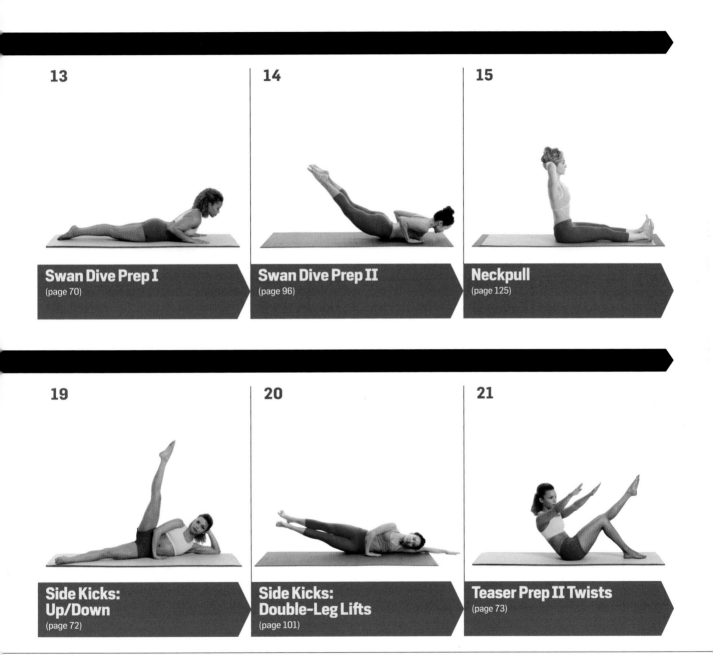

**13**

**Swan Dive Prep I**
(page 70)

**14**

**Swan Dive Prep II**
(page 96)

**15**

**Neckpull**
(page 125)

**19**

**Side Kicks:
Up/Down**
(page 72)

**20**

**Side Kicks:
Double-Leg Lifts**
(page 101)

**21**

**Teaser Prep II Twists**
(page 73)

# *Pilates by Purpose: Better Breathing and Endurance*

## Mains *cont'd*

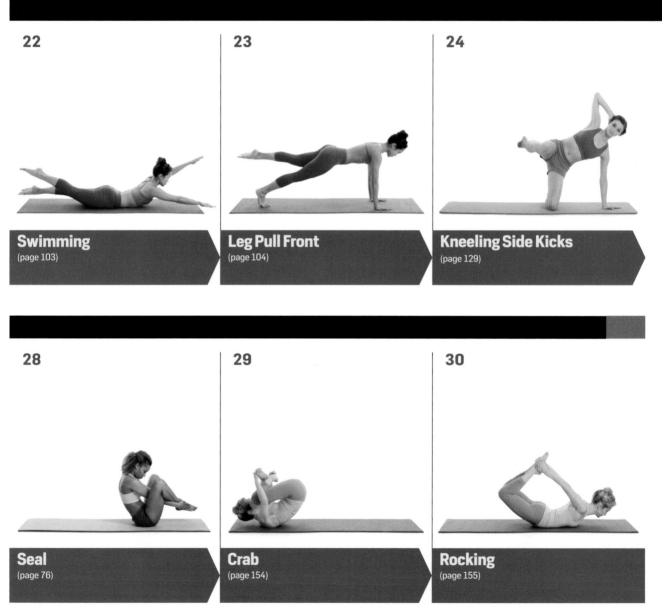

**22**

**Swimming**
(page 103)

**23**

**Leg Pull Front**
(page 104)

**24**

**Kneeling Side Kicks**
(page 129)

**28**

**Seal**
(page 76)

**29**

**Crab**
(page 154)

**30**

**Rocking**
(page 155)

**25**

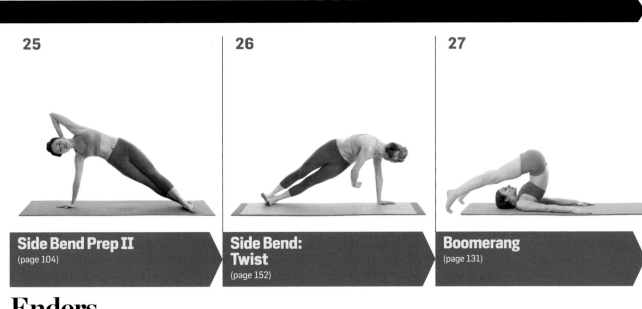

**Side Bend Prep II**
(page 104)

**26**

**Side Bend:
Twist**
(page 152)

**27**

**Boomerang**
(page 131)

# Enders

**1**

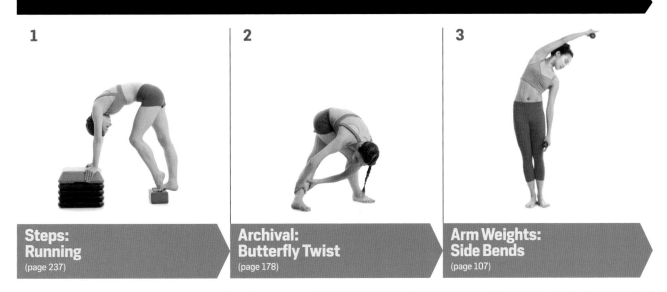

**Steps:
Running**
(page 237)

**2**

**Archival:
Butterfly Twist**
(page 178)

**3**

**Arm Weights:
Side Bends**
(page 107)

## Enders *cont'd*

**4**

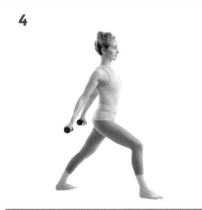

**Arm Weights:
Lunge Chest Expansion**
Twisting Arms (page 102)

**5**

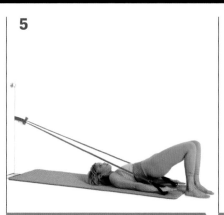

**Bands Lying Down:
Supine: Chest Expansion**
(page 188)

**6**

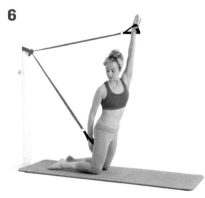

**Bands Kneeling Down:
Butterfly**
(page 200)

**7**

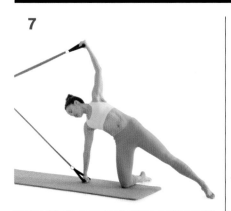

**Bands Kneeling Down:
Side Bend Arm Circles**
from Swakate Series (page 203)

**8**

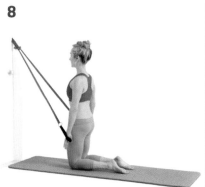

**Bands Kneeling Down:
Chest Expansion**
(page 198)

**9**

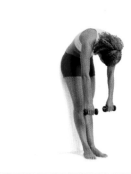

**Wall: Roll-Down**
(page 81)

# Better Flexibility and Mobility

These exercises heat your body from the inside out, increasing your range of motion, offering different types of stretching (static, dynamic, and more), and using unique methods of stretching to improve your overall flexibility. Bend away!

*"True flexibility can be achieved only when all muscles are uniformly developed."*—Joe Pilates

## TRAINING TIPS

* To best heat your body, a quicker pace may do; however, if you are very tight (such as first thing in the morning), you may want to hold back a bit.

* If your knees are bent, so be it! Don't push into positions that may strain. Work with what's available to you in the moment.

* Keep a band, strap, or towel nearby for assistance with some of the static stretches.

* After you feel you've outgrown "preps," take them to your rightful level.

## EXPERT VOICE

There are many factors that go into a healthy musculoskeletal system; however, the most important three are strength of musculature, flexibility of soft tissue, and proper neural control.

Muscle strength is often thought of in terms of how much weight we can lift or how fast or far we can run. However, there is another component to muscle strength that is much more important to health; that is how strong our "intrinsic" muscles are. Intrinsic muscles do not show on the outside; they are not the larger better-known muscles like the biceps or pectoralis major. Rather, they are smaller muscles located deeper in the body around the joints. Although it is important to strengthen all muscles of the body, strengthening the core intrinsic musculature is actually the most important because it protects and stabilizes our joints.

Soft tissue flexibility refers to having muscles, tendons, ligaments, and other fascial tissues that can lengthen out and be stretched. This is important because every time we contract a muscle to move our body, the muscles and other soft tissues located on the other side of the joint muscle lengthen to allow the motion to occur. Therefore, flexibility allows us to have mobility.

Stability and flexibility are antagonistic concepts: More of one is less of the other, and vice versa. However, they are both equally important to health; it is important to have a balance between them.

There is an old saying in the world of Pilates: "It is not how many; it is how." In other words, it is not the quantity of the movement that is important, but rather the quality of the movement pattern. This comes from our nervous system and is known as neural control. Each movement pattern that we create is actually the product of our nervous system ordering many muscles to contract together. In fact, when we say that a person is coordinated, what we are really saying is that the person's nervous system can co-order muscles to create efficient and graceful movements.

Putting together strength with flexibility and neural control is the key to not only a strong and graceful body but also a healthy one.

—JOE MUSCOLINO, DC,
global speaker and author of *Know the Body*
and *The Muscular System Manual*

# *Pilates by Purpose: Better Flexibility and Mobility*

## Starters

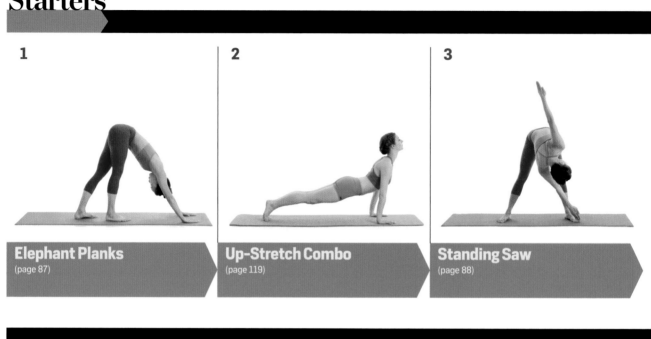

**1**

**Elephant Planks**
(page 87)

**2**

**Up-Stretch Combo**
(page 119)

**3**

**Standing Saw**
(page 88)

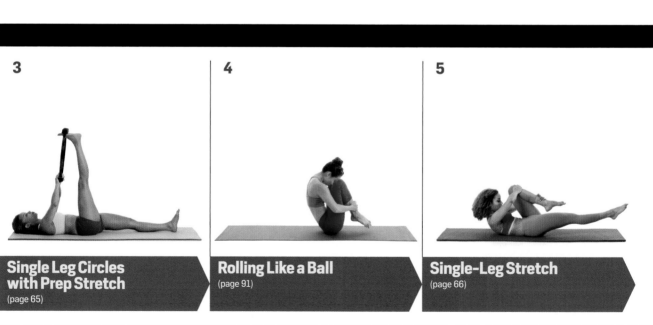

**3**

**Single Leg Circles with Prep Stretch**
(page 65)

**4**

**Rolling Like a Ball**
(page 91)

**5**

**Single-Leg Stretch**
(page 66)

# Mains

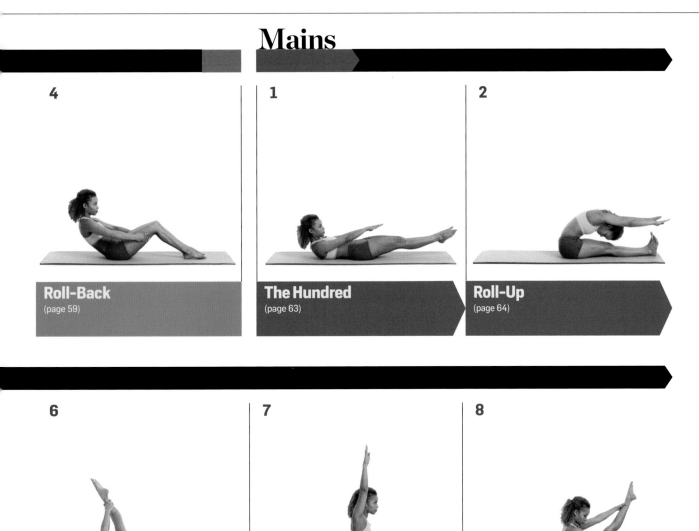

**4**

**Roll-Back**
(page 59)

**1**

**The Hundred**
(page 63)

**2**

**Roll-Up**
(page 64)

**6**

**Single Straight-Leg Stretch**
(page 92)

**7**

**Spine Stretch: With Arm Circles**
(page 68)

**8**

**Open-Leg Rocker Prep I**
(page 69)

## Mains *cont'd*

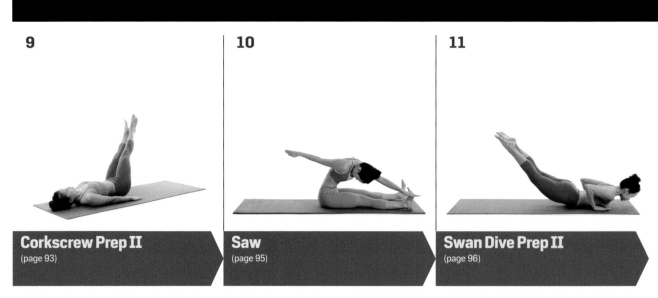

**9**

**Corkscrew Prep II**
(page 93)

**10**

**Saw**
(page 95)

**11**

**Swan Dive Prep II**
(page 96)

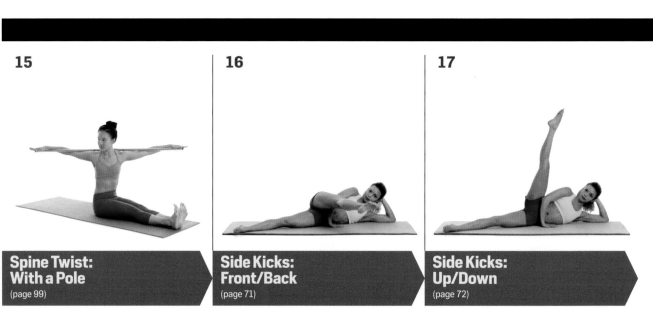

**15**

**Spine Twist:
With a Pole**
(page 99)

**16**

**Side Kicks:
Front/Back**
(page 71)

**17**

**Side Kicks:
Up/Down**
(page 72)

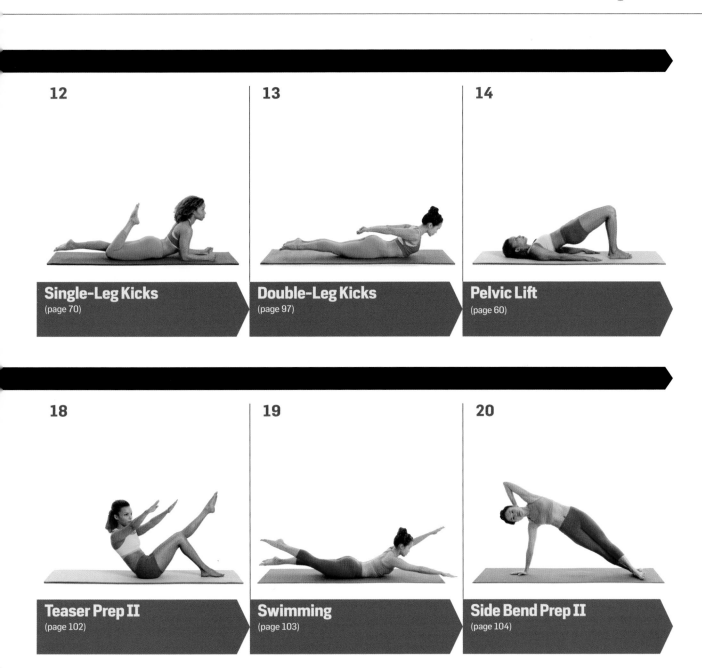

**12**

**Single-Leg Kicks**
(page 70)

**13**

**Double-Leg Kicks**
(page 97)

**14**

**Pelvic Lift**
(page 60)

**18**

**Teaser Prep II**
(page 102)

**19**

**Swimming**
(page 103)

**20**

**Side Bend Prep II**
(page 104)

# *Pilates by Purpose: Better Flexibility and Mobility*

## Mains *cont'd*

### Enders

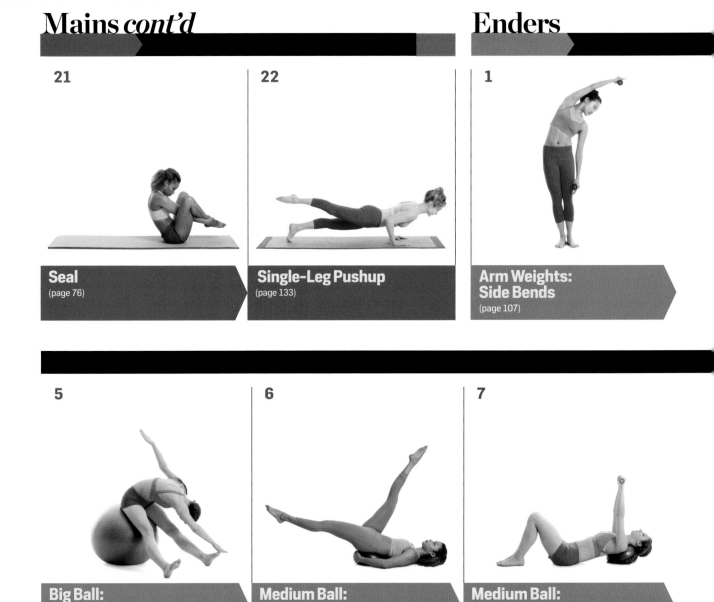

**21**

**Seal**
(page 76)

**22**

**Single-Leg Pushup**
(page 133)

**1**

**Arm Weights:
Side Bends**
(page 107)

**5**

**Big Ball:
Saw**
(page 215)

**6**

**Medium Ball:
Leg Series**
(all on pages 229–31)

**7**

**Medium Ball:
Arm Series**
(all on pages 227–28)

**2**

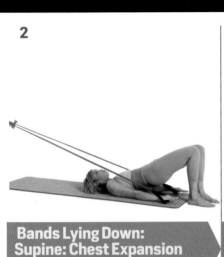

**Bands Lying Down:
Supine: Chest Expansion**
(page 188)

**3**

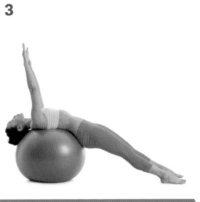

**Big Ball:
Back Stretch over Ball**
(page 224)

**4**

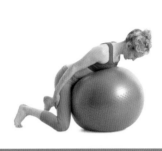

**Big Ball:
Swan**
(page 220)

**8**

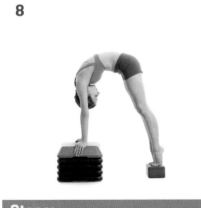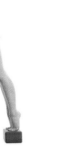

**Steps:
Footwork IV**
(page 236)

**9**

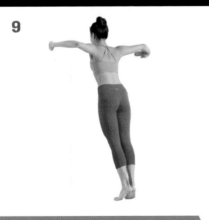

**Wall:
Corner Pushoffs**
(page 115)

**10**

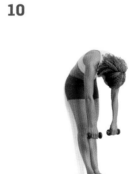

**Wall:
Roll-Down**
(page 81)

# Better Strength and Stability

According to research, if you do not strength train after age 20, you will lose (or have already lost!) between roughly $4^3/_4$ and 7 pounds of muscle *every decade*. Yikes! Adding weight and resistance to your workouts is a must. Your body weight counts as "weight" in strength training, so while you can add ankle weights or hold medicine balls, remember that exercises like planks and push-ups and lifting legs and arms all count, too! Strength means nothing without flexibility to accompany it. To maintain balance in the body, equal doses of both are required.

## TRAINING TIPS

- Extreme focus is the best way to build strength. Concentrate fully on each move to get the results you're seeking.

- Use your magic circle (page 239), Tensatoner (page 246), or resistance band (page 184) wherever possible to add strength and stability.

- Add unstable surfaces/ asymmetrical work (one leg or one arm).

- Add more load/weight/ resistance.

- Limit ROM.

# Starters

**1**

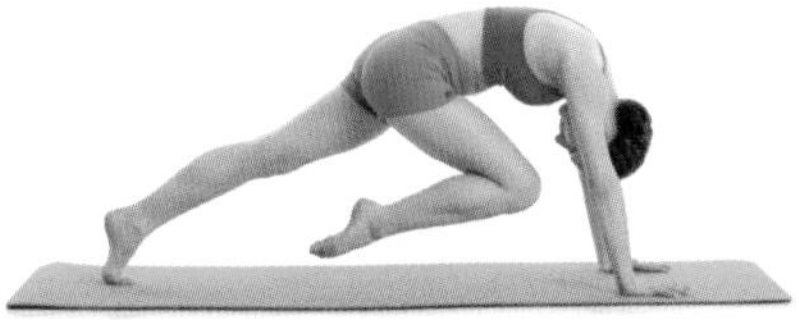

**Knee-Ins**
(page 169)

**2**

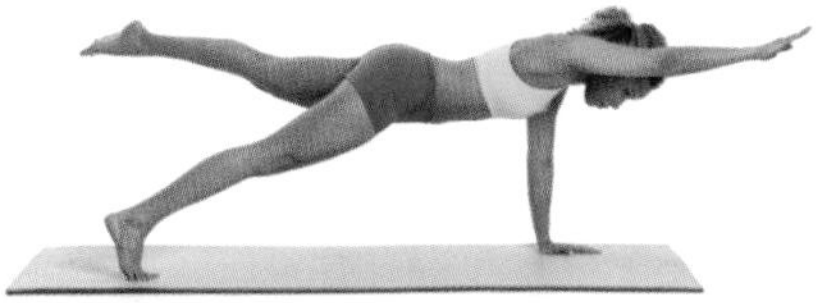

**Superman Planks**
(page 171)

**3**

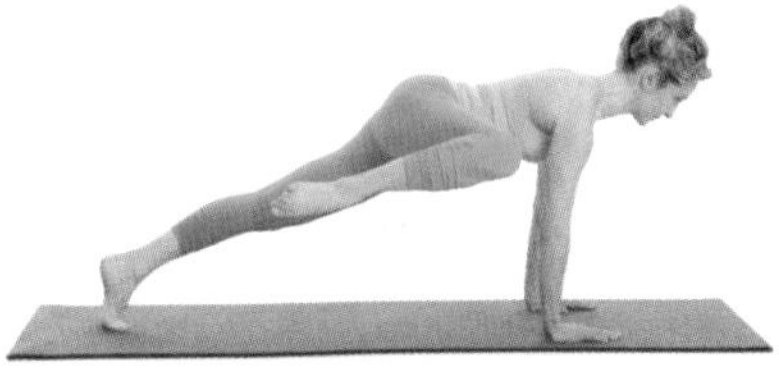

**Spider Planks**
(page 171)

# Mains

**1**

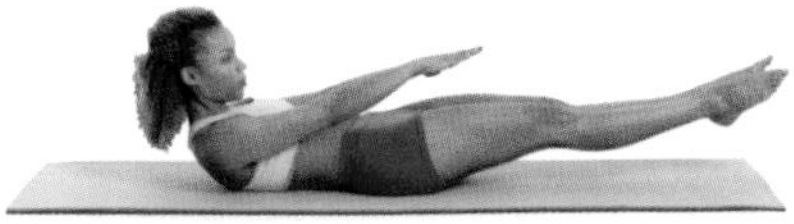

**The Hundred**
(page 63)

**2**

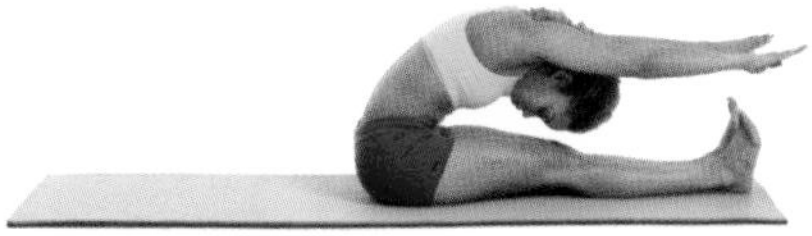

**Roll-Up**
(page 64)

**3**

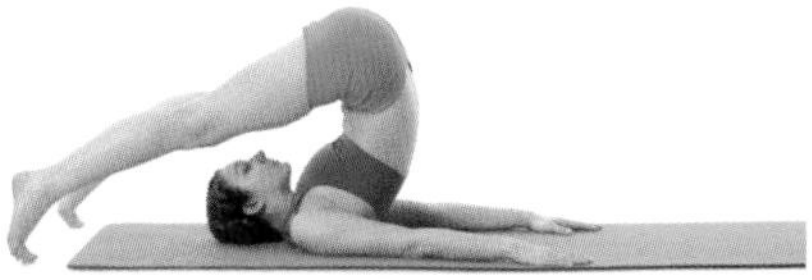

**Rollover I**
(page 121)

# Pilates by Purpose: Better Strength and Stability

## Mains *cont'd*

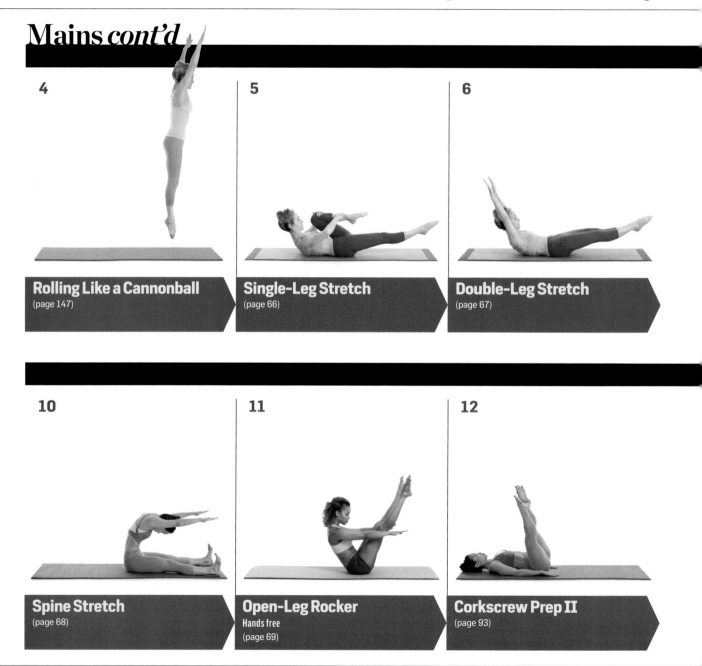

**4**

**Rolling Like a Cannonball**
(page 147)

**5**

**Single-Leg Stretch**
(page 66)

**6**

**Double-Leg Stretch**
(page 67)

**10**

**Spine Stretch**
(page 68)

**11**

**Open-Leg Rocker**
Hands free
(page 69)

**12**

**Corkscrew Prep II**
(page 93)

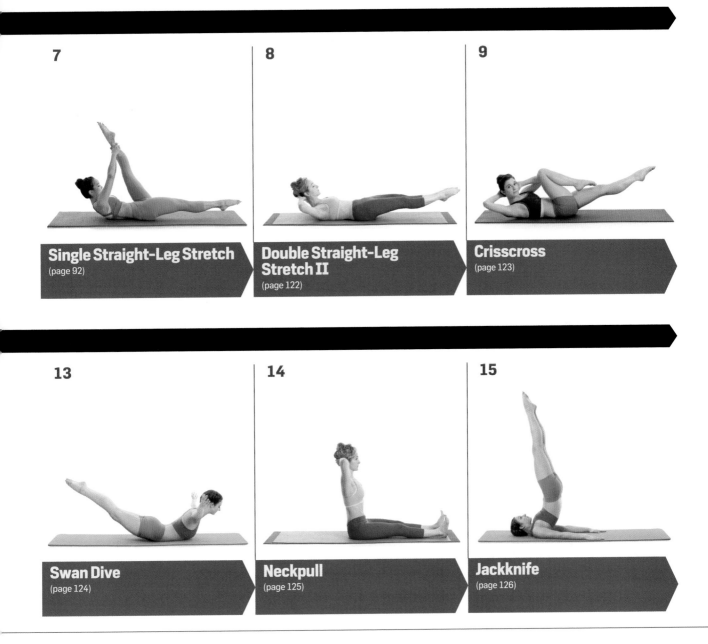

**7**

**Single Straight-Leg Stretch**
(page 92)

**8**

**Double Straight-Leg Stretch II**
(page 122)

**9**

**Crisscross**
(page 123)

**13**

**Swan Dive**
(page 124)

**14**

**Neckpull**
(page 125)

**15**

**Jackknife**
(page 126)

# *Pilates by Purpose: Better Strength and Stability*

## Mains *cont'd*

**16**

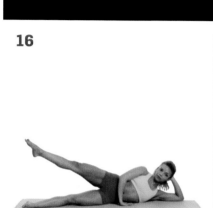

**Side Kicks: Circles**
(page 72)

**17**

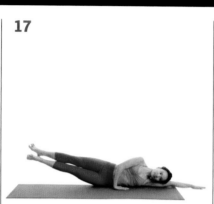

**Side Kicks: Double-Leg Lifts**
(page 101)

**18**

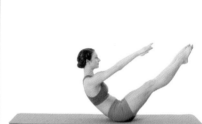

**Teasers**
(any or all on pages 102, 128, 151)

**22**

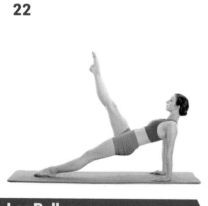

**Leg Pull**
(page 129)

**23**

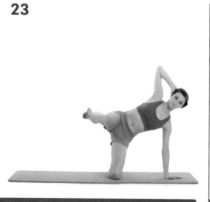

**Kneeling Side Kicks**
(page 129)

**24**

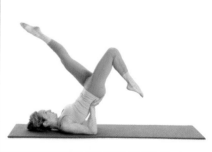

**Bicycle**
(page 150)

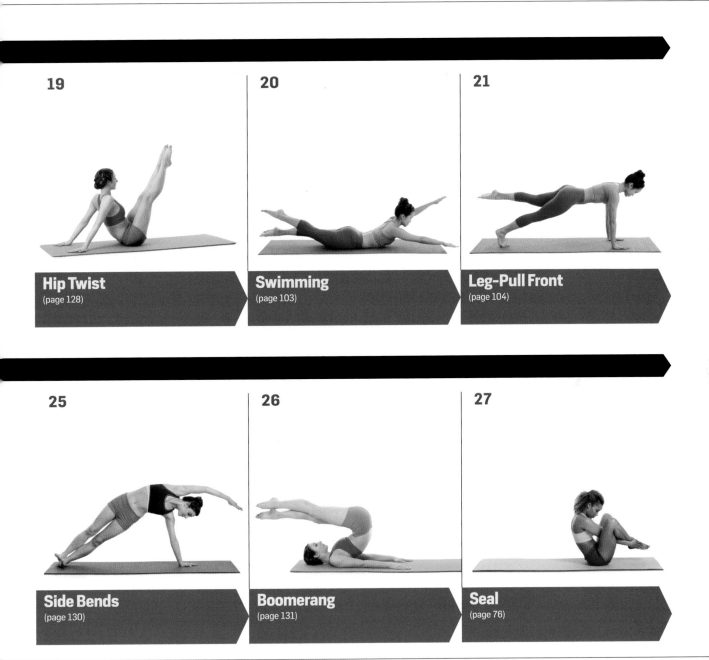

**19**

**Hip Twist**
(page 128)

**20**

**Swimming**
(page 103)

**21**

**Leg-Pull Front**
(page 104)

**25**

**Side Bends**
(page 130)

**26**

**Boomerang**
(page 131)

**27**

**Seal**
(page 76)

# *Pilates by Purpose: Better Strength and Stability*

## Mains *cont'd*

**28**

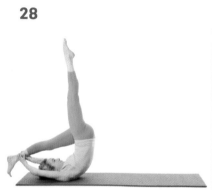

**Control Balance**
(page 156)

**29**

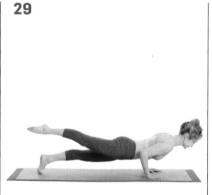

**Single-Leg Pushup**
Hold balance
(page 133)

## Enders

**1**

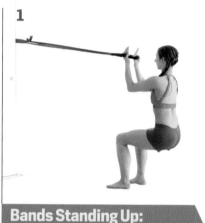

**Bands Standing Up:
Squats**
(page 210)

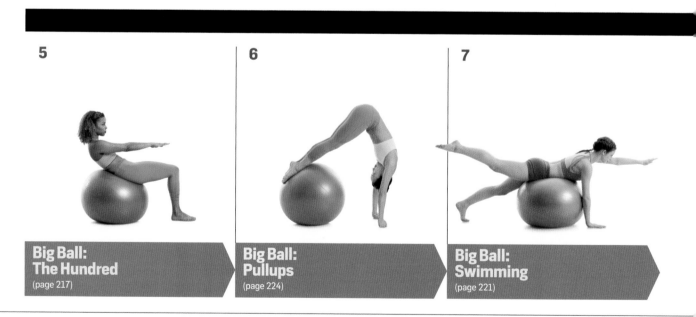

**5**

**Big Ball:
The Hundred**
(page 217)

**6**

**Big Ball:
Pullups**
(page 224)

**7**

**Big Ball:
Swimming**
(page 221)

**2**

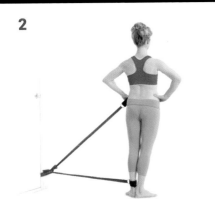

**Bands Standing Up:
Standing Side Kicks:
Inner Thighs** (page 211)

**3**

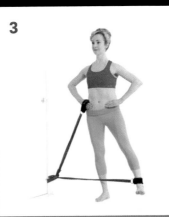

**Bands Standing Up:
Standing Side Kicks:
Outer Thighs** (page 211)

**4**

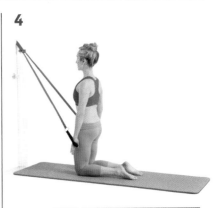

**Bands Kneeling Down:
Kneeling Arm Springs:
Chest Expansion** (page 198)

**8**

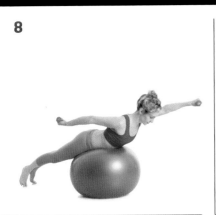

**Big Ball:
Arm Weights on the Ball**
(page 225)

**9**

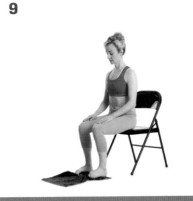

**Foot Corrector:
Tea Towel Exercise**
(page 255)

**10**

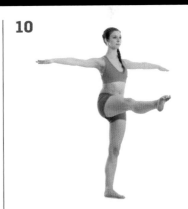

**Archival:
Single-Leg Balances to Front**
(page 178)

# *Pilates by Purpose: Better Strength and Stability*

## Mains *cont'd*

**11**

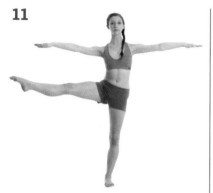

**Archival:**
**Single-Leg Balances to Side**
(page 178)

**12**

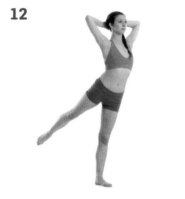

**Archival:**
**Single-Leg Balances to Back**
(page 178)

**13**

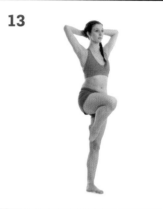

**Archival:**
**Standing Bicycle**
(page 177)

**14**

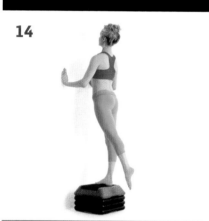

**Steps:**
**Going Up Front**
(page 233)

**15**

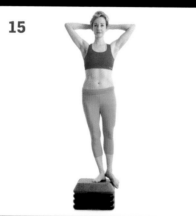

**Steps:**
**Going Up Side**
(page 234)

**16**

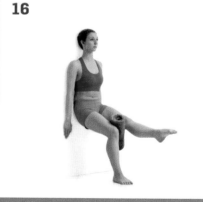

**Wall:**
**Single-Leg Squats**
(page 139)

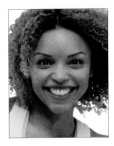

Belissa is a current trainee of Brooke Siler's re:AB Pilates Teacher Training Program.

# Belissa Savery

"My introduction to Pilates came in 2001 during my freshman year of college when I purchased a set of Pilates videotapes. However, it wasn't until 2010, when I stumbled into Brooke's studio, that I truly discovered the essence of this method. Years of weight training, boxing, and dance had provided only temporary changes to my body, accompanied by many aches, pains, and injuries.

*I saw a drastic change in my body after only two weeks, and then I knew Pilates would be in my life forever.*

The changes to my mind, body, and spirit have been astounding. In the future, I plan to share my Pilates expertise in urban communities to give back to communities that lack resources and education in the areas of health and fitness."

# CHAPTER 11

# Pilates by Pursuit

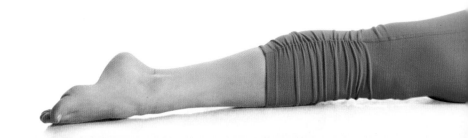

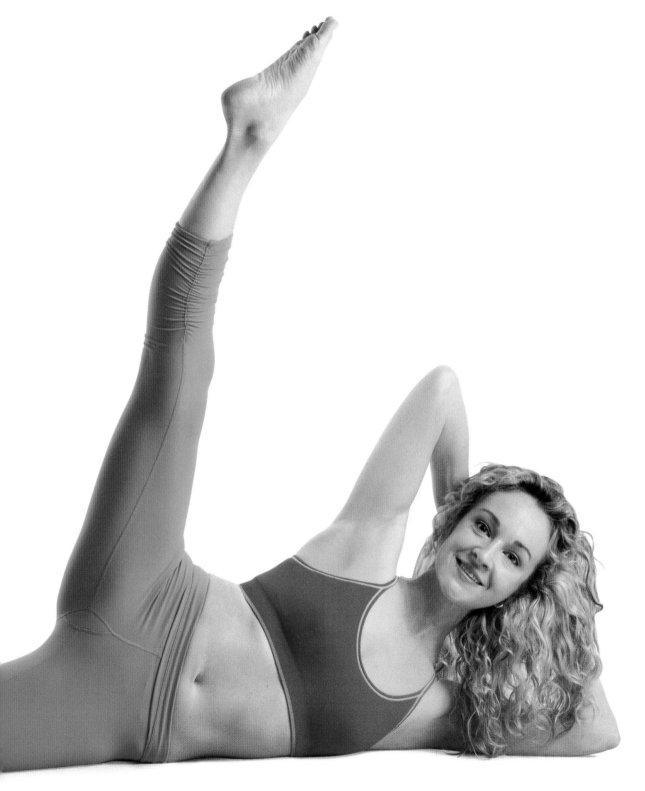

# Up Your Athletic Game

Sports require specific demands from your body that normal, everyday activities may not. Sports like tennis and golf are generally one-sided activities (you favor one arm when you swing); therefore, proper body awareness is critical to ensure you are not developing imbalances that may lead to injury down the line.

According to physical therapist Dr. Robert Donatelli, muscle is the best force offsetter in the body. Our joints are surrounded by muscle that initiates movements, slows down movements, and controls movements of bones. In other words, muscles are our best shock absorbers. To accomplish these functions, Dr. Donatelli explains, one group of muscles initiates movement and the other muscle group controls movement. This relationship is referred to as agonist and antagonist. Muscle imbalance results from weakness, poor flexibility, and inadequate endurance in either the agonist or the antagonist.

You can address an imbalance by choosing a series from an earlier chapter best suited to your needs by level and/or purpose (flexibility, strength, or endurance), then add in the following moves recommended for your sport of choice.

## Athletic Awareness Test

**1.** What directional movements does my sport require from me?

**2.** What parts of the body are getting the most stressed in my sport?

**3.** What can I do to balance my muscles to make myself more efficient and injury-proof?

# Running

There are upward of 75 million runners in the United States.

Twenty-six bones, 33 joints, 112 ligaments, and a network of tendons, nerves, and blood vessels—all in the feet—have to work together when we run. Obviously, we need to make sure that our feet are properly readied for the task by keeping them strong and supple. But reducing the ground-pounding effects of running takes more than just your feet, it takes a muscular village. This is where Pilates comes in.

Your new powerhouse muscles will help keep you upright without strain and facilitate complete breathing. Pilates teaches you the art of tension and relaxation so that you can pour power into your abs, hips, and thighs while simultaneously keeping your trunk, shoulders, and neck tension free.

## TRAINING TIPS

- Stabilize and strengthen the abs, glutes, feet, foot-knee-hip alignment, and obliques (torso rotation).

- Mobilize the hips and respiratory muscles.

- See page 253 for a refresher on "Meet Your Feet."

*"When all your muscles are properly developed, you will, as a matter of course, perform your work with minimum effort and maximum pleasure.'* —Joe Pilates

# Pilates by Pursuit: Running

## Moves to Improve

**1**

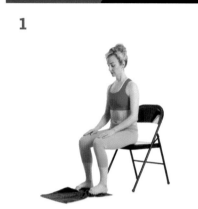

**Foot Corrector:**
**Tea Towel Exercise**
(page 255)

**2**

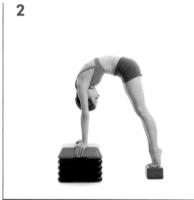

**Steps:**
**Footwork IV**
(page 236)

**3**

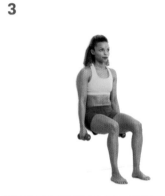

**Wall:**
**Squats**
(add any arm combos you like on page 139)

**7**

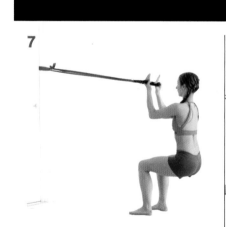

**Bands Standing Up:**
**Squats**
(page 210)

**8**

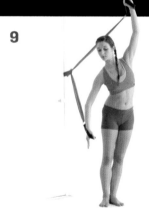

**Bands Lying Down:**
**Hamstring Curls**
(page 193)

**9**

**Bands Standing Up:**
**Butterfly**
(page 207)

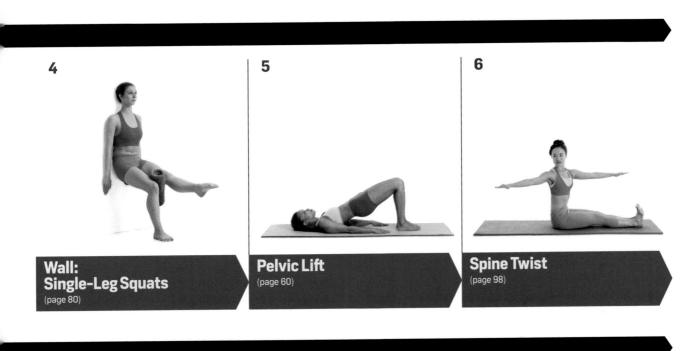

**4**

**Wall:**
**Single-Leg Squats**
(page 80)

**5**

**Pelvic Lift**
(page 60)

**6**

**Spine Twist**
(page 98)

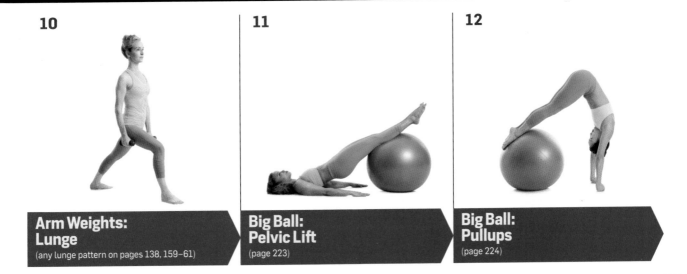

**10**

**Arm Weights:**
**Lunge**
(any lunge pattern on pages 138, 159–61)

**11**

**Big Ball:**
**Pelvic Lift**
(page 223)

**12**

**Big Ball:**
**Pullups**
(page 224)

## Moves to Improve *cont'd*

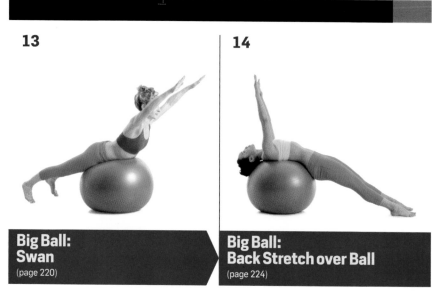

**13**

**Big Ball:
Swan**
(page 220)

**14**

**Big Ball:
Back Stretch over Ball**
(page 224)

# Cycling

When I was a kid, my dad once tried to get me to ride my bike to Central Park through the traffic-heavy streets. I got out 1 block and froze up. I couldn't do it. Fast-forward to my midtwenties and the amazing Gary Fisher hybrid cycle my boyfriend bought me for my birthday. That bike and I never parted. I weaved through traffic wearing everything from skirts and heeled boots to leather pants. Fast-forward again—20 years older, two kids richer, and 20 pounds heavier—I broke the bike out of storage and had it tuned up. I've learned a lot from these recent rides. Namely, that cycling takes serious powerhouse and loads of "in and up" abs if you want to do it right! Cycling is a stable, low-impact exercise that increases joint mobility and stability. Plus, it's fun!

## TRAINING TIPS

- Stabilize and strengthen the obliques, glutes, neck flexors, thoracic spine.

- Mobilize the quads, flexors, hamstrings, gastrocnemius, and soleus. (See also the kyphotic posture series, page 268.)

# *Pilates by Pursuit: Cycling*

## Moves to Improve

**1**

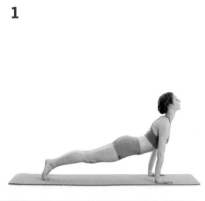

**Up-Stretch Combo**
(page 119)

**2**

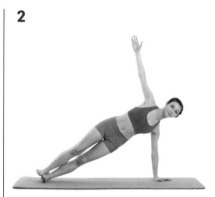

**Side Planks**
(page 171)

**3**

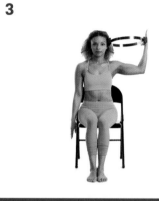

**Magic Circle:
Against the Head Isometric
Series** (any or all on page 241)

**7**

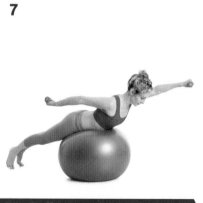

**Big Ball:
Arm Weights on the Ball**
(choose one on page 225)

**8**

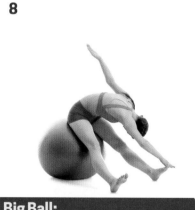

**Big Ball:
Saw**
(page 219)

**9**

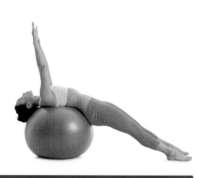

**Big Ball:
Back Stretch over Ball**
(page 224)

**4**

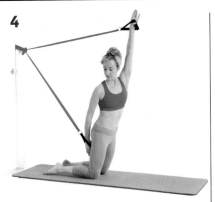

**Bands Kneeling Down:
Kneeling Arm Springs:
Butterfly** (page 200)

**5**

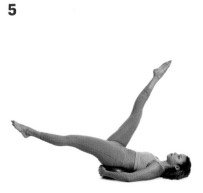

**Medium Ball:
Leg Series**
(page 229–30)

**6**

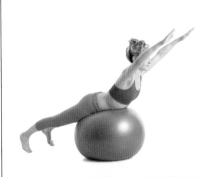

**Big Ball:
Flying Swan**
(page 220)

**10**

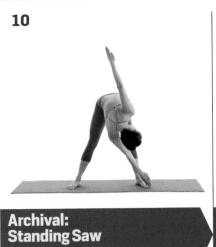

**Archival:
Standing Saw**
(page 179)

**11**

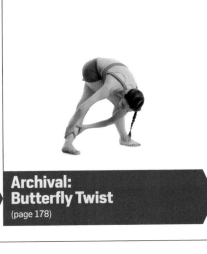

**Archival:
Butterfly Twist**
(page 178)

**12**

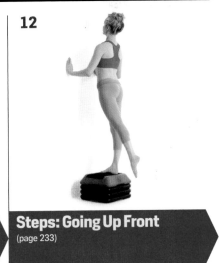

**Steps: Going Up Front**
(page 233)

# *Pilates by Pursuit:* Cycling

## Moves to Improve *cont'd*

**13**

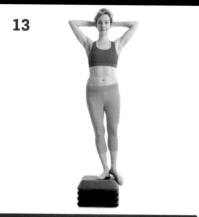

**Steps:**
**Going Up Side**
(page 234)

**14**

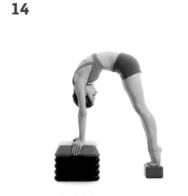

**Steps:**
**Footwork IV**
(page 237)

**15**

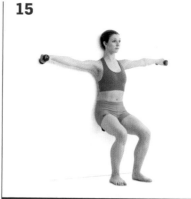

**Wall:**
**Squats with Wings**
(page 138)

**16**

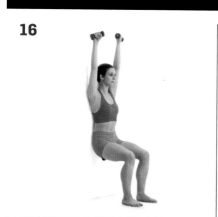

**Wall:**
**Squats with Levers**
(page 139)

**17**

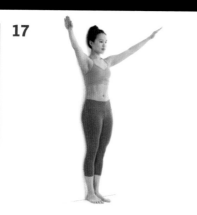

**Wall:**
**Flush with Circles**
(page 110)

**18**

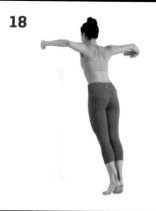

**Wall:**
**Corner Pushoff**
(page 113)

# Swimming

Every year, I renew my local gym membership for one reason and one reason only: the pool! Swimming is easily one of my favorite pastimes and undeniably one of my preferred workouts.

The benefits of swimming are plentiful, particularly as an asthmatic. It provides a tremendous and unique advantage to strengthening my cardiovascular system because of its ability to train the lungs both aerobically and anaerobically. I swam while pregnant, pre- and post-heart surgery, and every time I go into "training mode."

When you swim, as with Pilates, you're working so many muscles in harmony that the cross-section of beneficiaries is even more abundant than with most other sports.

## TRAINING TIPS

- Stabilize and strengthen your chest, lats and shoulders, shoulder blades, lower back, and abs. "You want to pull with your body and not your arms."

- Strengthen the glutes and quads for the push-off phase.

- Mobilize the chest and shoulders, back line of the legs, and inner thighs and use rotation for mobilizing lats.

*"A lot of our attention in dry land training goes towards our swimmer's core. The core is what transfers energy, and we want to make sure that there aren't any energy leaks between the power areas of the upper and lower body."*

—Jason Dierking, assistant director of Olympic sports performance at the University of Louisville

# *Pilates by Pursuit: Swimming*

## Moves to Improve

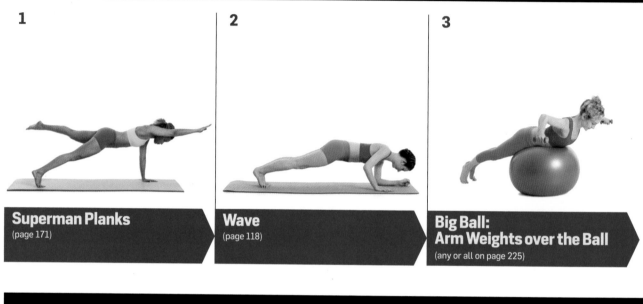

**1**

**Superman Planks**
(page 171)

**2**

**Wave**
(page 118)

**3**

**Big Ball:
Arm Weights over the Ball**
(any or all on page 225)

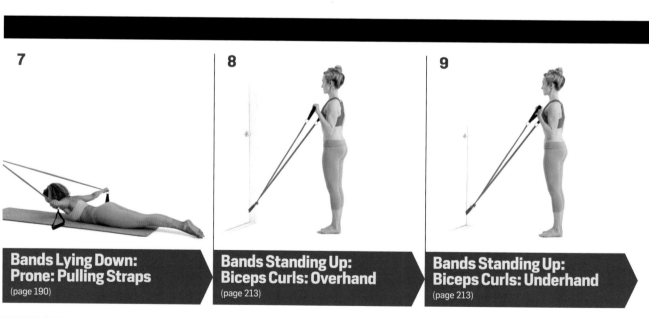

**7**

**Bands Lying Down:
Prone: Pulling Straps**
(page 190)

**8**

**Bands Standing Up:
Biceps Curls: Overhand**
(page 213)

**9**

**Bands Standing Up:
Biceps Curls: Underhand**
(page 213)

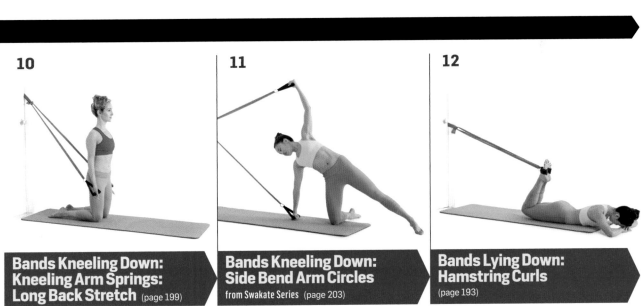

**4**

**Big Ball:
Pullups**
(page 224)

**5**

**Big Ball:
Swimming**
(page 221)

**6**

**Bands Standing Up:
Squats**
(page 210)

**10**

**Bands Kneeling Down:
Kneeling Arm Springs:
Long Back Stretch** (page 199)

**11**

**Bands Kneeling Down:
Side Bend Arm Circles**
from Swakate Series (page 203)

**12**

**Bands Lying Down:
Hamstring Curls**
(page 193)

## Moves to Improve *cont'd*

**13**

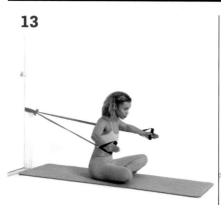

**Bands Sitting Up:
Rowing Hug**
(page 196)

**14**

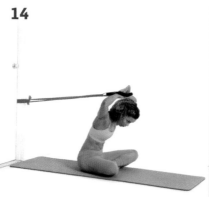

**Bands Sitting Up:
Rowing Shave**
(page 195)

**15**

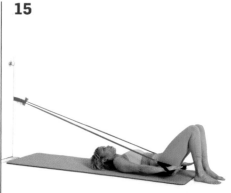

**Bands Lying Down:
Supine: Triceps Extensions**
(page 189)

**18**

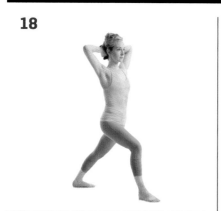

**Arm Weights:
Lunge Shaving**
(page 161)

**19**

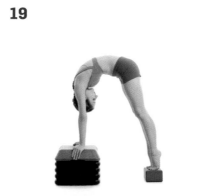

**Steps:
Footwork IV**
(page 236)

**20**

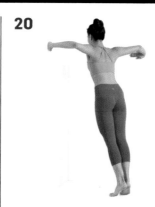

**Wall:
Corner Pushoff**
(page 113)

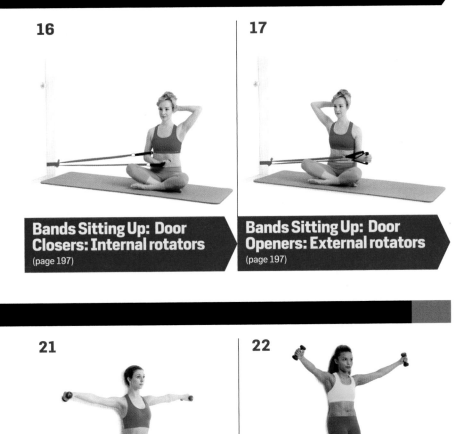

**16**

**Bands Sitting Up: Door Closers: Internal rotators**
(page 197)

**17**

**Bands Sitting Up: Door Openers: External rotators**
(page 197)

**21**

**Wall: Squats with Wings**
(page 140)

**22**

**Wall: Arm Circles**
(page 79)

# CHAPTER 12
# *Pilates Rx*

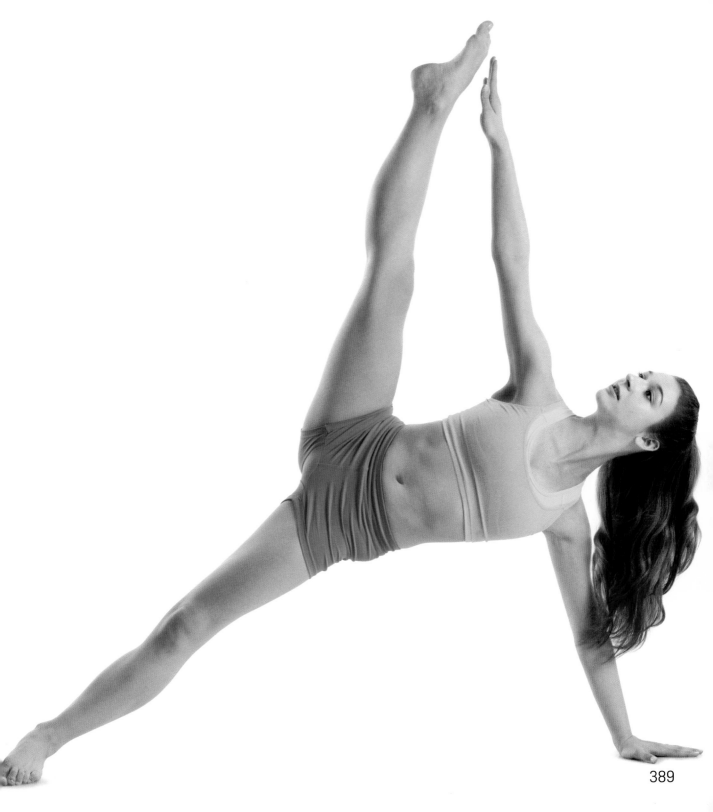

# Ease Chronic Aches and Pains

Most chronic pain is a result of imbalance in our bodies. Joe asserted that "incorrect habits are responsible for most of our ailments—if not all of them." Think about the habits we almost all assume: carrying shoulder bags on only one shoulder; standing with weight on the same leg; wearing the same shoes day after day; crossing the same leg over the other; talking on the phone on the same side; carrying children, groceries, etc., on the same hip over and over. These add up.

Dr. Steve Young, author of *Body Solutions*, says that the definition of injury from a physiological level is "failure of the body to adapt." We can train our bodies to adapt by building strength progressively from the inside out, utilizing all muscles (large and small), and gradually adding more and more challenges through differing patterns of movement, coordination, and breath. We are not trying to trick our bodies but to direct them with the practice of an intelligent movement system.

Pilates is rehabilitative, but it's not physical therapy! It's so important to understand this. As a Pilates teacher, I know many ways of rehabilitating the body, but isolating injury is not one of them. Instead, these workouts are crafted to consider the *whole* body in a way that looks for causes, not symptoms. Since we are not working in a fully equipped studio, I've made some suggestions of

*"I must be right. Never an aspirin. Never injured a day in my life. The whole country, the whole world, should be doing my exercises."*
—Joe Pilates

*"If one joint is restricted in motion, an adjacent joint will usually compensate by moving more. In the spine, the compensation might be above or below. In the extremities, the compensation can be on the same or opposite side of the body. In time, because the compensation moves more, it is often overused and becomes painful."*
—Dr. Joe Muscolino

moves using props that you may find helpful. Your job is to use these moves in conjunction with your chosen mat series, modifying as needed to keep you safe and pain free while getting you back on track to progress.

Sometimes, pain is a useful way to learn about yourself. What is your body trying to tell you about the way you stand or sit or play? Which directions of movement hurt? Which feel good? Stick with what feels good.

If this chapter is where you are actually beginning your Pilates journey, I would like to take a moment to differentiate between *chronic aches* and *acute pain*. According to WebMD, "Acute pain starts suddenly and usually doesn't last long. Chronic pain lasts for weeks, months, even years. In some cases, the pain comes and goes." This distinction is tricky because you have to know how to discern between "I shouldn't be moving this" type of pain and "this is always bothering me" discomfort. If you are in acute pain, please seek the help of a medical professional. When you are cleared for movement, come back to this Pilates program. (I'll wait!) If your pain is of the achy, nagging nature, proceed with intelligence, intuition, and caution. Remember: Nothing in Pilates should hurt! Go slow and listen to your body.

# Shoulders

Your shoulder is a ball-and-socket joint, which makes it your most moveable kind of joint in the body. But with all that mobility comes the potential for instability and injury as well. Since the ball of the upper arm bone is twice the size of the shoulder-blade socket, like a golf ball on a tee, in order for the ball to be stable the shoulder needs help from the surrounding muscles and tendons. That's where the rotator cuff comes in. The rotator cuff is a muscle tendon unit made up of four deep muscles that connect the "ball" of the upper arm to your shoulder blade. As your shoulder blade moves back, so does the whole socket, which lessens your chance of injury. So "wings down and back" should produce stability and allow for more range from the proper places of your shoulder.

## TRAINING TIPS

- When in doubt . . . leave it out! (Nothing should ever hurt!)

- Limit your ROM (range of motion).

- Do not go below your elbow on pushups.

- Keep your "wings" on your back.

# To Stabilize

**1**

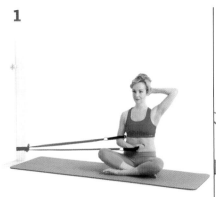

**Bands Sitting Up:
Internal Rotators and
External Rotators** (page 197)

**2**

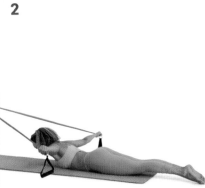

**Bands Lying Down:
Pulling Straps**
(page 190)

**3**

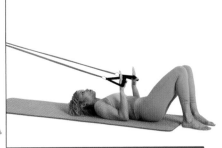

**Bands Lying Down:
Supine: Triceps Extensions**
(page 189)

**4**

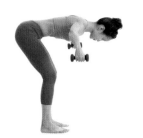

**Arm Weights:
The Bug**
(page 109)

**5**

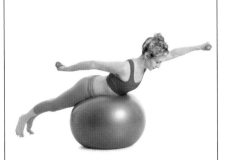

**Big Ball: Arm Weights
on the Ball** (choose any or all bug, boxing,
triceps extensions  on page 225)

**6**

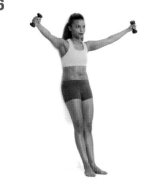

**Wall:
Arm Circles**
(page 79)

# *Pilates Rx: Shoulders*

## To Stabilize *cont'd*

## To Mobilize

**7**

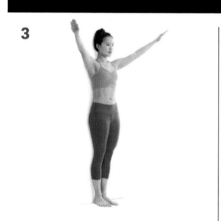

**Wall:
Pushoffs**
(page 112)

**1**

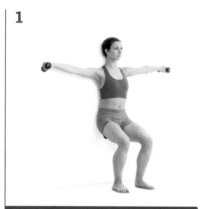

**Wall:
Squats with Wings**
No weight  (page 140)

**2**

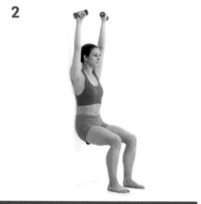

**Wall:
Squats with Levers**
No weight  (page 141)

**3**

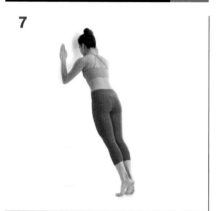

**Off the Wall:
Flush with Circles**
No weight  (page 110)

**4**

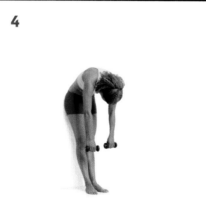

**Wall:
Roll-Down**
(page 81)

**5**

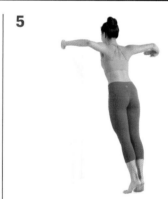

**Wall:
Corner Pushoffs**
(page 113)

# Back

The psoas muscle connects from the sides of your lumbar spine to the inside of your thigh bone. When contracted it will want to bring your lower back forward and can "lock" your back down into a lordotic posture. If constant, this compression of the lumbar disks causes degeneration and makes them more susceptible to injury.

If it's only short and tight on one side, the psoas will pull the spine or pelvis into imbalance, which can cause a host of other issues including some postural scoliosis.

Since the glutes are one of the muscle groups that oppose the psoas, a deficient derriere can force other back muscles to overcompensate.

The moral of the story is: Balance your strength multidimensionally so that your abs, back, and glute muscles all share the load.

## TRAINING TIPS

- When in doubt . . . leave it out! (Nothing should ever hurt!)

- Start with exercises that keep your back flat.

- Bend your knees when needed.

- Support your lower back with your hands or props as needed.

- Make sure your power-house muscles are supporting your movements (abs in and up, tight seat, inner thigh muscles turned on and glued together).

# Pilates Rx: Back

## To Stabilize

**1**

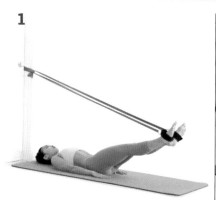

**Bands Lying Down:
Leg Spring Series**
(any on pages 192–93)

**2**

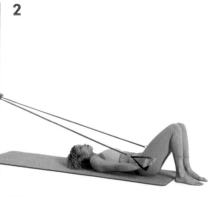

**Bands Lying Down:
Arm Spring Series**
(all on pages 188–90)

**3**

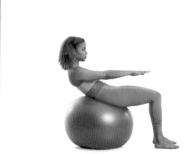

**Big Ball:
Roll-Back**
(page 216)

## To Mobilize

**7**

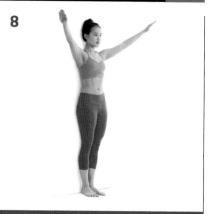

**Wall:
Squats with Circles**
(page 111)

**8**

**Wall:
Flush with Circles**
(page 110)

**1**

MODIFIED
VERSION
- With your head
  down, gently pull
  one knee toward
  your chest, using
  your hands to hold
  your knee to the
  chest.
- Allow your extended
  leg to rest on the
  mat, opening the
  muscles over the
  front of your hip.

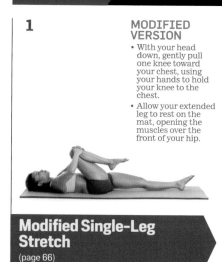

**Modified Single-Leg
Stretch**
(page 66)

**4**

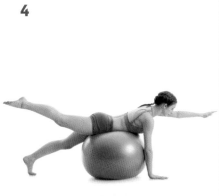

**Big Ball:
Swimming**
(page 221)

**5**

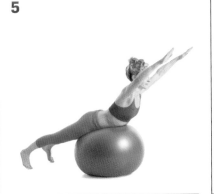

**Big Ball:
Flying Swan**
(page 220)

**6**

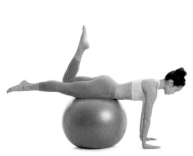

**Big Ball:
Single-Leg Kicks**
(page 221)

**2**

**MODIFIED
VERSION**

- Tight, shortened hamstrings can also contribute to lower-back pain.
- You can use a towel, a band, or the magic circle to support the weight of your leg and help guide the movement.

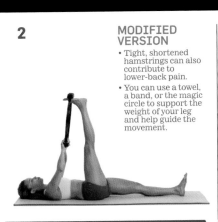

**Modified Single-Leg Circle**
(page 65)

**3**

**MODIFIED
VERSION**

- Lie on your back with your knees bent and your feet flat on the floor.
- With your knees together, bring them to one side.
- Your feet should stay on the floor.

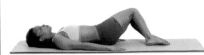

**Modified Hip Twist**
(page 103)

**4**

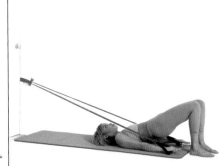

**Bands Lying Down:
Supine Chest Expansion**
(page 188)

# Pilates Rx: Back

## To Mobilize *cont'd*

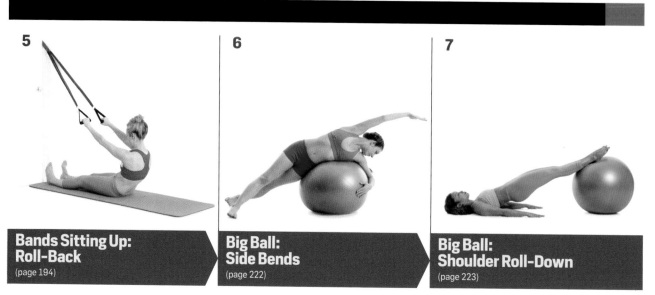

**5**

**Bands Sitting Up:
Roll-Back**
(page 194)

**6**

**Big Ball:
Side Bends**
(page 222)

**7**

**Big Ball:
Shoulder Roll-Down**
(page 223)

# Neck

There are 33 joints in your neck, making it wonderfully mobile. But limited neck-muscle support asks the joints to support the weight of your head, and that's an unfair load for such a small set of bones and tissues. Believe it or not, strengthening your abdominals (to hold you upright) and practicing more complete breathing (to support your shoulder structure) will help relieve postural neck pain. Stress, emotional tension, and prolonged work intensity can cause some of the muscles that connect the head, neck, and shoulders to tighten and contract, resulting in pain and stiffness.

In general, neck pain is caused by keeping your head or your shoulders in compromising positions (computer overload, anyone?). So check your bad habits and don't stick your neck out for nobody!

## TRAINING TIPS

- When in doubt . . . leave it out! (Nothing should ever hurt!)

- Place a pillow ot towel under the head or the nape of the neck.

- Exercise with your head down instead of lifted.

- Do not start upper-body lifts from the floor (for example, instead of Roll-Ups, do Roll-Backs).

- Press the back of your tongue to the roof of your mouth before lifting your head to strengthen the deep neck flexors.

- Take the postural awareness test again on page 264 to identify possible issues.

# *Pilates Rx: Neck*

## To Stabilize

**1**

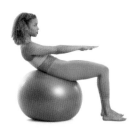

**Big Ball:
Roll-Back**
(page 216)

**2**

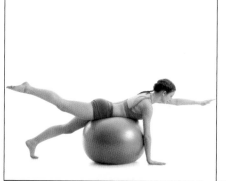

**Big Ball: Swimming**
Make sure your head is in line with your spine
(page 221)

**3**

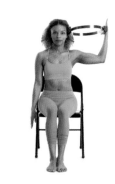

**Magic Circle: Against
the Head** (Isometric Series) Direction depends
on where discomfort is (page 241)

## To Mobilize

**1**

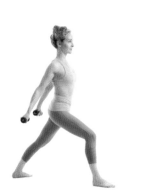

**Arm Weights:
Chest Expansion**
(page 137)

**2**

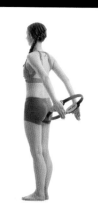

**Standing: Magic Circle
between the Heels of Hands:
Back** Add slow and steady head turns (page 242)

**3**

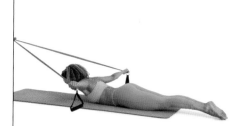

**Bands Lying Down:
Prone: Pulling Straps**
Keep head in line with spine (page 190)

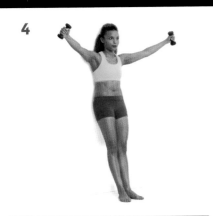

**4**

**Wall:
Arm Circles**
No weights (page 79)

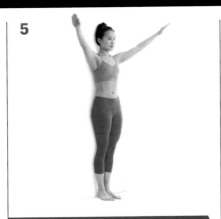

**5**

**Wall:
Flush with Circles**
No weights (page 110)

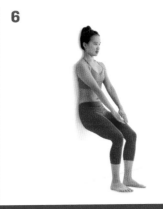

**6**

**Wall:
Squats with Circles**
No weights (page 112)

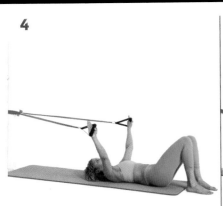

**4**

**Bands Lying Down:
Supine: Arm Circles**
(page 190)

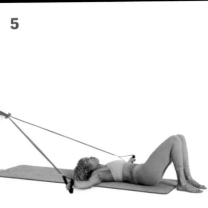

**5**

**Bands Lying Down:
Supine: Wings**
(page 190)

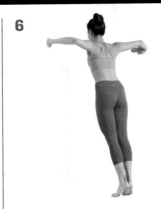

**6**

**Wall: Corner Pushoffs**
Add slow head turns, and make sure the head
is in line with your spine (page 113)

# Knees

The knee is susceptible to overuse injuries due to, you guessed it, muscle imbalance! What can make your knees most cranky is weakness in your quads paired with tightness in your hamstrings, which increases the compressive forces to the kneecap (patella). Additionally, a broad sheet of connective tissue running along the outside of your thigh, the iliotibial band (or ITB), can shorten as a result of too much sitting or from weak outer hip muscles, and then the quad shuts off.

These imbalances can change the patella's ability to track effectively. Over time, the result is cartilage damage and pain. Pulling your abs in and up, and aligning your knees with your hips and heels, are the training tricks to eliciting proper knee tracking.

## TRAINING TIPS

- When in doubt . . . leave it out! (Nothing should ever hurt!)

- Limit knee flexion (for instance, place a pillow or ball between your heels and bottom for Sit to Heels; place your hands behind your knees rather than on top for knee-to-chest exercises).

- Do not squat below 90 degrees.

- Do not lock knees.

- Strengthen any weakness in hip abductors (outside of the hip) and hip external rotators (glutes).

- Do not allow your knees, ankles, and arches of your feet to droop inward or it is nearly impossible for the kneecap to move smoothly.

- The majority of Pilates matwork is non-weight bearing so naughty knees are particularly safe.

# To Stabilize

**1**

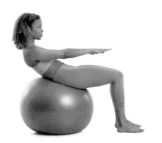

**Big Ball: Roll-Back**
You can alternate lifting one heel off the floor or the whole foot (page 216)

**2**

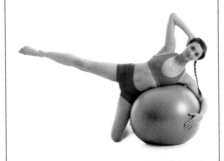

**Big Ball:
Kneeling Side Kicks**
(page 222)

**3**

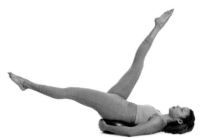

**Medium Ball:
Leg Series: Helicopter**
(page 230)

# To Mobilize

**4**

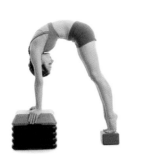

**Steps:
Footwork IV**
(page 236)

**5**

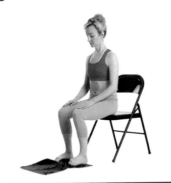

**Foot Corrector:
Tea Towel Exercise**
(page 255)

**1**

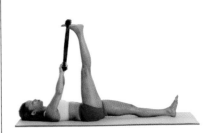

**Modified Single-Leg Circle**
Use a towel, band, or magic circle to help guide the leg across the midline to mobilize the ITB. (page 65)

# Pilates Rx: *Knees*

## To Mobilize *cont'd*

**2**

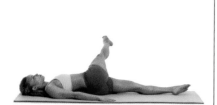

**Single-Leg Circles I: Hip Off**
Do not let the thigh rotate inward in the hip joint
(page 65)

**3**

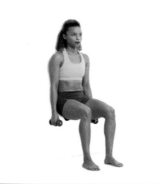

**Wall: Squats**
Pay extra attention to the tracking of your knees!
(page 80)

**4**

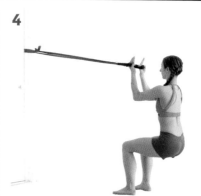

**Bands Standing Up: Squats** Pay extra attention to the tracking of your knees! (page 210)

**5**

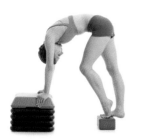

**Steps: Running**
(page 237)

**6**

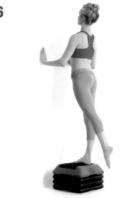

**Steps: Going Up Front**
(page 233)

**7**

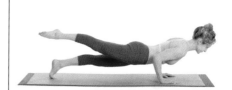

**Single-Leg Pushup**
(page 133)

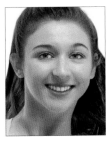

Zoe is the daughter and life-long student of distinguished Pilates teacher Kathryn Ross-Nash.

# Zoe Ross-Nash

"Pilates has always been a part of my life. Since my mother is an instructor, I grew up in the studio (as a child, I would fall asleep in the barrel or pretend it was a boat). I dance classical ballet and as my career progressed, I realized that Pilates was the perfect type of training to take me to the next level. It helped me become a better dancer, even during the times I was injured. When I tore the ligaments in my ankle, I used the foot corrector to build strength again. More important, *Pilates changed my body, helping me create healthy movement habits that are healthy for everyday activities."*

# Resources

## How to reach Brooke:

Twitter: **@BSilerPilates**
Facebook: **Brooke Siler Pilates**
Train with me: **www.reABnyc.com**

## Teacher Listings

**www.ClassicalPilates.net** is a directory of classically trained teachers worldwide who are within one to three generations of Joe and Clara Pilates. This free directory has served as a key resource for the classical community and public at large since 2002.

**www.AuthenticPilatesUnion.com** The APU was established in 2012 as a nondiscriminatory organization dedicated to preserving the authentic work and philosophy of Joseph H. Pilates. Its listings show members' commitment to continuing education by tracking the number of continuing education courses completed annually by each teacher. Members represent all different backgrounds of Pilates.

## Continuing Education

**www.reABnyc.com** I started the teacher training program at my New York studio in 2005 and work a very limited number of potential teachers through a rigorous 700+ hour course. Think you've got what it takes? Reach out to us at Training@reABnyc.com

**www.jaygrimes.com** Jay Grimes is one of the most sought-after teachers in the world and teaches conferences abroad as well as lessons at his Los Angeles studio.

**www.romanaspilates.com** Romana Kryzanowska no longer teaches but her daughter and granddaughter continue Romana's Pilates program.

**www.Pilates-gratz.com** More than just a manufacturer, Gratz Pilates hosts events worldwide where you can work out with the pros and experience the body-changing effects of Contrology on the equipment as it was meant to be practiced.

## Online Pilates Workouts

**www.Pilatesology.com** Pilatesology offers unlimited streaming of Classical Pilates workouts with some of the world's best teachers and is dedicated to recording, preserving, and spreading Joseph Pilates' pure, original work worldwide.

**www.Pilatesanytime.com** Pilates Anytime is an online offering of Pilates classes, showcasing many different styles of Pilates teachings.

## Symbiotic Somatic Specialties

**The Art and Science of Kinesiology**
*http://www.learnmuscles.com*
Dr. Muscolino is a licensed chiropractic physician and teaches anatomy, physiology, and nutrition at Purchase College, State University of New York (SUNY). Dr. Muscolino is the author of eight major publications with Mosby of Elsevier Science.

**The Breathing Project**
*http://www.breathingproject.org*
At the Breathing Project, Leslie Kaminoff and Amy Matthews teach principles of human structure and movement based on experiences of body, breath, and mind. These principles can be integrated with any style or technique.

**Myofascial Meridians**
*http://www.anatomytrains.com*
Tom Myers' Anatomy Trains® maps the whole-body fascial and myofascial linkages and leads to new holistic strategies for health professionals, movement teachers, and athletes to resolve complex postural and movement patterns.

**Yoga Anatomy**
*http://www.yogatuneup.com*
Jill Miller's Yoga Tune Up® is a health and fitness system combining yoga, corrective exercise, and self-massage.

**Connective Tissue Rejuvenation**
*http://www.meltmethod.com*
Sue Hitzmann's MELT® Method is a self-treatment system that restores the supportiveness of the body's connective tissue.

## Clothing

**www.rogiani.com** Elisabetta Rogiani's made-to-order lines of couture fitness make the best leggings in the business. I've had the same three pairs for ten years!

**www.Zohba.com** This yogawear line with its own foundation for charitable giving makes great pieces and supports Pilates as well.

**www.Activewearusa.com** A veritable one-stop-shop for high-performance women's activewear, footwear, and accessories with a social mission of sponsoring women's fitness-focused groups nationwide.

## Books

***Pilates' Return to Life Through Contrology: Revised Edition for the 21st Century*** by Joseph Pilates, Judd Robbins, and Lin Van Heuit-Robbins (Presentation Dynamics, 2012). Originally published in 1945, this book is a critical must-read for anyone wishing to learn Joe's original matwork. Available on Amazon.

***Your Health*** by Joseph Pilates (Presentation Dynamics, 1998). Originally published in 1934, this book is what I call "Joe's manifesto." It sheds much light into the thinking behind the Contrology method and its master. Available on Amazon.

***The Pilates Body*** by Brooke Siler (Harmony, 2000). The *New York Times* bestseller that launched my career. Available on Amazon.

***Voices of Classical Pilates*** by Peter Fiasca (2013). This book showcases essays by 28 classical Pilates teachers about their lives and work in the world of Pilates. Available on Amazon.

***Fix Your Feet Using the Pilates Method*** by Kathryn Ross-Nash (2009). This 40-page pictorial, from a Pilates great, offers solutions to prevent pain, relieve pain, or move you forward with strength and alignment. Available on Amazon.

## DVDs and Audio

***Classical Pilates Technique: The Complete Mat Workout Series***, Peter Fiasca (Classical Pilates, Inc., 2002). Available on Amazon.

***Element: Pilates Weight Loss for Beginners***, Brooke Siler (Anchor Bay, 2008). A combination of Pilates-conscious cardio and mat Pilates, this low-impact workout will strengthen and tone your whole body. Available on Amazon.

***The Pilates Body Kit*** (St. Martin's Griffin, 2003). This kit was a follow-up to my first book and includes two 70-minute audio CDs, containing eight complete classes, plus 70 flash cards and a workbook. Great for your iPod or MP3 player. Available on Amazon.

## Accessories and Apparatus

**The Tensatoner™** is currently in production and requests can be sent to orders@tensatoner.com.

Original strength **Magic Circles** can be purchased through www.Pilates-Gratz.com and lighter Stamina-brand Magic Circles through Amazon or WalMart.

**Resistance bands** by TheraBand, a trusted name in the industry. These latex-free bands come in multiple tensions identifiable by color. The colors used in the book (red, blue, green) represent medium through extra heavy. Available on Amazon.

**Door Anchor Strap** by FIT CORD Durable, high-density nylon strap attaches into your door jamb for use with resistance band exercises. Available on Amazon.

**Exercise Balls** by Natural Fitness—Burst Resistance up to 300 lbs. and manufactured using a nontoxic/phthalate-free material. This company takes into account your health as well as the planet's. www.naturalfitnessinc.com.

**The TriadBall** This latex-free ball can be customized to support your individual comfort level and ability in order to help you build more core strength. Available at www.zenirgy.com or www.optp.com.

# *Index*

Boldface page references indicate photographs.
Underscored page references indicate boxed text.